PSYCHIATRIC
CARE PLANNING

Second Edition

Susan L.W. Krupnick, RN, MSN, CARN, CS
Psychiatric Liaison Nurse Specialist
Baystate Healthcare System
Baystate Medical Center
Springfield, Massachusetts
Adjunct Lecturer
University of Massachusetts
Amherst

Andrew Wade, RN, MSN
Psychiatric Clinical Nurse Specialist
Thomas Jefferson Hospital
Adjunct Lecturer
Thomas Jefferson University
School of Nursing
Philadelphia

Springhouse Corporation
Springhouse, Pennsylvania

Staff

Vice President
Matthew Cahill

Clinical Director
Judith Schilling McCann, RN, MSN

Art Director
John Hubbard

Managing Editor
David Moreau

Clinical Consultants
Patricia Kardish Fischer, RN, BSN; Beverly Ann Tscheschlog, RN

Editors
Karen Diamond, Peter Johnson, Carol Munson

Copy Editors
Cynthia C. Breuninger (manager), Deborah Arnold, Brenna H. Mayer, Pamela Wingrod

Designers
Arlene Putterman (associate art director), Mary Ludwicki

Manufacturing
Deborah Meiris (director), Patricia K. Dorshaw (manager), Otto Mezei (book production manager)

Editorial Assistants
Beverly Lane, Marcia C. Mills, Liz Schaeffer

Printed in the United States of America.
PSYCP2- D
02 01 00 99   10 9 8 7 6 5 4 3 2

℞ A member of the Reed Elsevier plc group

Library of Congress Cataloging-in-Publication Data

Psychiatric care planning/[edited by] Susan L.W. Krupnick, Andrew Wade. — 2nd ed.
    p.   cm.
    Includes bibliographical references and index.
    1. Psychiatric nursing. 2. Nursing care plans. I. Title
[DNLM: 1. Mental disorders — nursing. 2. Patient Care Planning — nurses' instruction. 3. Nursing Process. 4. Psychiatric Nursing — methods. WY 160P9717 1999]
RC440.P7298 1999
610.73'68—dc21

DNLM/DLC   98-38122
ISBN 0-87434-953-2 (alk. paper)   CIP

Contents

Consultant, contributors, and reviewers

Consultant

Jean A. Haspeslagh, RN, DNSC
Associate Professor
University of Southern Mississippi
School of Nursing
Hattiesburg

Contributors

Suzanne M. Brennan, RN, MSN, CS
Private Nurse Psychotherapist and Family Therapist
Doctoral Candidate
University of Pennsylvania
Philadelphia

Lisa Field, RN, MSN
Nurse Clinician
Adult Inpatient Psychiatric Unit
Hospital of the University of Pennsylvania
Philadelphia

Martha G. Horton, RN, MSN, CS
Psychiatric Clinical Nurse Specialist
Thomas Jefferson University Hospital
Philadelphia

Lynette W. Jack, RN, PhD, CARN
Assistant Professor
University of Pittsburgh
School of Nursing

Catherine Knox-Fischer, RN, MSN
Mental Health Clinical Nurse Specialist
Philadelphia

Tona Leiker, RN,C, MN, ARNP-CNS, CARN, NCAC-II
Certified School Nurse Practitioner
Andover, Kans.

Patricia Long, RN, EdD, CARN, CS, NPP
Professor and Chair
Department of Community and Mental Health Nursing
School of Nursing, State University of New York at Stonybrook
Private Psychotherapist
Selden, N.Y.

Mimi Meiselman, RN, MSN, CAC
Nurse Psychotherapist
Rush North Shore Medical Center
Skokie, Ill.

Alfred J. Moyer, RN, MSN, CS
Psychiatric Clinical Nurse Specialist
Hospital of the University of Pennsylvania
Adjunct Clinical Lecturer
Psychiatric Mental Health Division
School of Nursing
University of Pennsylvania
Philadelphia

Nancy Vanore-Black, RN, MSN, CS
Nurse Psychotherapist
Bryn Mawr, Pa.

Reviewers

Elizabeth Bonham, RN, MSN, CS
Family Support Services Program Director
Indiana Juvenile Justice Task Force
Indianapolis

Linda Carmen Copel, RN, PhD, CS, CGP, DAPA
Associate Professor
Villanova (Pa.) University

Donna Iszler, RN,C, MSN, MA
Associate Professor
University of North Dakota
Statewide Psychiatric Nursing Program
Jamestown

Elizabeth Kaiser, RN, PhD, CS
Director of Psychiatric Mental Health Services
University of Pennsylvania Health Care System
Philadelphia

Gretchen LaGodna, RN, PhD, CS, FAAN
Professor Emeritus
University of Kentucky
Lexington

Acknowledgments

This project has been accomplished by enlisting and marshaling the assistance, talent, and support of many individuals. We wish to acknowledge the outstanding work that each contributor and reviewer provided in strengthening the fabric of this book. We also are grateful to our families for their emotional backing, nurturance, and general support throughout the course of our work. We are most appreciative of our friends and colleagues who generously supported us through this endeavor.

Heartfelt thanks are extended to Rob Krupnick for his wise comments, support, and guidance during many long hours of revising, editing, and searching out evidence-based tools to enhance this edition. We also are grateful to Judy McCann and Beverly Tscheschlog at Springhouse for their guidance and encouragement during some challenging moments.

We want to acknowledge all of the nurses, client-consumers of mental health services, and families who struggle with psychiatric–mental health and addiction disorders. We wish them continued success in their endeavors in learning to use, helping to improve, and challenging our country's mental health system and associated research foundations to develop effective care and treatments for individuals suffering from mental illness.

Finally, we wish to applaud each other for our resilience, persistence, occasional emergence of our humor, and consistent commitment to enhancing the mental health of individuals, families, organizations, and communities as we engage in our daily work.

DEDICATION

We dedicate this book to the memory of Dr. Melva Jo Hendrix, RN, DNSc, FAAN. During her professorship at the University of Kentucky, "Jo" worked tirelessly to develop systems and educate nurses to provide more effective care to persistently mentally ill individuals living in both urban and rural settings. During her presidency of the Society of Education and Research in Psychiatric Nursing, she worked collaboratively with the presidents of the Association of Child and Adolescent Psychiatric Nursing and the International Society of Psychiatric Consultation Liaison Nurses to forge an alliance that has greatly enhanced communication and cooperation within the specialty of psychiatric–mental health nursing. Although Jo is greatly missed, her spirit, ideals, and ability to join people together to reach a more inclusive goal will be carried on by all who were taught, mentored, or otherwise inspired by her. Many clients and their families have benefited from her commitment to excellent psychiatric and mental health care for all who need it.

S.L.K.
A.W.

Preface

Psychiatric nursing has undergone tremendous growth, development, and change as a nursing specialty in the last decade. As psychiatric–mental health nurses' roles and responsibilities have expanded, so has their need for resources that address all aspects of client- and family-focused care. This second edition of *Psychiatric Care Planning* continues to serve as a comprehensive reference for psychiatric–mental health nurses who work in clinical practice environments across the continuum of care, including inpatient psychiatric units, outpatient clinics, psychiatric emergency or crisis intervention units, long-term treatment programs, and extended-care facilities. Nurses practicing in medical-surgical or subacute units and home care will also find this manual useful when caring for the client with an illness-related emotional problem, a coexisting psychiatric diagnosis, or both.

Part 1 of this new edition offers a multifaceted overview of psychiatric–mental health nursing. A brief history of psychiatric and mental health care provides a context for discussions of nursing roles and functions, treatment modalities, and the nursing process as it applies to psychiatric nursing.

Parts 2 to 13 present comprehensive plans of care, grouped according to psychiatric diagnostic categories. The plans are based on the nurse's role as both an independent and collaborative practitioner and address both levels of practice. The plans offer classifications from the American Psychiatric Association's *Diagnostic and Statistical Manual,* 4th ed., revised *(DSM-IV)* in conjunction with focused nursing diagnoses. Each plan begins with an introduction to the disorders, followed by latest findings about etiology, precipitating factors, and potential complications. Next, assessment guidelines cover nursing history and physical findings. The guidelines are followed by appropriate nursing diagnoses (approved by the North American Nursing Diagnosis Association [NANDA]), with nursing priorities, outcome criteria for each diagnosis, and interventions with associated rationales. Each plan concludes with a list of discharge criteria to facilitate evaluation and documentation and a current list of selected references.

Part 14 provides evidence-based assessment tools, interview guides, and evaluation scales to enhance the nurse's ability to perform comprehensive assessments and to evaluate care. These assessment tools will help the nurse to focus care according to individualized responses and clinically measurable information. The appendices provide additional information of interest to the psychiatric nurse, including the *DSM-IV* classification categories and codes, NANDA diagnostic categories arranged by Gordon's functional health patterns, commonly prescribed medications associated with sexual adverse effects, managing adverse drug reactions, and resources for clients and their families, including community agencies, hotlines, and Internet sites.

Psychiatric Care Planning is an up-to-date, reliable source of practical, clinically focused information for planning, implementing, and evaluating care in any clinical practice setting. Psychiatric nurses will find it an invaluable reference and indispensable care-planning tool.

Part 1

Overview of psychiatric nursing

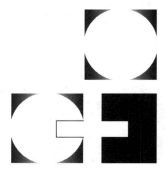

Today's psychiatric nursing roles

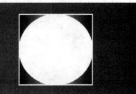

Psychiatric nursing uses an interpersonal process to promote, maintain, restore, and rehabilitate individual, family, and community mental health and functioning. Psychiatric nurses accept individuals, families, groups, and communities as clients, using skills that draw on the psychosocial and biophysical sciences and on theories of personality and human behavior. The American Nurses Association (ANA) considers psychiatric nursing a specialized area of nursing practice that employs the theories of human behavior as its science and "powerful use of self" as its art; the National Institute of Mental Health (NIMH) recognizes it as a core mental health discipline.

Psychiatric nurses practice in diverse settings, including psychiatric hospitals, community mental health centers, general hospitals, community health agencies, outpatient clinics, homes, schools, prisons, health maintenance organizations, primary care practices, private practices, crisis units, and industrial centers. In those settings, a psychiatric nurse can assume the role of staff nurse, administrator, consultant, in-service educator, clinical practitioner, researcher, program evaluator, primary care provider, and liaison between the client and other members of the health care delivery system.

LEVELS OF PRACTICE

Various factors determine the level at which a psychiatric nurse practices, including state nurse practice acts, education and experience, certification, practice setting, personal initiative, and professional practice standards.

Nurse practice acts

Nurse practice acts regulate entry into the profession and define the legal limits of nursing practice. Some state nurse practice acts also address advanced practice and require a second licensure at that level. Each state nurse practice act defines whether the advanced practice psychiatric nurse can apply for prescriptive authority in that particular state.

Education and experience

Education and experience determine whether a psychiatric nurse practices as a generalist or a specialist. The *psychiatric nurse generalist* has received basic nursing preparation, typically a baccalaureate degree, and meets the profession's standards of knowledge, experience, and quality of care. The psychiatric nurse generalist provides most of the nursing care to patients in inpa-

tient settings, offering direct and indirect care through the nurse-client relationship; however, the generalist is not prepared to conduct psychotherapy. The *advanced practice psychiatric nurse* may be a *primary psychiatric nurse practitioner* or *psychiatric clinical nurse specialist;* in either case, the advanced practice psychiatric nurse has a master's degree and has had supervised clinical experience. The clinical nurse specialist has in-depth knowledge, competence, and skill in psychiatric nursing practice and is certified at the clinical nurse specialist level by the American Nurses Credentialing Center (ANCC). Clinical nurse specialists provide individual, family, and group psychotherapy in inpatient, outpatient, and community health settings and in private practice; they also provide indirect services, teaching, and client-focused or system-focused consultation to the institutional administration.

The psychiatric consultation-liaison nurse specialist possesses specific knowledge and skills for providing psychiatric–mental health consultation to other nurses, clients, and families in the general hospital setting. As earlier hospital discharges become the rule, psychiatric consultation-liaison nurse specialists are moving into consultations in the home care, sub-acute, and long-term care settings. In the institutional setting, their knowledge of organizational systems enables these specialists to act as project leaders, focusing on improving psychosocial care to clients and their families. They also assist in addressing the mental well-being of health care workers, especially if the institution lacks employee assistance program services.

The recent trend toward integrating behavioral health care with primary care has created some opportunities for psychiatric–mental health nurses to expand into new practice arenas. However, this has also led to disagreements about who is best educated to be the primary behavioral or psychiatric health care provider. To remedy this, psychiatric nurses at the advanced practice level have teamed with innovative faculty to develop university-based educational programs to prepare the primary psychiatric nurse practitioner to be the provider in these integrated primary care practices and clinics. A primary psychiatric nurse practitioner has a master's degree in psychiatry and is also a nurse practitioner.

Certification

Psychiatric nurses may be certified by professional organizations. ANA certification requires a formal review, including a written test. Certification provides credentials for clinical practice as a psychiatric nurse generalist or a clinical nurse specialist. Presently, several psychiatric nursing leaders and nursing organizations (Association of Child and Adolescent Psychiatric Nursing, American Psychiatric Nurses Association [APNA], International Society of Psychiatric Consultation Liasion Nurses, and Society for Education and Research in Psychiatric Mental Health Nursing) collaborating with the ANCC to determine the best manner in which to provide certification for the primary psychiatric nurse practitioner to ensure that these nurses have the appropriate credentials to allow them full practice privileges based on their education and clinical practice.

Practice setting
A health care organization's philosophy of mental health and mental illness and its approach toward treatment shape the nurse's and client's expectations. Administrative policies will either foster or limit the full use of the psychiatric nurse's practice abilities and expertise.

Personal initiative
The psychiatric nurse's willingness to act as an agent of change, coupled with a thorough knowledge of his or her personal strengths and weaknesses, and his or her realization of clinical competence will influence the level at which the psychiatric nurse performs.

Professional practice standards
Professional standards define nursing practice and performance. The ANA first developed standards for adult psychiatric and mental health nursing in 1973 and revised them in 1982 and 1994. Standards for child and adolescent psychiatric and mental health nursing were established in 1985; standards for psychiatric consultation-liaison nursing were established in 1990. (See *Selected practice standards,* pages 4 to 6.)

PSYCHIATRIC NURSING FUNCTIONS

Psychiatric nursing functions involve direct and indirect care. The ANA defines psychiatric nursing functions to include:
• maintaining a therapeutic milieu
• working to solve the client's current problems
• fulfilling a surrogate parent role
• using somatic therapies to alleviate the client's health problems
• educating consumers about factors that influence mental health
• promoting change to improve socioeconomic conditions
• providing leadership and clinical supervision to colleagues

• conducting psychotherapy
• engaging in social and community mental health efforts.
In addition, the psychiatric nurse participates in continuing education, in-service, and nursing administration and engages in consultation and research.

Nursing functions occur on three levels of prevention: primary, secondary, and tertiary. When the psychiatric nurse is involved in *primary prevention,* the functions include conducting health education, improving socioeconomic conditions, offering consumer education about normal growth and development, providing referrals before symptoms develop, supporting family members, and engaging in community and political activities. In *secondary prevention,* the functions include screening and evaluating clients promptly; providing emergency treatment, crisis intervention, and a therapeutic milieu; supervising medication administration; preventing suicide; counseling on a time-limited basis; conducting psychotherapy; and initiating community and organization interventions such as helping to set up shelters for the homeless. In *tertiary prevention,* nursing functions include establishing vocational training, psychosocial rehabilitation, and aftercare programs and participating in partial hospitalization.

MEETING LEGAL STANDARDS
Legal issues also shape psychiatric nursing roles. Psychiatric nurses are held to the same standards of reasonable and prudent behavior expected of other professionals with the same education in similar circumstances and must provide care that meets with professional standards established by the ANA. Psychiatric nurses must know and abide by statutory provisions concerning client admissions into psychiatric care. Obtaining informed consent is the admitting provider's responsibility, but the nurse should supply the client with relevant information about consent and document whether or not the consent was valid. A nurse who must violate a client's rights, for whatever reason, should carefully document all signs and symptoms, treatments, and treatment effects as a precaution against litigation. Interventions, such as the legal use of restraints or seclusion if deemed clinically necessary to protect a client's safety, are performed within the institutional policies that are guided by and in compliance with external regulatory boards and statutes and based on the principle of least restrictive interventions to provide safety. Indeed, the nurse has an obligation to protect a client from self-harm, even against the client's wishes.

(Text continues on page 6.)

Overview of
psychiatric nursing

Selected practice standards

This chart outlines the American Nurses Association (ANA) standards for general psychiatric–mental health nursing practice and performance. These standards consist of two sections. The first section includes those standards related to the direct clinical care the client receives, as demonstrated through the nursing process. The second section addresses professional performance, which describes a competent level of behavior in the professional role.

Professional practice standards

"Standards of Care" pertain to professional nursing activities that are demonstrated by the nurse through the nursing process. These involve assessment, diagnosis, outcome identification, planning, implementation, and evaluation. The nursing process is the foundation of clinical decision making and encompasses all significant action taken by nurses in providing psychiatric–mental health care to all clients.

Standard I. Assessment

The psychiatric–mental health nurse collects client health data.

Rationale

The assessment interview — which requires linguistically and culturally effective communication skills, interviewing, behavioral observation, database record review, and comprehensive assessment of the client and relevant systems — enables the psychiatric–mental health nurse to make sound clinical judgments and plan appropriate interventions with the client.

Standard II. Diagnosis

The psychiatric–mental health nurse analyzes the assessment data in determining diagnoses.

Rationale

The basis for providing psychiatric–mental health nursing care is the recognition and identification of patterns of response to actual or potential psychiatric illnesses and mental health problems.

Standard III. Outcome identification

The psychiatric–mental health nurse identifies expected outcomes individualized to the client.

Rationale

Within the context of providing nursing care, the ultimate goal is to influence health outcomes and improve the client's health status.

Standard IV. Planning

The psychiatric–mental health nurse develops a plan of care that prescribes interventions to attain expected outcomes.

Rationale

The plan of care is used to guide therapeutic intervention systematically and achieve the expected client outcomes.

Standard V. Implementation

The psychiatric–mental health nurse implements the interventions identified in the plan of care.

Rationale

In implementing the plan of care, psychiatric–mental health nurses use a wide range of interventions designed to prevent mental and physical illness and promote, maintain, and restore mental and physical health. Psychiatric–mental health nurses select interventions according to their level of practice. At the basic level, the nurse may select counseling, milieu therapy, self-care activities, psychobiological interventions, health teaching, case management, health promotion and health maintenance, and a variety of other approaches to meet the mental health needs of clients. In addition to the intervention options available to the basic-level psychiatric–mental health nurse, at the advanced level the certified specialist may provide consultation, engage in psychotherapy, and prescribe pharmacologic agents where permitted by state statutes or regulations.

Standard Va. Counseling

The psychiatric–mental health nurse uses counseling interventions to assist clients in improving or regaining their previous coping abilities, fostering mental health, and preventing mental illness and disability.

Standard Vb. Milieu therapy

The psychiatric–mental health nurse provides, structures, and maintains a therapeutic environment in collaboration with the client and other health care providers.

Standard Vc. Self-care activities

The psychiatric–mental health nurse structures interventions around the client's activities of daily living to foster self-care and mental and physical well-being.

Standard Vd. Psychobiological interventions

The psychiatric–mental health nurse uses knowledge of psychobiological interventions and applies clinical skills to restore the client's health and prevent further disability.

Standard Ve. Health teaching

The psychiatric–mental health nurse, through health teaching, assists clients in achieving satisfying, productive, and healthy patterns of living.

Standard Vf. Case management

The psychiatric–mental health nurse provides case management to coordinate comprehensive health services and ensure continuity of care.

Standard Vg. Health promotion and health maintenance

The psychiatric–mental health nurse employs strategies and interventions to promote and maintain mental health and prevent mental illness.

Selected practice standards *(continued)*

Standard Vh. Psychotherapy

The certified specialist in psychiatric–mental health nursing uses individual, group, and family psychotherapy, child psychotherapy, and other therapeutic treatments to assist clients in fostering mental health, preventing mental illness and disability, and improving or regaining previous health status and functional abilities.

Standard Vi. Prescription of pharmacologic agents

The certified specialist uses prescription of pharmacologic agents in accordance with the state nursing practice act to treat symptoms of psychiatric illness and improve functional health status.

Standard Vj. Consultation

The certified specialist provides consultation to health care providers and others to influence the plans of care for clients, and to enhance the abilities of others to provide psychiatric and mental health care and effect change in systems.

Standard VI. Evaluation

The psychiatric–mental health nurse evaluates the client's progress in attaining expected outcomes.

Rationale

Nursing care is a dynamic process involving change in the client's health status over time, giving rise to the need for new data, different diagnoses, and modifications in the plan of care. Therefore, evaluation is a continuous process of appraising the effect of nursing interventions and the treatment regimen on the client's health status and expected health outcomes.

Professional performance standards

"Standards of Professional Performance" describe a competent level of behavior in the professional role, including activities related to quality of care, performance appraisal, education, collegiality, ethics, collaboration, research, and resource utilization. All psychiatric–mental health nurses are expected to engage in professional role activities appropriate to their education, position, and practice setting. Therefore, some standards or measurement criteria identify these activities.

While "Standards of Professional Performance" describe the roles of all professional nurses, there are many other responsibilities that are hallmarks of psychiatric–mental health nursing. These nurses should be self-directed and purposeful in seeking necessary knowledge and skills to enhance career goals. Other activities — such as membership in professional organizations, certification in specialty or advanced practice, continuing education, and further academic education — are desirable methods of enhancing the psychiatric–mental health nurse's professionalism.

Standard I. Quality of care

The psychiatric–mental health nurse systematically evaluates the quality of care and effectiveness of psychiatric–mental health nursing practice.

Rationale

The dynamic nature of the mental health care environment and the growing body of psychiatric nursing knowledge and research provide both the impetus and the means for the psychiatric–mental health nurse to be competent in clinical practice, to continue to develop professionally, and to improve the quality of client care.

Standard II. Performance appraisal

The psychiatric–mental health nurse evaluates own psychiatric–mental health nursing practice in relation to professional practice standards and relevant statutes and regulations.

Rationale

The psychiatric–mental health nurse is accountable to the public for providing competent clinical care and has an inherent responsibility as a professional to evaluate the role and performance of psychiatric–mental health nursing practice according to standards established by the profession and regulatory bodies.

Standard III. Education

The psychiatric–mental health nurse acquires and maintains current knowledge in nursing practice.

Rationale

The rapid expansion of knowledge pertaining to basic and behavioral sciences, technology, information systems, and research requires a commitment to learning throughout the psychiatric–mental health nurse's professional career. Formal education, continuing education, certification, and experiential learning are some of the means the psychiatric–mental health nurse uses to enhance nursing expertise and advance the profession.

Standard IV. Collegiality

The psychiatric–mental health nurse contributes to the professional development of peers, colleagues, and others.

Rationale

The psychiatric–mental health nurse is responsible for sharing knowledge, research, and clinical information with colleagues, through formal and informal teaching methods, to enhance professional growth.

Standard V. Ethics

The psychiatric–mental health nurse's decisions and actions on behalf of clients are determined in an ethical manner.

Rationale

The public's trust and its right to humane psychiatric–mental health care are upheld by professional nursing practice. The foundation of psychiatric–mental health nursing practice is the development of a therapeutic relationship with the client. The psychiatric–mental health nurse engages in therapeutic interactions and relationships which promote and support the healing process. Boundaries need to be established to safeguard the client's well-being and to prevent the development of intimate or sexual relationships.

(continued)

Selected practice standards (continued)

Standard VI. Collaboration

The psychiatric–mental health nurse collaborates with the client, significant others, and health care providers in providing care.

Rationale

Psychiatric–mental health nursing practice requires a coordinated, ongoing interaction between consumers and providers to deliver comprehensive services to the client and the community. Through the collaborative process, different abilities of health care providers are used to solve problems, communicate, and plan, implement, and evaluate mental health services.

Standard VII. Research

The psychiatric–mental health nurse contributes to nursing and mental health through the use of research.

Rationale

Nurses in psychiatric–mental health nursing are responsible for contributing to the further development of the field of mental health by participating in research. At the basic level of practice, the psychiatric–mental health nurse uses research findings to improve clinical care and identifies clinical problems for research study. At the advanced level, the psychiatric–mental health nurse engages and/or collaborates with others in the research process to discover, examine, and test knowledge, theories, and creative approaches to practice.

Standard VIII. Resource utilization

The psychiatric–mental health nurse considers factors related to safety, effectiveness, and cost in planning and delivering client care.

Rationale

The client is entitled to psychiatric–mental health care which is safe, effective, and affordable. As the cost of health care increases, treatment decisions must be made in such a way as to maximize resources and maintain quality of care. The psychiatric–mental health nurse seeks to provide cost-effective quality care by using the most appropriate resources and delegating care to the most appropriate, qualified health care provider.

Adapted with permission from *A Statement of Psychiatric–Mental Health Clinical Nursing Practice and Standards of Psychiatric–Mental Health Clinical Nursing Practice.* Washington, D.C.: American Nurses Association, 1994.

care. Obtaining informed consent is the admitting provider's responsibility, but the nurse should supply the client with relevant information about consent and document whether or not the consent was valid. A nurse who must violate a client's rights, for whatever reason, should carefully document all signs and symptoms, treatments, and treatment effects as a precaution against litigation. Interventions, such as the legal use of restraints or seclusion if deemed clinically necessary to protect a client's safety, are performed within the institutional policies that are guided by and in compliance with external regulatory boards and statutes and based on the principle of least restrictive interventions to provide safety. Indeed, the nurse has an obligation to protect a client from self-harm, even against the client's wishes.

A FINAL WORD

Today's psychiatric–mental health nurse needs to be a life-long learner who is constantly challenged by new evidence-based practices and who looks for ways to improve on the standard way of doing things. More than ever, psychiatric–mental health nurses need to collaborate with their colleagues in the neurosciences and

medical-surgical practice areas to gain fuller understanding of how physical illness often manifests itself as a primary psychiatric disorder. This collaboration is equally beneficial to nonpsychiatric nursing colleagues, because they too are often challenged with behaviors that are difficult to sort out and manage on medical, surgical, and critical care units. Psychiatric nurses can no longer isolate themselves from other health care practitioners. Otherwise, they risk isolating themselves out of jobs, thereby eroding the specialty.

Psychiatric–mental health nurses also need to understand managed health cost strategies and their impact on mental health care reimbursement. They also need to be active in a psychiatric nursing organization that best meets their practice, educational, and legislative needs. We often remind clients to stay connected to with individuals who can support and guide them in times of crisis, which is exactly what psychiatric–mental health nurses need to do. We need to build partnerships and alliances with health care colleagues, clients, families, and advocacy groups to obtain the best care for easily disenfranchised clients.

SELECTED REFERENCES

Andrews, M. M., and Boyle, J.S. *Transcultural Concepts in Nursing Care,* 2nd ed. Philadelphia: Lippincott-Raven Pubs., 1995.

Boyd, M.A., and Nihart, M.A. *Psychiatric Nursing: Contemporary Practice.* Philadelphia Lippincott-Raven, Pubs., 1998.

Burgess, A.W. *Advanced Practice Psychiatric Nursing.* Stamford, Conn.: Appleton & Lange, 1998.

Cummings, N.A., et al. *Behavioral Health in Primary Care.* Madison, Conn.: Psychosocial Press, 1997.

Dyer, J., et al. "The Psychiatric-Primary Care Nurse Practitioner: A Futuristic Model for Advanced Practice," *Archives of Psychiatric Nursing* 11:2, 1997.

Haber, J., and Billings, C.V. "Primary Healthcare: A Model for Psychiatric-Mental Health Nursing," *Journal of American Psychiatric Nurses Association* 1(5):154-63, 1995.

Johnson, B.S. *Adaptation and Growth: Psychiatric-Mental Health Nursing,* 4th ed. Philadelphia: Lippincott-Raven Pubs., 1997.

Knesper, D.J., et al. *Primary Care Psychiatry.* Philadelphia: W.B. Saunders Co., 1997.

Levin, B., and Petrila, J., eds. *Mental Health Services: A Public Health Perspective.* New York: Oxford University Press, 1996.

Lutzen, K., et al. "Moral Sensitivity in Psychiatric Practice," *Nursing Ethics: An International Journal for Health Care Professionals* 4(6):472-83, 1997.

A Statement of Psychiatric-Mental Health Clinical Nursing Practice and Standards of Psychiatric-Mental Health Clinical Nursing Practice. Washington, D.C.: American Nurses Association, 1994.

Trygstad, L. "The Need to Know: Biological Learning Needs Identified by Practicing Psychiatric Nurses," *Journal of Psychosocial Nursing* 32(2):13-18, 1994.

Varcarolis, E.M. *Foundations of Psychiatric Mental Health Nursing,* 3rd ed. Philadelphia: W.B. Saunders Co., 1998

Walker, L. "Perceptions of Psychiatric Nurse's Role: A Pilot Study," *Nursing Standard* 12(16):7-13, 35-38, January 1998.

Wilbur, S., et al. "Psychosocial Rehabilitation Nurses: Taking Our Place on the Multidisciplinary Team," *Journal of Psychosocial Nursing and Mental Health Services* 36(4):33-41, 47-48, April 1998.

Overview of
psychiatric nursing

Treatment modalities

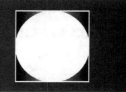

Various treatment modalities, including psychotherapy, crisis intervention, group therapy, family therapy, milieu therapy, behavioral therapy, psychobiological therapies, and psychopharmacology, are used with psychiatric and mental health clients. Each treatment modality can be used alone or in combination with another modality.

PSYCHOTHERAPY

In psychotherapy, a client enters into an explicit or implicit agreement to interact with a psychotherapist within preestablished boundaries. General goals of psychotherapy may include personal growth, resolving lifestyle problems, and alleviating or relieving symptoms. Individual psychotherapy has changed greatly during the last decade under the influence of economic strictures and recent psychoanalytical research. Traditional long-term psychoanalysis has not been found to be any more effective than the short and brief psychotherapy models that are currently being practiced, and third-party payers are not reimbursing for long-term psychotherapy. However, individuals who want and can afford the traditional approach can still find specialists who continue to utilize many of the tools of psychoanalysis, such as free association, analysis of dreams, transference, and countertransference.

Presently, psychotherapy tends to concentrate more on the client's behavior in current relationships and situations so that corrective actions and interventions can be made in the here and now. The current psychotherapeutic mode is brief individual psychotherapy, which comes in many forms, such as brief supportive psychotherapy (BSP), short-term psychodynamic therapy (STPD), cognitive-behavioral therapy (CBT), interpersonal therapy (IPT), strategic therapy (STP), solution-focused psychotherapy (SFP), or single-session therapy (SST). SST is commonly used in psychiatric consultation-liaison nursing and medical practice and for some individuals in psychosocial crisis, but it is not usually appropriate for clients with chronic mental disorders.

In BSP, the therapist encourages the client to express feelings, explore choices, and make decisions in a safe, caring relationship. Existing coping mechanisms are reinforced and no new means of coping are introduced. STPD, CBT, and IPT typically aim at reeducation.

Reeducative therapy introduces the client to new ways of perceiving and behaving; alternatives are examined in a planned, systematic manner. Reeducative therapy takes somewhat longer than supportive psychotherapy, since the goal involves changing established behaviors and trying out new behaviors. By changing specific behaviors, the client may change his self-perception. Reconstructive therapies, such as psychoanalytic and insight-oriented psychodynamic (not BSP) therapies, involve a long-term interaction that explores all aspects of the client's life, including both cognitive and emotional components. Ultimately, the client increases his understanding of the self and others, and gains emotional freedom, the potential for new abilities, and renewed capacity for love and work.

CRISIS INTERVENTION

During a crisis, stress overwhelms an individual's coping mechanisms. Predisposing factors include a disastrous event, threatened loss of a basic need, failure to cope with stress, or a perceived absence of support. Confronting a problem or threat (real or perceived), the individual uses strategies that have worked previously. When these methods fail, disorganization and disequilibrium result, with an increase in general anxiety. A sense of emergency occurs and may result in emotional decompensation, which could include psychosis, violence, or even suicide. Given adequate support and resources, however, a crisis is typically self-limiting and resolves within 4 to 6 weeks.

Crisis intervention attempts to resolve the emergency positively. Interventions offer immediate help by reestablishing equilibrium. The goal is to restore the client to precrisis functioning by teaching new ways of problem solving and by minimizing the negative effects of the crisis situation on the individual, family, and community.

Crisis intervention involves a step-wise approach. Initially, the therapist assesses the nature of the crisis, its effect on the client, and the client's coping mechanisms and support systems. Then the therapist identifies a step-by-step plan of action. Next, interventions (environmental manipulation) provide direct support or remove stress and reassure the client that the therapist understands and will help (general support measures). The therapist can use a generic approach, using standard interventions for a given crisis, or an individual approach, tailoring interventions to a particular client. Finally, evaluation determines whether the crisis has been resolved.

Techniques of crisis intervention include taking an active role in exploring the client's problem; maintaining the client's orientation; encouraging expression of feelings and an awareness of the relationships among events, current feelings, and behavior; persuading the client to view the therapist as a helper; promoting and reinforcing adaptive behavior; supporting the client's defenses; increasing the client's self-esteem; and exploring solutions to the cause of the crisis.

GROUP THERAPY

A group is a gathering of three or more individuals in which each individual influences and is in turn influenced by the other group members as they work together to accomplish a common task. Typically, the group is facilitated by a qualified group therapist. Because humans are social and desire interaction with others, groups can offer a safe environment for sharing emotional experiences. Many forces can influence the group's goals, including intrapersonal and interpersonal characteristics, needs, the physical environment, and the unique interaction of the group.

Group therapy can alleviate intrapsychic stress, reduce anxiety, and provide clients with opportunities to explore and practice new behaviors in a structured and controlled environment. Inpatient groups generally use a short-term treatment model, have open membership, and meet daily to accommodate a constantly fluctuating clientele. Outpatient groups have longer treatment periods, may meet once or twice a week, and have closed membership. Client candidates for group therapy must be cognitively and behaviorally capable of participating; therefore, the inclusion of an individual who is acutely psychotic, manic, or demented in a psychotherapy-focused group is usually contraindicated.

A group proceeds through three stages of development; in each stage, conflicts may arise, but these can further emotional bonding within the group. In the initial stage, the conflict issues are dependency and authority. This stage involves superficial communication, where the members become acquainted and search for personal similarities. Norms of behavior, roles, and responsibilities may be established during this time. In the middle or working stage, the conflict issues are intimacy, cooperation, and productivity. The group approaches problems and possible solutions and makes decisions through sharing and discussion. In the final or termination stage, the conflict issues are disengagement and dissolution. The group evaluates the experience and explores the members' feelings about the experience and impending separation.

For group therapy to be effective, the leader must adopt a style that is most effective for that group. Generally, the leader adopts one of three styles: autocratic (maintains control over decision making), democratic (encourages all members to participate in decision mak-

ing), or laissez-faire (relinquishes control over decision making and provides minimal guidance or direction). The effective group leader is skilled in techniques and interventions that foster interaction and shape behavior.

A group may be one of several types, including milieu groups (multifamily, community meeting, transition), social skills growth groups, age-related groups, support groups (quality of life, caregiver, bereavement), self-help groups, gender-specific groups, and multicultural groups. Psychotherapy groups can include T-groups (training groups) and psychoanalytic, psychodynamic, cognitive-behavioral, psychodrama, marathon, and encounter groups.

FAMILY THERAPY

Family therapy identifies a problem within a context, explores how family members relate to the problem, and focuses on how family interaction perpetuates the problem. The entire family is viewed as the client; the goal of therapy is to expand the family members' knowledge and skills for managing the complexities of daily living within their family structure.

The three predominating models of family therapy include Bowen's levels of differentiation model (family systems), structural (Minuchin), and strategic (Haley) therapies. Psychodynamic family therapy regards family pathology as a result of internal intrapsychic forces manifested in these intimate interactions. Bowen's levels of differentiation model (an individual's ability to identify his differences) proposes that family pathology results from a lack of differentiation and high levels of anxiety. Bowen advocated a healthy differentiation of self in relation to one's family. Differentiation is the individual's ability to learn how to develop a separate identity with a social (family) content.

Structural family therapy examines the individual within the family's social context. Family pathology is believed to result from the family's inability to nurture its members due to a faulty social organization and structure and due to dysfunctional interactions among members. Structural family therapy also explores the issues of power, influence, relationships, and boundaries within the family and aims to transform family structural patterns by challenging the family's ideas of where the problem lies and how it can be solved.

Strategic therapy, also known as problem-solving or brief family therapy, has its roots in communication theory. This model explores a behavior's function rather than its meaning. Consequently, treatment focuses on the presenting problem and the behaviors that maintain it, not on the problem's history or the motivation behind it. The therapist takes an active and deliberate role in promoting the reframing and redistribution of power and responsibility in resolving the family problems.

MILIEU THERAPY

Milieu (environment or social setting) therapy is a group therapy approach that uses a total living experience to achieve its therapeutic objectives; it draws on recreational, occupational, psychosocial, psychiatric, nursing, medical, and mental health therapies. It focuses on the client's interaction with the environment, creating a secure atmosphere in which the client can develop appropriate responses to people and situations. It is deliberately planned and structured to modify maladaptive behaviors and to promote positive insights and coping skills.

Milieu therapy operates through five principles: containment, support, structure, involvement, and validation. Containment sustains the physical well-being of clients and those around them while setting limits and external controls on unacceptable behaviors. Containment is a primary focus of an acute inpatient psychiatric unit whose clients are hospitalized with severe symptoms that could endanger their health or well-being. Support promotes clients' well-being and self-esteem through encouragement, alternative coping recommendations with rehearsal and feedback, positive reenforcement, general praise for attempts to change, and reality testing, and it gives clients an overall sense of hope that things will be different in their lives with the use of new coping strategies. Structure relates to all the aspects in the milieu that provide an organized, predictable environment, including a daily schedule of events, providing a safe and secure environment, and general rules of conduct. Involvement means active participation in milieu activities and interaction between the client, staff, and family members. Validation gives the client opportunities to be affirmed as a unique individual.

Milieu therapy is utilized by customized client- and family-focused treatment plans rather than by a standardized plan for a client with a specific mental disorder. Shorter inpatient stays have required nurses (who historically were the managers of the milieu) to become very creative in maintaining these milieu principles in the face of 5- to 10-day hospitalizations for clients with acute psychiatric disturbances or severe exacerbations of chronic mental illnesses.

BEHAVIORAL THERAPY

Also known as behavior modification, behavioral therapy aims to alleviate overt symptoms, without regard for the client's experience or inner conflicts. Assuming that most behaviors are learned, behavioral therapy teaches the client to substitute adaptive behaviors for maladaptive ones. Techniques used include generalization, dis-crimination, extinction, prompting and fading, shaping, modeling, imagery, and progressive muscle relaxation.

Behavioral therapy relies on classical conditioning and operant conditioning. In classical conditioning, an unconditioned stimulus elicits an unconditioned response. When a conditioned stimulus is paired with an unconditioned stimulus, a conditioned response may result. The original unconditioned response, whether positive or negative, reinforces the conditioned stimulus and response. Operant conditioning, also called operant reinforcement therapy, uses reinforcement to increase the probability of a desired response. The unconditioned stimulus is paired with a conditioned stimulus, and the combination acts as a reinforcer. The reinforcer must meet a need and be goal directed. A positive reinforcer strengthens desired behavior; a negative reinforcer encourages avoidance of undesirable behavior.

PSYCHOBIOLOGICAL THERAPIES

Although psychobiological therapies have been used for treating mental disorders for a long time, they have really come into their own only in the last 10 years. Psychobiological therapies include psychopharmacologic medications, electroconvulsive therapy (ECT), psychosurgery, light therapy (phototherapy), and rapid rate transcranial magnetic stimulation therapy (RTMS). Insulin coma therapy is no longer used because of its numerous adverse effects and because psychotropic drugs have made it obsolete. Also, hydrotherapy is no longer used because newer targeted therapies have replaced this generally soothing and containing therapy.

Before the advent of effective psychotropic drugs, psychosurgery, in the form of prefrontal lobotomy, had been used to control aggression. This technique has been superseded by modern stereotactic surgical techniques (for example, producing lesions of the cingulum bundle or anterior limb of the internal capsule) to control severe, medication- and treatment-resistant obsessive-compulsive disorder.

ECT, once stigmatized as "shock therapy," has been greatly refined. Typically, a brief electrical current is passed through the brain to produce generalized seizures lasting 25 to150 seconds. ECT can be administered either unilaterally or bilaterally to the side of the head. Although it produces rapid improvement of depressive symptoms, its exact antidepressant mechanism is unclear. It down-regulates beta-adrenergic receptors in a manner similar to pharmacologic antidepressants, but it also up-regulates serotonin. ECT must be used cautiously according to clinical practice guidelines for depression.

RTMS, a treatment in which electrical stimulation is applied to the cerebral cortex on one side, is a new innovation that is currently undergoing research. Phototherapy, or light therapy, is another recently researched and developed somatic therapy. It can be used alone or in combination with psychopharmacology. In phototherapy, the patient is exposed to an artificial light, which is about 200 times brighter than usual indoor lighting, during the winter months to alleviate seasonal affective disorder. The patient sits approximately 3′ (0.9 m) in front of the lights, glancing directly into the light every few minutes. Exposure each day for 1 to 2 hours is usually sufficient. The antidepressant response usually begins in 1 to 4 days; a full response occurs after about 2 weeks. It is postulated that artificial light triggers a shift in the patient's circadian rhythm to an earlier time.

PSYCHOPHARMACOLOGY

Drug treatment for psychiatric disorders is relatively new — chlorpromazine was not used to treat schizophrenia until the 1950s — but has dramatically improved the client's prognosis. Clients with schizophrenia, for example, may leave inpatient care sooner, live in the community, and take part in other therapies previously unavailable to them.

In the past 40 years, additional drugs have become available to treat psychiatric disorders. Antianxiety agents such as diazepam and antidepressants such as amitriptyline are prescribed commonly. Although medications may be used alone, they are usually used in conjunction with other therapeutic modalities, such as psychotherapy.

Drugs that alter behavior are likely to be prescribed for intermediate to long-term therapy, while drugs that promote sleep are usually prescribed for short-term therapy. Consequently, the client should be monitored closely for adverse reactions and signs of noncompliance. Because some psychoactive drugs are addictive, the health care professional must watch for signs of dependence or increasing tolerance and, when the medication is discontinued, abstinence withdrawal syndrome.

Antianxiety agents

Also called anxiolytics, antianxiety agents include some of the most commonly prescribed drugs in the United States. They are used primarily to treat anxiety disorders. The two primary categories of antianxiety medications are the benzodiazepines (alprazolam, chlordiazepoxide, clonazepam, clorazepate, diazepam, halazepam, lorazepam, oxazepam, and prazepam) and azaspirodecanedione (buspirone). Benzodiazepines have replaced barbiturates for treating anxiety because they interact with fewer drugs and cause fewer adverse reactions. Benzodiazepines do interact with other central nervous system (CNS) depressants, causing additive effects. The most common adverse reactions affect the CNS, producing drowsiness, motor incoordination, and increased reaction time.

Antidepressant and mood stabilizing agents

Mood disorders respond to antidepressant and mood stabilizing agents. The antidepressants include monoamine oxidase (MAO) inhibitors, tricyclic antidepressants, tetracyclics, triazolopyridines, aminoketones, selective serotonin reuptake inhibitors (SSRI), and selective serotonin-norepinephrine reuptake inhibitors (SSNRI). Psychostimulants can be used in treating depression in the medically ill and in the elderly when they exhibit a failure to thrive, although they are no longer used as a single agent in long-term treatment of depression. Psychostimulants include dextroamphetamine, methylphenidate (Ritalin), and pemoline (Cylert). They may be used to augment another antidepressant and then discontinued after a brief period of stabilization.

Mood stabilizing agents include lithium (lithium carbonate or lithium citrate), anticonvulsants (carbamazepine, clonazepam, valproic acid), calcium channel blockers, alpha-adrenergic blockers, and beta-adrenergic blockers.

Antidepressants are indicated to treat the following: bipolar disorder (depressed), depression in the medically ill and elderly, dysthymic disorder, major depression, obsessive-compulsive disorder, panic attacks, schizoaffective disorder (depressed), and treatment-resistant depression (refractory depression).

Antipsychotic agents

Antipsychotic agents control psychotic symptoms that can occur with schizophrenia, mania, and other psychoses. Antipsychotic agents have also been called major tranquilizers, because they can reduce agitation, but the label is inaccurate and seldom used now. They are also called neuroleptics, because of their neurologic effects. Antipsychotic agents are classified according to their structure, as follows: phenothiazines, thioxanthenes, butyrophenones, benzisoxazoles, dihydroindolones, dibenzepines, and phenylbutypiperidines.

These agents act on a variety of brain neurotransmitter receptor sites, specifically dopamine, histamine, norepinephrine, and serotonin. They act on both the CNS (limbic, reticular activation, and extrapyramidal systems) and peripheral nervous system. The newer antipsychotic agents (clozapine, risperidone, olanzapine, and quetiapine fumarate) have much more specific receptor blockading action, and thus fewer adverse effects, than earlier phenothiazines.

Antipsychotic agents help to alleviate the following symptoms: agitation (severe), anorexia related to psychosis, blunted affect, combativeness, confusion, delusions, feelings of unreality, hallucinations, ideas of reference, insomnia related to psychosis, paranoia, terror, unclear or racing thoughts, uncontrollable hostility, and verbal threats and aggressiveness.

Hypnosedative agents

Hypnosedative agents are used for insomnia. The three main classes of hypnosedative agents are benzodiazepines, barbiturates, and nonbarbiturates. Benzodiazepines include five primary hypnosedative agents: flurazepam (Dalmane), estazolam (ProSom), quazepam (Doral), temazepam (Restoril), and triazolam (Halcion). These agents are widely used because they cause fewer adverse reactions, less CNS depression, and less toxic risk from potential overdose than the barbiturates and nonbarbiturates.

Barbiturates include amobarbital (Amytal), aprobarbital (Alurate), butabarbital (Butisal), pentobarbital (Nembutal), phenobarbital (Barbital, Luminal), and secobarbital (Seconal). Barbiturates are nonspecific CNS depressants that act on the reticular formation linked to arousal, and they produce effects ranging from sedation to hypnosis, anesthesia, or coma. These agents have a high potential for physical and psychological dependence, abuse, and life-threatening toxicity with overdose. Adverse reactions are common and include CNS and respiratory depression. Therefore, barbiturates are no longer a first choice for treating insomnia.

Nonbarbiturate agents include chloral hydrate (Noctec), ethchlorvynol (Placidyl), glutethimide (Doriden), methyprylon (Noludar), and paraldehyde (Paral). Their mechanisms of action are not clear, and they carry a higher risk of brain damage or death than other hypnosedatives. Currently, they are rarely prescribed for insomnia because more effective medications with fewer (and less harmful) adverse effects are available. Adverse effects include gastrointestinal distress, some hangover effects, and possible respiratory depression.

SELECTED REFERENCES

Aguilera, D.C. *Crisis Intervention: Theory and Methodology,* 8th ed. St. Louis: Mosby–Year Book, Inc., 1998.

Boyd, M.A., and Nihart, M.A. *Psychiatric Nursing: Contemporary Practice.* Philadelphia: Lippincott-Raven Pubs., 1998.

Burgess, A.W. *Advanced Practice Psychiatric Nursing.* Stamford, Conn.: Appleton & Lange, 1998.

Gelenberg, A.J., and Bassuk, E.L. *The Practitioner's Guide to Psychoactive Drugs,* 4th ed. New York: Plenum Publishing Corp., 1997.

Haber, J., et al. *Comprehensive Psychiatric Nursing,* 5th ed. St. Louis: Mosby–Year Book, Inc., 1997.

Haley, J. *Learning and Teaching Therapy.* New York: Guilford Press, 1996.

Harway, M. *Treating the Changing Family.* New York: John Wiley & Sons, 1996.

Krupnick, S.L.W. "Psychopharmacology," in *Psychiatric Nursing: A Comprehensive Reference,* 2nd ed. Edited by Lego, S. Philadelphia: Lippincott-Raven Pubs., 1996.

Stuart, G.W., and Laraia, M.T. *Principles and Practices of Psychiatric Nursing,* 6th ed. St. Louis: Mosby–Year Book, Inc., 1998.

Teicher, M., et al. "The Phototherapy Light Visor. More to It Than Meets the Eye," *American Journal of Psychiatry* 152:1197, 1995.

Varcarolis, E.M. *Foundations of Psychiatric Mental Health Nursing,* 3rd ed. Philadelphia: W.B. Saunders Co., 1998.

The nursing process in psychiatric nursing

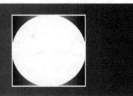

The nurse's relationship with a client is documented through the nursing process — a system for making nursing decisions that includes assessment, nursing diagnosis, planning, implementation, and evaluation. The nursing process guides the nurse in providing quality care to the client and family in any setting. By following this process and supporting it with thorough documentation, the nurse can develop effective strategies for responding to the client's and family's current and potential needs while promoting mental health.

ASSESSMENT

The first step in the nursing process involves the orderly collection and careful interpretation of information about a client's health status. Information comes from subjective data derived from interviews with the client or family members and from objective data, such as physical examination, medical records, diagnostic test results, and other medical or nursing sources. Together, subjective and objective data give the nurse information essential to developing an effective plan of care.

Psychiatric assessment is the scientific process of identifying a client's psychosocial problems, strengths, and concerns. Besides serving as a basis for psychiatric care, psychiatric assessment has broad nursing applications. Recognizing psychosocial problems and how they affect health is important in any clinical setting. Psychiatric assessment involves the psychiatric interview, mental status examination, physical examination, and diagnostic testing.

Psychiatric interview

A systematic psychiatric interview provides information about the client's behavioral disturbances, emotional and social history, and mental status. With this information, the nurse can assess psychological functioning, understand coping methods and their effect on psychosocial growth, build a therapeutic relationship that encourages open communication, and develop a plan of care.

The client must feel comfortable enough in the interview to discuss problems. Before beginning the interview:
• explain the interview's purpose
• reassure the client that privacy will be maintained
• ask the client if a family member or friend should be present
• ask how the client wishes to be addressed
• find out what outcome the client expects from the treatment.

The interview's success hinges on the nurse's ability to listen objectively and respond with empathy. Use these guidelines when interviewing psychiatric clients:
• Have clearly set goals — the interview is not a random discussion.
• Control personal values so that they do not compromise professional judgment.
• Pay attention to the client's reactions and any unspoken signals; observe for signs of anxiety and distress.
• Identify and discuss the client's cultural values and beliefs.
• Avoid making assumptions about how past events affected the client emotionally.
• Monitor personal reactions; watch for interference with interview goals.

Determine the chief complaint — who or what prompted the client to seek treatment. Some clients may not have a chief complain; some identify several small problems, while others will insist nothing is wrong. A client with a medical problem may fail to recognize concurrent depression or anxiety. When possible, discuss the client's complaint, including when the symptoms began, their severity, and their onset (insidious or abrupt).

During the interview, obtain psychosocial, psychiatric, and family histories. The psychosocial history provides information about the client's mental and social status and function. Such a history includes information about the client's beliefs, relationships, lifestyle, coping skills, diet, and sleeping patterns as well as the use of alcohol and drugs, including tobacco, caffeine, nicotine. The history should describe school, work, religious practices, community life, hobbies, and sexual activity. The psychosocial history also should explore how the client has coped with any significant changes such as a recent divorce or death. Numerous assessment tools are available to help the nurse gather information about the client's psychosocial history. (See Section III of this book for samples.)

The psychiatric history explores previous psychological disorders; any episodes of violence, delusions, or attempts at suicide; and previous psychiatric treatment and its results. The family history explores family customs, child-rearing practices, and emotional support during childhood. It also includes information about family members' physical and emotional health, such as a history of substance abuse, alcoholism, suicide, violence, diabetes mellitus, or thyroid disorders.

Throughout the interview, gather information about the client's personality, including level of maturity; ego functioning, such as ability to control impulses, cope with stress, and maintain a sense of identity; strengths, such as talents and accomplishments; and ability to find emotional support.

Mental status examination

Usually part of the psychiatric interview, the mental status examination provides a means of assessing psychological dysfunction and identifying the causes of psychopathology. The nurse needs to understand the components of the examination to be able to interpret the doctor's findings as well as plan appropriate nursing interventions. Various tools are available for mental status assessment. (See *Folstein Mini-Mental State Examination.*)

The mental status examination assesses the client's level of consciousness, general appearance, behavior, speech, mood and affect, intellectual performance, judgment, insight, perception, and thought content.

Level of consciousness helps determine basic brain function: the client's response to stimulation, including the degree and quality of movement; content and coherence of speech; and level of eye opening and eye-to-eye contact. An impaired level of consciousness may indicate a tumor or abscess, an electrolyte or acid-base imbalance, or toxicity from liver or kidney failure or alcohol or drug use.

Appearance, including weight, coloring, skin condition, odor, body build, and obvious physical impairments, indicates the client's overall mental status. Note any discrepancies between objective observation and the client's feelings about his health. A disheveled appearance may indicate self-neglect or a preoccupation with other activities. Posture and gait also may reveal physical and emotional disorders—for example, a slumped posture may indicate depression, fatigue, or suspiciousness.

Behavior includes the client's demeanor and way of relating to others. Note whether the client is cooperative, mistrustful, embarrassed, hostile, or too revealing when responding to questions. Body language, such as tenseness, rigidity, or restlessness, may be significant. An inability to sit still may indicate anxiety. Also watch for any extraordinary behavior, such as disconnected gestures that may indicate hallucinations.

Speech is observed for content and quality. Note any incoherence, illogical or irrelevant replies, speech defects, excessively slow or fast speech, sudden interruptions, excessive volume, altered tone or modulation, slurring, excessive number of words, or minimal monosyllabic responses.

Mood and affect refer to an individual's pervading feeling and how it is expressed. Ask how the client feels and evaluate facial expression and posture.

Intellectual performance involves the ability to reason abstractly, make judgments, or solve problems. Various simple tests can be used to characterize the client's intellectual abilities, such as tests that evaluate orientation, immediate and delayed recall, recent and remote memory, attention level, comprehension, concept formation, and general knowledge.

Judgment is the ability to evaluate choices and draw a conclusion. *Insight* is the capacity for realistic self-assessment. *Perception* involves interpreting reality and using the senses.

Thought content is assessed throughout the mental status examination in terms of connection to reality, clarity, and progression in a logical sequence. Observe for indications of morbid thoughts and preoccupations; abnormal beliefs; suicidal, self-destructive, violent, or superstitious thoughts; recurring dreams; distorted perceptions of reality; and feelings of worthlessness or persecution.

Besides using information from the interview and the mental status examination, observe the client for significant behavior changes. Identify any departures from usual behavior patterns and compare them with the results of the interview and the client's history. Key signs and symptoms include changes in appetite, energy level, motivation, hygiene, self-image, self-esteem, sleep, sex drive, and competence.

Also assess for any signs of self-destructive behavior, including suicide attempts or threats. Keep in mind that not all self-destructive behavior is suicidal in intent. Some clients engage in self-destructive behavior such as self-mutilation. A client who has lost touch with reality may commit self-harm, such as cutting or mutilating, to focus on physical pain, which may be less overwhelming than emotional distress. If the psychosocial interview or observation reveals any signs of hopelessness, assess the risk of suicide and protect the client from self-harm.

Physical examination

Because psychiatric problems may stem from organic causes or medical treatments, the nurse should conduct a physical assessment of all body systems, employing inspection, palpation, percussion, and auscultation. Although the extent of physical assessment depends on the client's needs, the health care setting, the nurse's level of training, and other factors, every client should be examined to obtain basic physiologic data. During any physical assessment, pay particular attention to areas associated with current complaints and past problems identified during the health history.

For the psychiatric client, assessment of the cranial nerves, cerebellar function, and sensory and motor systems is essential. A defect in perception may indicate cranial nerve dysfunction. A neurologic assessment will

Folstein Mini-Mental State Examination

The Folstein Mini-Mental State Examination is the preferred tool for assessing the mental status of a client with suspected cognitive impairment. To perform the examination, ask the client to follow a series of simple commands that test the ability to understand and perform cognitive functions. Award a designated point value for successful completion of each instruction; then total the scores to determine the client's mental status. Scores of 26 to 30 indicate that the client has normal function; 22 to 25, mildly impaired; and less than 22, significantly impaired.

Client instructions	Maximum score	Actual score
Orientation		
• Ask the client to name the year, season, date, day, and month. (Score one point for each correct response.)	5	_____
• Ask the client to name his state, city, street, and house address, and the room in which he is standing. (Score one point for each correct response.)	5	_____
Comprehension		
Name three objects, pausing 1 second between each name. Then ask the client to repeat all three names. (Score one point for each correct response.) Repeat this exercise until the client can correctly name all three objects. (The client will be tested on his ability to recall this information later in the examination.)	3	_____
Attention and calculation		
Ask the client to count backward by sevens, beginning at 100; have him stop after counting out five numbers. Alternatively, ask the client to spell "World" backward. (Score one point for each correct response.)	3	_____
Recall		
Ask the client to restate the name of the three objects previously identified in the examination. (Score one point for each correct response.)	5	_____
Language		
• Point to a pencil and a watch. Ask the client to identify each object. (Score one point for each correct response.)	3	_____
• Ask the client to repeat "No ifs, ands, or buts." (Score one point for a correct response.)	2	_____
• Ask the client to take a paper in the right hand, then fold the paper in half, then put the paper on the floor. (Score one point for each correct response to this three-part command.)	3	_____
• Ask the client to read and obey the written instruction "Close your eyes." (Score one point for a correct response.)	3	_____
• Ask the client to copy the following design. (Score one point for a correct response.)	1	_____
	1	_____
	TOTAL SCORE	_____

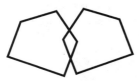

From Folstein, M.F., et al. "Mini-Mental State: A Practical Method for Grading the Cognitive State of Patients for the Clinician," Journal of Psychiatric Research 12:196-97, 1975. Adapted with permission from Mini-Mental LLC, Boston. © 1998 M. Folstein.

help determine whether a sensory defect results from a damaged nerve or a somatoform disorder (a physical condition with no apparent organic cause).

The cerebellum controls equilibrium and muscle function, ensuring smooth, steady, and coordinated movement. An abnormality in cerebellar function may cause the client to depend on other people or mechanical devices for simple tasks, such as walking, bathing, or cooking. Loss of these abilities may create intense loneliness, sadness, or feelings of uselessness.

The sensory system carries impulses from various areas of the body to the central nervous system, which registers and interprets them. Sensory functions include simple touch, pain, temperature, stereognosis, and two-point discrimination. The client with a sensory disturbance experiences severe psychological stress, becoming alternately demanding and withdrawn. A sensory disorder occurring along the distribution pathway of a nerve is apt to have an organic cause; otherwise, suspect a somatoform disorder.

In the motor system, neurons carry impulses from the cerebrum to the skeletal muscles through the pyramidal and extrapyramidal motor tracts. Impulses traveling along the pyramidal tract stimulate individual muscles; those traveling along the extrapyramidal tract stimulate muscle groups. Motor system assessment includes observation of muscle tone, size, and strength. A client with a somatoform disorder may exhibit tics, tremors, or various paralyses with no apparent physiologic cause.

Diagnostic testing

Performing common diagnostic tests for the client with a suspected psychiatric disorder serves five purposes: it assists in accurate diagnosis, investigates any underlying physiologic disorders, establishes normal renal and hepatic function before the client takes prescribed psychotropic medications, monitors for therapeutic medication levels, and determines if the client is using a psychoactive substance. Diagnostic tests include invasive and noninvasive laboratory tests as well as psychological tests.

Laboratory tests may include a complete blood count (CBC), hemoglobin and hematocrit levels, and routine urinalysis. A CBC and hemoglobin and hematocrit help assess for an underlying condition, such as infection, anemia, and dehydration, that might cause or increase psychiatric symptoms. For example, an elevated hemoglobin value might indicate dehydration, which can cause delirium in an elderly or debilitated client. In addition, psychotropic medications may cause such conditions as aplastic anemia or leukopenia; consequently, regular blood counts are important. Urinalysis determines basic kidney function, an important consideration before the doctor prescribes psychotropic medica-

tions because these drugs are excreted through the kidneys.

Toxicologic screening of the blood or urine commonly are ordered as part of the initial assessment. Such tests help determine the presence and level of drugs and can monitor blood levels of prescribed medications, such as lithium, to ensure therapeutic dosage.

Serum electrolyte levels may be checked because electrolyte disturbances can cause symptoms of mental confusion. Abnormal serum electrolyte levels may be a sign of certain psychiatric disorders. For example, an alcoholic client may have an elevated chloride level resulting from renal disease or metabolic acidosis, whereas an anorexic client may have a low chloride or potassium level from excessive vomiting. Some psychotropic medications can cause thirst; a client may have a low sodium level from excessive fluid intake.

Thyroid function tests may be ordered because signs of thyroid dysfunction are very similar to those of anxiety disorder, panic disorder, and depression. Thyroid studies are ordered before lithium is prescribed because the drug may induce hypothyroidism.

Liver function tests are ordered routinely for clients at high risk for liver disease (such as alcoholics and I.V. drug users) as well as to determine the liver's ability to filter medications from the blood.

Serologic evaluation for sexually transmitted diseases and human immunodeficiency virus (HIV) testing may be ordered for clients who exhibit high-risk behaviors, such as multiple sexual partners, I.V. drug use, and unprotected sex. HIV-positive clients also may present with symptoms of depression.

Routine testing for most clients usually includes a chest X-ray and an electrocardiogram to rule out cardiopulmonary abnormalities or disease. An electroencephalogram may be performed to rule out neuroelectrical abnormalities. The following diagnostic procedures also may be ordered to rule out physical causes, such as lesions, abscesses, atrophy, or arteriovenous abnormalities, for abnormal behavior:
• computed tomography, which provides a study of tissue density through radiologic and computer analysis
• magnetic resonance imaging, which provides detailed pictures of body structures on multiple planes
• positron emission tomography, which uses radioactive isotopes to map the brain's metabolic activity (this is useful in detecting such conditions as transient ischemia attacks, seizures, and head trauma as well as the effects of medication therapy)
• single photon emission computed tomography, used primarily to measure regional cerebral blood flow.

In addition to routine diagnostic tests, a client presenting with symptoms of depression may undergo a dexamethasone suppression test. Although not completely diagnostic for depression, this test can reveal if low corticotropin levels may be the cause of the depression.

Additional assessment tools used specifically for the diagnosis of depression include rating scales, such as the Beck Depression Inventory (a 21-item self-rating scale, in which high scores indicate severe depression), the 20-item Zung Self-Rating Depression Scale, and the Geriatric Depression Scale (designed specifically for use with elderly individuals). Other psychological tests include the Stanford-Binet test, the Wechsler Adult Intelligence Scale (revised), and the Minnesota Multiphasic Personality Inventory.

Noninvasive diagnostic tests specifically related to alcohol and drug abuse include:
• CAGE, a four-question tool in which two or three positive responses indicate alcoholism
• Michigan Alcoholism Screening Test, a 24-item timed test in which a score of 5 or better classifies the client as alcoholic
• Drug Use Questionnaire, used when drug use is suspected
• Cocaine Addiction Severity Test and Cocaine Assessment Profile, used when cocaine use is suspected.

NURSING DIAGNOSIS

After completing the assessment step, the nurse analyzes the subjective and objective data and formulates nursing diagnoses. In psychiatric nursing, the nurse uses diagnoses based on the North American Nursing Diagnosis Association (NANDA) taxonomy and the medical diagnoses in the American Psychiatric Association's *Diagnostic and Statistical Manual of Mental Disorders,* 4th ed. *(DSM-IV).*

A nursing diagnosis is a statement of an actual or potential health problem that a nurse can and is licensed to treat. Determining one or more applicable nursing diagnoses for a client provides the basis for an individualized, effective nursing plan of care. Each diagnosis must be supported by clinical information obtained during assessment. Complete care involves collaborative treatment.

Nursing diagnoses provide a common language to convey the nursing management necessary for each client to any nurse involved in that client's care. To help ensure standardized nursing diagnosis terminology and usage, NANDA has formulated and classified a series of nursing diagnostic categories based on nine human response patterns:
• exchanging (mutual giving and receiving)
• communicating (sending messages)
• relating (establishing bonds)
• valuing (assigning worth)
• choosing (selecting alternatives)
• moving (activity)

• perceiving (receiving information)
• knowing (meaning associated with information)
• feeling (subjective awareness of information).
Within each pattern are NANDA-approved nursing diagnostic categories. For example, the human response pattern devoted to relating includes such diagnostic categories as *sexual dysfunction* and *parental role conflict.* The complete list of NANDA diagnostic categories, arranged by human response pattern, is called the *nursing diagnosis taxonomy.* (For the complete list, see appendix B, NANDA diagnostic categories arranged by Gordon's functional health patterns.) Assigning specific nursing diagnoses involves several steps, including grouping assessment data, choosing the appropriate category, and adding specific client information.

To help nurses classify psychiatric disorders, the American Nurses Association's (ANA) Division of Psychiatric and Mental Health Nursing Practice supported a project to identify and develop a working list of the specific phenomena that concern psychiatric and mental health nurses. A panel of specialists in specific age and diagnostic client groups convened to develop a conceptual classification system. The classification system is called the *ANA Classification of Phenomena of Concern to Psychiatric and Mental Health Nursing,* also referred to as *Psychiatric Nursing Diagnoses,* 1st ed.

The standard interdisciplinary psychiatric diagnosis serves the mental health team in labeling a client's disorder. (The nursing diagnosis assists the nurse in conceptualizing the client's human response that nursing can address.) The official guide to psychiatric classification is the *DSM-IV.* This classification system reflects the medical model, but also includes descriptive, behavioral, and social understandings of mental disorders. Because interdisciplinary health care teams, managed mental health payors, and other insurance payors use *DSM-IV,* it is important for psychiatric–mental health nurses to understand the classification system.

PLANNING

After formulating appropriate nursing diagnoses, the nurse develops a plan of care appropriate for the client and family. Effective planning focuses on the client's specific needs, considers strengths and weaknesses, encourages the client's participation in setting achievable goals and in the care itself, includes feasible interventions, and is within the scope of applicable nursing practice acts. Planning involves three basic steps: setting and prioritizing goals, formulating nursing interventions, and developing a plan of care.

The nurse sets one or more goals for each applicable diagnosis. A goal — the desired client outcome after nursing care — states what the nurse and client will do to minimize or eliminate a problem. Appropriate goals help the nurse select nursing interventions and also serve as criteria for evaluating the interventions. Goals should relate directly to the nursing diagnoses and reflect the desires of the client, family, and nurse, who work together to formulate them. Setting goals with the client and family helps ensure appropriate and realistic care planning, encourages client involvement, and gives the client a sense of control.

An effective goal statement, or outcome criterion, is measurable, realistic, and stated so that the client and family understand it. It should include the desired client behavior and predicted outcome, measurement criteria, a specified time for attainment or reevaluation, and any other conditions under which the behavior will occur. After goals are formulated, the nurse works with the client and family to prioritize them. Goals may be short-term or long-term. Short-term goals may take priority over long-term ones. When prioritizing goals, the nurse and client should account for possible effects of the client's ethnic and cultural background, socioeconomic status, and other factors that might influence goal achievement.

The nurse formulates interventions to achieve each short- and long-term goal. Effective nursing interventions must be based on both sound nursing practice and research. Such a knowledge base provides the proper rationales to support nursing interventions. These interventions will include strategies, actions, or activities that help the client reach established goals by diminishing or resolving problems identified in the nursing diagnoses. The nurse and client should work together to formulate interventions, analyzing possible strategies and choosing those best suited to the client's circumstances. Interventions may be collaborative, including nursing and medical care, physical therapy, nutritional counseling, and social services.

The nurse develops a plan of care by integrating each step of the nursing process: collecting and analyzing health history and physical assessment data, selecting nursing diagnoses, setting and prioritizing goals, formulating interventions, and evaluating outcomes. The plan of care, which can be revised and updated as needed, acts as a written guide for and documentation of the client's care. Also, it helps ensure continuity of care when the client interacts with other members of the health care team.

The format of nursing plans of care varies among health care facilities and sometimes among units in the same facility. All plans of care, however, include written nursing diagnoses, goals, interventions, and evaluation criteria. Standardized care plans have evolved as a time-saving and efficient method of ensuring accurate documentation. A standardized care plan incorporates the major aspects of nursing care required by clients with a similar problem, while allowing alterations to reflect individual differences.

IMPLEMENTATION

Implementation involves working with the client and family to accomplish the designated interventions and move toward the desired outcomes. Effective implementation requires a sound understanding of the plan of care and collaborative interactions among the client, family, and other members of the health care team, as needed. The implementation phase begins as soon as the plan of care is completed and ends when the established goals are achieved. Before and during implementation of any intervention, the nurse reassesses the client to ensure that planned interventions continue to be appropriate. Periodic reassessment helps ensure a flexible, individualized, and effective plan of care.

To implement nursing interventions effectively, the nurse will use four types of skills:
• cognitive skills, based on knowledge of current clinical practice and basic sciences
• affective skills, including verbal and nonverbal communication and empathy
• psychomotor skills, involving both mental and physical activity and encompassing traditional nursing actions (such as taking vital signs and administering medications) and more complex procedures
• organizational skills, such as counseling, managing, and delegating.

EVALUATION

Through evaluation, the nurse obtains additional subjective and objective assessment data relating to the goals identified in the planning stage. The nurse uses these data to determine whether goals have been met totally, met partially, or remain unmet. Although evaluation is the final step in the nursing process, it actually occurs throughout, particularly during implementation, where the nurse continually reassesses the effect of interventions. The nurse is responsible for monitoring the client's progress based on established and measurable expected outcomes. Evaluation is directly linked to and must be based on the goals developed from each nursing diagnosis.

When all goals for a particular nursing diagnosis have been met, the nurse and client may decide that the diagnosis is no longer valid. The nurse then documents when and how the goals were met and may delete the diagnosis from the nursing plan of care. Alternatively, the nurse and client may judge a goal met but still feel that the nursing diagnosis requires other goals; they then would retain it in the plan of care.

If goals have been met only partially or remain unmet by the target date, the nurse must reevaluate the plan of care. Reevaluation involves deciding whether the initial plan was appropriate, whether the assigned time frame was realistic, whether the goals were realistic and measurable, and whether other factors interfered. Based on this information, the nurse can clarify or amend the assessment data, reexamine and correct the nursing diagnoses as necessary, establish new goals reflecting the revised diagnoses, and devise new interventions for achieving these goals. The nurse then adds the revised plan of care to the original document and records the rationale for these revisions in the nursing notes.

SELECTED REFERENCES

Boyd, M.A., and Nihart, M.A. *Psychiatric Nursing: Contemporary Practice.* Philadelphia: Lippincott-Raven Pubs., 1998.

Carpenito, L. *Nursing Diagnosis: Application to Clinical Practice,* 7th ed. Philadelphia: Lippincott-Raven Pubs., 1997.

Folstein, M.F., et al. "Mini-Mental State: A Practical Method for Grading the Cognitive State of Patients for the Clinician," *Journal of Psychiatric Research* 12(3):189-98, 1975.

Gordon, M. *Manual of Nursing Diagnosis: 1997-1998.* St. Louis: Mosby–Year Book, Inc., 1997.

Varcarolis, E.M. *Foundations of Psychiatric Mental Health Nursing,* 3rd ed. Philadelphia: W.B. Saunders Co., 1998.

Part 2

Anxiety disorders

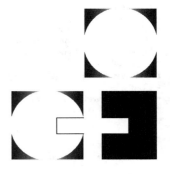

Organic-related anxiety disorders

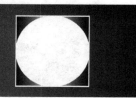

DSM-IV classifications
293.89 Anxiety disorder due to a general medical condition
291-292 Substance-induced anxiety disorder

INTRODUCTION

Description
Anxiety disorder due to a medical condition, also called secondary anxiety, is characterized by clinically significant anxiety that is caused by the direct physiologic effects of one or more general medical conditions. Symptoms can include prominent generalized anxiety symptoms, panic attacks, or obsessions or compulsions. These symptoms produce clinically significant distress, which impairs social and occupational function. The history, physical assessment, and laboratory findings must show that the anxiety is the direct physiologic consequence of the client's general medical condition.

A comprehensive psychophysiologic assessment should confirm that the client's anxiety symptoms are due to a general medical condition. Many medical conditions may cause anxiety symptoms. (*See Medical conditions presenting with anxiety.*)

Substance-induced anxiety disorder is characterized by anxiety symptoms that arise from direct physiologic effects of a prescription drug, an over-the-counter (OTC) drug, or a controlled substance. Clinical presentation depends on the effects of the substance and the context in which the symptoms occur (for example, intoxication or withdrawal). Many drugs have been reported to cause anxiety symptoms. (*See Medications associated with anxiety.*)

Etiology and precipitating factors
The etiologic factors that lead to these disorders are summarized in the two charts on the following pages.

Potential complications
Anxiety may exacerbate undiagnosed medical conditions. Additionally, undiagnosed or misdiagnosed anxiety due to a medical or substance-induced condition can worsen the underlying condition. Such clients often have low thresholds of discomfort, and anxiety can

Medical conditions presenting with anxiety

Anxiety may result from medical conditions or exacerbate preexisting medical conditions. The following are some common examples to consider when making the diagnosis of anxiety.

Cardiovascular disorders
• Arrhythmias (such as supraventricular tachycardia, ventricular tachycardia)
• Cardiomyopathies
• Heart failure
• Coronary insufficiency
• Mitral valve prolapse
• Myocardial infarction or angina

Endocrine disorders
• Adrenal insufficiency
• Carcinoid syndrome
• Cushing's syndrome
• Hyperparathyroidism
• Hyperthyroidism or hypothyroidism
• Hypoglycemia, hyperinsulinemia
• Thyroiditis

Gastrointestinal disorders
• Colitis
• Irritable bowel syndrome
• Peptic ulcer disease

Metabolic disorders
• Hypocalcemia or hypercalcemia
• Hypokalemia
• Hyponatremia

Neurologic disorders
• Central nervous system infections, masses
• Essential tremor
• Huntington's chorea
• Multiple sclerosis
• Parkinson's disease
• Postconcussion syndrome
• Seizure disorders (such as temporal lobe epilepsy, complex partial seizures)
• Vestibular dysfunction

Pulmonary disorders
• Asthma
• Chronic obstructive pulmonary disease
• Hyperventilation syndrome
• Pneumothorax
• Pneumonia
• Primary pulmonary hypertension
• Pulmonary edema
• Pulmonary embolism

progress to a panic state or panic attacks, possibly requiring emergency room care.

ASSESSMENT GUIDELINES

Nursing history (functional health pattern findings)

Health perception–health management pattern
• Extreme concern over health, worried about "getting worse"
• Worry over medication compliance, follow-up visits and inability to follow through on health related plans
• Increased focus on somatic complaints related to their medical conditions
• Increased use of health care system due to exacerbations of medical conditions
• Worry over inability to control feelings
• Fear of "going crazy"

Nutritional-metabolic pattern
• Concern about eating behaviors, such as overeating or undereating to decrease anxiety
• Eating foods with poor nutritional value
• Increased intake of caffeine and salt
• Weight fluctuations

Elimination pattern
• Concern over gastrointestinal system disturbances
• Frequent urination
• Concern over increased sweating, cold and clammy skin, or both

Activity-exercise pattern
• Concern about being easily fatigued
• Difficulty in accomplishing normal daily activities
• Concern about inability to participate in and enjoy leisure activities
• Withdrawn or apathetic behavior
• Concern about any limitations and restrictions of activity caused by disease or condition

Sleep-rest pattern
• Concern about falling or staying asleep and nightmares
• Experiencing nighttime "suffocation"
• Feeling fatigued after sleep
• Concern about use or abuse of sleep aids, such as alcohol, benzodiazepines, and hypnotics

Cognitive-perceptual pattern
• Difficulty concentrating
• Difficulty with understanding and reacting to external stimuli
• Concern about memory and concentration changes
• Worry over inability to think clearly
• Distorted perceptions

Anxiety disorders

Medications associated with anxiety

Anxiety can result from prescribed or over-the-counter medications. Consider these drugs when assessing the client's medication regimen for possible causes.

• Amphetamines
• Analgesics
• Anesthetics
• Anticholinergics
• Antidepressants (tricyclics, selective serotonin reuptake inhibitors, bupropion)
• Antihistamines
• Antihypertensives
• Antimicrobials
• Appetite suppressants
• Asthma medications (bronchodilators)
• Caffeine preparations
• Calcium-blocking agents
• Cholinergic-blocking agents
• Central nervous system depressants (withdrawal syndrome)
• cocaine
• estrogen

• ethosuximide
• Heavy metals
• hydralazine
• insulin
• levodopa
• Muscle relaxants
• Nasal decongestants
• Neuroleptics
• Nonsteroidal anti-inflammatory agents
• procaine
• procarbazine
• Steroids
• Sympathomimetics
• theophylline
• Thyroid preparations
• tranylcypromine

Self-perception–self-concept pattern
• Concern over being indecisive and dependent
• Perception of self as being highly anxious
• Perception of self as incompetent and powerless
• Concerns about body image, self-esteem, and self-worth

Role-relationship pattern
• Concern about how community members and neighbors may respond to the disease or condition
• Concern over the lack of response to or support of lifestyle changes from family and friends
• Concern about a distressful work situation
• Concern about perceived inability to fulfill role responsibilities (home, work, community)

Sexual-reproductive pattern
• Dissatisfaction with sexual relations
• Concern about poor self-image due to medical condition
• Difficulty with intimacy
• Experiencing sexual dysfunction due to medical condition or treatment

Coping–stress tolerance pattern
• Constant irritability, feeling on edge or keyed up
• Constant shakiness, trembling, or twitching
• Belief that medical condition and subsequent lifestyle changes are contributing to feeling out of control
• Inability to identify those persons or measures that alleviate rather than exacerbate the condition

Value-belief pattern
• Desire to decrease or increase involvement in spirituality or religion
• Concern over impaired ability to believe in anything or anyone
• Disbelief about present and immediate future situation; unable to believe that they will get better and are not hopeful about immediate future
• Feeling powerless to achieve life goals

Physical findings
Cardiovascular
• Cold, clammy skin
• Elevated blood pressure
• Hot and cold flashes
• Increased heart rate
• Palpitations
• Sweating
• Tingling sensation

Respiratory
• Choking sensation
• Increased respiratory rate
• Shortness of breath
• Smothering sensation
• Wheezing (may be related to underlying pulmonary disorder)

Gastrointestinal
• Abdominal distress
• Diarrhea
• Difficulty swallowing
• Dry mouth
• Nausea
• Vomiting

Genitourinary
• Frequent urination

Musculoskeletal
• Increased muscle fatigue
• Muscle aches, pains, or soreness
• Muscle tension
• Restlessness
• Shakiness
• Trembling
• Twitching

Neurologic
• Dilated pupils
• Dizziness or faintness
• Insomnia
• Light-headedness
• Paresthesias
• Restlessness
• Syncope

Psychological
• Feeling keyed up or on edge
• Inability to concentrate
• Difficulty remembering (forgetting to take medications or taking too many)
• Increasing anxiety to panic level, causing decompensation of medical condition

Nursing diagnosis

Anxiety (moderate to severe) related to physiologic impact of medical condition or medications

Nursing priority

Help the client and primary health care provider identify causative factors of the anxiety and minimize or alleviate the impact of these factors.

Patient outcome criteria

As treatment progresses, the client, family, or both should be able to:
• monitor intensity of anxiety
• seek out information to reduce anxiety
• use relaxation techniques
• maintain concentration and improve ability to focus
• maintain medication regimen.

Interventions

1. Identify the pattern and presentation of anxiety.

2. Review all medications the client is taking (prescribed or otherwise).

3. Identify stressors in the client's life that contribute to anxiety.

4. Collaborate with prescribing and treating health care providers to evaluate the client's response to treatment and explore the client's continued needs for medications that may be causing anxiety.

5. Teach and practice with the client the use of relaxation techniques, such as guided imagery, meditation, muscle relaxation, and self-hypnosis.

6. Administer prescribed antianxiety medication and monitor the client's response using subjective and objective information.

7. Instruct the client about prescribed antianxiety medication. Assess the client's self-administration, and provide written instructions. Point out management strategies for adverse effects.

Rationales

1. Careful observations by the client, family members, and the nurse yield knowledge of causes and exacerbating and alleviating factors.

2. Some medications may cause intense anxiety; perhaps they can be replaced by another drug category or merely a different brand. An OTC medication or an herbal remedy may be interacting with the client's prescription and causing symptoms.

3. Identifying stressors and determining their relevance and significance helps the client understand which stressors have positive and negative impact on one's physical and mental well-being.

4. Collaboration with all relevant health care providers is key to understanding the root causes of the client's anxiety and in warding off potential problems. For example, the client (especially if elderly) may be taking several medications prescribed by different providers, thus running the risk of serious drug incompatibilities.

5. Relaxation techniques can help reduce emotional and physical distress that accompanies anxiety and may decrease other anxiety-related symptoms.

6. Antianxiety medications can relieve physical symptoms and promote a calming effect, thereby helping the client participate in stress-reduction exercises and other forms of therapy.

7. Adequate drug information enables the client and family to take appropriate action if adverse reactions occur.

NURSING DIAGNOSIS

Social isolation related to effects of medical and corresponding treatments

Nursing priority

Identify and activate social supports to decrease self-imposed or system-imposed social isolation.

Patient outcome criteria

As treatment progresses, the client, family, or both should be able to:
- interact with family, significant others, and friends
- interact with other members of a support group
- report time and emotional assistance provided by others
- verbalize willingness to call others for assistance.

Interventions

1. Explore with the client the quality and availability of social supports. Assess the individuals in the client's network regarding their reliability and accessibility. Determine if the client feels that they are supportive.

2. Determine which local agencies and resources would be useful and available to the client, especially in regard to the underlying medical condition.

3. Encourage the client to verbalize or, if unable to speak, write about concerns and fears and to ask questions.

Rationales

1. Social support can buffer the effects of physical and psychological stress and illness.

2. Clients are often unaware of where they can get specific information, help, and emotional support. Joining in may alleviate their sense of being alone in their plight. Groups, such as an Automated Internal Cardiac Defibrillation (AICD) support group, Heart Menders, or AIDS support groups, can provide the client with resources that can assist with aspects of the medical condition. Checking Internet sites for additional information may also be helpful.

3. Showing genuine concern and interest helps the client by decreasing the sense of alienation, thereby decreasing isolation.

Nursing diagnosis

Sleep pattern disturbance related to physiologic disturbance (medical condition, effects of medication or other medical treatments)

Nursing priority

Help the client recognize the relationship between the medical condition, medication, and anxiety and sleep disturbance.

Patient outcome criteria

As the treatment progresses, the client, family, or both should be able to:
- report an increase in the amount of hours of sleep
- demonstrate an improved sleep pattern
- report more uninterrupted sleep time
- report feeling refreshed after a sleep cycle.

Interventions

1. Identify the sleep pattern disturbance and assess the client's usual sleep rituals.

2. Encourage the client to restrict or abstain from stimulants and depressants before bedtime.

3. Teach the client relaxation techniques to use at bedtime.

4. Teach the client specific sleep hygiene methods.

5. Encourage the client to increase daytime activity, participate in an exercise program, and avoid exercise two hours before bedtime.

6. Teach the client about the prescribed sedative-hypnotic medication. Encourage the client to use the medication only as directed and to keep a journal (sleep record) describing responses to the behavioral interventions and the medication and how both are affecting sleep.

Rationales

1. Identifying a client's usual sleep rituals can help isolate causative factors and assist selection of focused interventions to manage the sleep disturbance. The client may be eating large meals late in the evening along with caffeine-containing coffee, they may be taking a diuretic late in the evening that could be causing them to awaken to urinate, or they may have had to sleep during the day and work at night.

2. Stimulants (for example, caffeine, nicotine, psychostimulants, some selective serotonin reuptake inhibitors) and depressants (for example, alcohol) interfere with the normal sleep cycle and can produce a sleep pattern disturbance.

3. Relaxation techniques can reduce anxious feelings and muscle tension and may restore the client's previous ability to sleep. However, these techniques usually need to be coupled with other treatments.

4. Having a concrete and focused plan can help the client by alleviating indecisiveness and feelings of incompetence and by enhancing the sleep pattern. Sleep hygiene methods focus on identifying causes of sleep deprivation and on developing a focused plan to decrease the impact of the causative factors.

5. Regular activity and light to moderate exercise (within the individual's functional limitations) increases body fatigue and the desire to rest and sleep, without overstimulating the client before bedtime.

6. Sedative-hypnotic medications can interfere with non-rapid eye movement (NREM) and rapid eye movement (REM) sleep and the quality of rest. A significant problem of rebound insomnia, characterized by intense dreaming, nightmares, and increased sleep disruptions, can develop.

DISCHARGE CRITERIA

Nursing documentation indicates that the client:
• has demonstrated an increased ability to recognize the impact of the medical condition or treatment on anxiety
• has demonstrated an increased ability to recognize anxiety symptoms
• understands the diagnosis, treatment, and expected outcomes
• is aware and has made contact with available group, family, or marital therapy and group resources
• has demonstrated an improved ability to utilize sleep hygiene methods.

SELECTED REFERENCES

Barry, P.D. *Psychosocial Nursing: Care of Physically Ill Patients and Their Families,* 3rd ed. Philadelphia: Lippincott-Raven Pubs., 1996.

Diagnostic and Statistical Manual of Mental Disorders, 4th ed. Washington, D.C.: American Psychiatric Association, 1994.

Johnson, M., and Maas, M. *Nursing Outcomes Classification (NOC).* St. Louis: Mosby–Year Book, Inc., 1997.

Knesper, D.J., et al. *Primary Care Psychiatry.* Philadelphia: W.B. Saunders Co., 1997.

Lishman, W.A. *Organic Psychiatry: The Psychological Consequences of Cerebral Disorder,* 3rd ed. London: Blackwell Science, 1998.

Moore, D.P., and Jefferson, J.W. *Handbook of Medical Psychiatry.* St. Louis: Mosby–Year Book, Inc., 1996.

Rundell, J.R., and Wise, M.G. *Textbook of Consultation Liaison Psychiatry.* Washington, D.C.: American Psychiatric Association, 1996.

Wyszynski, A.A., and Wyszynski, B. *A Case Approach to Medical-Psychiatric Practice.* Washington, D.C.: American Psychiatric Association, 1996.

Phobic and panic disorders

DSM-IV classifications
Phobic disorders
300.22	Agoraphobia without history of panic disorder
300.23	Social phobia
300.29	Specific phobia (Identify)

Panic disorders
300.01	Panic disorder without agoraphobia
300.21	Panic disorder with agoraphobia

INTRODUCTION

Description
Phobic disorders
Phobic disorders are characterized by a persistent, irrational fear of a specific activity, object, or situation. These disorders, which affect about 5% of the population, are classified as agoraphobia without history of panic disorder, social phobia, and specific phobia. A diagnosis of phobia is generally made when the avoidance behavior is extreme or the problem so pervasive that it interferes with the individual's normal functioning at home, work, or school.

Agoraphobia without history of panic disorder is relatively rare because agoraphobia usually is accompanied by panic. Less severely affected individuals may experience remissions and exacerbations of symptoms, whereas those more severely affected may suffer lifetime disability. Generally, agoraphobic individuals, who often have a history of generalized anxiety as well, limit travel and social activity. They may venture out only with a companion.

Social phobia is characterized by a persistent fear of and excessive anxiety about being exposed to the scrutiny of others (that is, in a classroom, when speaking in public, and at social events). Individuals with social phobias may avoid eating, drinking, or speaking in public.

Specific phobia (also called simple phobia) is marked by overwhelming anxiety due to exposure to a specific object (such as a snake, spider, dog, or germ) or a situation (such as flying, seeing blood, or receiving an injection). Common phobias include the fear of heights, thunder, lightning, closed spaces, and certain animals. Although a specific phobia usually causes minimal impairment, it can become incapacitating with prolonged or frequent exposure to the feared object or activity. Specific phobias that develop in adulthood usually require treatment before they are alleviated.

Panic disorders
Panic is an extreme and overwhelming form of anxiety often experienced when an individual is in a life threatening situation. In such situations panic is a normal and expected reaction. However, in panic disorder, persons experience panic in situations that do not pose any real danger or threat to them Therefore, panic disorders are characterized by recurrent, unpredictable attacks of intense apprehension or terror. Such panic attacks can render an individual unable to control a situation or to perform even simple tasks. Behavior can be further complicated by an anticipatory fear of helplessness or of losing control. In its most severe state, a panic attack can produce such symptoms as chest pain, numbness, and shortness of breath, which are typically associated with a heart attack. (See *Recognizing a panic attack*.)

Sometimes, panic attacks occur during sleep, manifesting as a sudden awakening with apprehension or fear. There is usually no recall of dream content and sleep panic attacks do not appear to be dependent on rapid eye movement (REM). They do tend, however, to be associated with late stage 2 and early stage 3 sleep. Individuals with sleep panic attacks often develop a fear of falling asleep.

Panic disorders occur with or without agoraphobia. Panic disorders with agoraphobia are especially debilitating because they typically lead to severe social, work, and travel restrictions. Individuals with the disorder become severely restricted in their ability to socialize and suffer from social isolation.

Women are much more likely to experience panic disorder than men. The National Comorbidity Survey discovered no difference in the prevalence of panic disorder in whites and blacks. However, the Epidemology Catchment Area (ECA) study did find lower lifetime rates of panic disorder among Hispanics. The usual age of individuals when they experience the onset of symptoms of panic disorder is between 20 and 29 years; however, some individuals develop symptoms after age 40.

Etiology and precipitating factors
Explanations of etiology and precipitating factors for phobic and panic disorders continue to be the focus of research. Current research focuses on neurobiology, brain imaging, and neuroanatomy to clarify the impact of genetic predisposition, in conjunction with biological and psychological causes of panic.

Current research evidence supports a substantial familial predisposition. There is an estimated lifetime risk for panic disorder as high as 25% among first-degree relatives of individuals diagnosed with panic disorder. Additional evidence has been found in studies of twins where the occurrence of panic attacks was as much as five times more frequent in monozygotic than dizygotic twins. Although no specific gene has been identified as yet, the studies are promising and can be useful in educating families about their mental health risks and in planning mental health prevention strategies.

Magnetic resonance imaging (MRI) studies have detected specific neurologic abnormalities in patients diagnosed with panic disorder. The abnormalities include focal areas of abnormal activity in the medial portion of the temporal lobe in the parahippocampal area, usually on the right side, and significant asymmetrical atrophy of the temporal lobe. However, it is not clear whether these findings indicate a genetic predisposition to panic disorder or represent a result of the disorder.

Biochemical research has identified certain neurotransmitters that are believed to be involved in panic disorder. Studies of the action of norepinephrine are inconclusive but suggest that dysfunctional regulation in the norepinephrine system exists in individuals with panic disorder. Serotonin (5-HT) may also interact with norephinephrine, and preliminary findings are providing some insight into the mechanisms by which selective serotonin reuptake inhibitors (SSRIs) have their effect in the treatment of panic disorder.

Gamma-aminobutyric acid (GABA) is the primary inhibitory neurotransmitter in the brain. GABA receptor stimulation produces anxiolytic, sedative, cognitive, anticonvulsant, and muscle relaxant effects. The benzodiazepine receptor exists in the same molecular complex as the GABA receptors; therefore, benzodiazepines bind to these receptors and potentiate GABA effects. Abnormalities in the benzodiazepine-GABA interaction have been implicated in panic disorder. Further studies with positron emission tomography (PET) scans and single photon emission computed tomography (SPECT) are beginning to provide more direct information about these receptors.

Corticotropin-releasing factor (CRF), a neuropeptide, is important in the function of the hypothalamus-pituitary-adrenal (HPA) axis. CRF and CRF receptors are found outside the hypothalamus and are distributed in the forebrain (frontal cortex, amygdala and hippocampus), and the brain stem (including the locus ceruleus). Severe and persistent stressors cause increased CRF concentrations in the hippocampus, amygdala, and locus ceruleus. Recent research has found that traumatic events in early life stages can produce persistent alterations in CRF.

Cholecystokinin (CCK) is a neuropeptide that has been implicated in the etiology of panic disorder. The cerebral cortex, amygdala, and hippocampus have high concentrations of CCK. When administered in challenge studies, CCK tetrapeptide (CCK-4) induces panic attacks in patients with panic disorder. Several other neuropeptides, including growth hormone (GH), growth hormone releasing factor (GRF), and somatostatin (SRIF), also appear to be involved in the etiology of panic disorder. Individuals with panic disorder exhibit blunted GH responses to several pharmacologic, biochemical, and neuropeptide challenge tests. Unfortunately, the exact mechanism for this finding has not yet been established.

Additional challenge studies have been conducted employing various panicogenic agents, including sodium bicarbonate, sodium lactate, and carbon dioxide (CO_2). Individuals with panic disorder may be hypersensitive to CO_2; they experience a "false suffocation alarm" response and subsequently the CO_2 increases the locus ceruleus firing, which promotes a sense of panic in the individual. Dysfunction in the norepinephrine system may be secondary to CO_2 hypersensitivity. Studies of cerebral blood flow patterns in patients with panic disorder show abnormalities during panic attacks. For example, individuals with the disorder who experience panic during an intravenous challenge of sodium lactate exhibit asymmetry of blood flow to the parahippocampal regions.

Psychological theorists regard anxiety as an outward sign of internal conflict. Currently the psychoanalytic

Recognizing a panic attack

A panic attack is a brief period of intense apprehension or fear; it may last from minutes to hours. It may be a result of another disorder and not necessarily panic disorder; however, a history of four attacks within 4 weeks that are not related to physical exertion, exhaustion, presence of life-threatening situations, or phobias does confirm a panic disorder.

During a panic attack, the client will display four or more of these signs and symptoms:

- chest pains, palpitations
- choking
- depersonalization or derealization
- diaphoresis
- dyspnea
- faintness, light-headedness
- fear of going crazy, fear of dying, fear of losing control during the attack
- hot and cold flashes
- nausea, abdominal distress
- shakiness or trembling.

theories initiated by Freud and his colleagues are no longer universally supported as causative factors for panic disorder. And the movement into psychiatric illnesses as brain disorders and the support for research funding in this area has decreased the acceptance of the psychoanalytic theories that have not been subject to scientific rigor.

Psychodynamic theories identify factors that include a history of childhood separation anxiety, sudden loss of a family member or loved one, and a series of stressful life events that occur in a cumulative manner. Additional research in the area of psychodynamic theories has proposed that negative feelings of low self-esteem and powerlessness make the individual feel vulnerable to the stress of daily life events. Consequently, further avoidance of negative feelings, and the powerlessness to control them, escalates into fear and dread, and, thereby, precipitates the start of panic attacks.

Behavioral theories have limitations in adequately explaining the development of panic disorder, based on learning theory or classic conditioning theory because many individuals studied were unable to identify an adverse or fear provoking event(s).

Research based on behavioral theories has demonstrated that controlled exposure and cognitive restructuring techniques can reduce symptoms of panic disorder. Unfortunately, these theories do not explain nonrapid eye movement (REM) sleep panic attacks, and often individuals are unaware of their own catastrophic interpretations of events and therefore may not be able to attend to these feelings until their awareness is enhanced.

Effective treatment requires an integrated biopsychosocial model of panic disorder. This model of a panic disorder cycle involves three distinct stages: the panic attack which is biologically generated; anticipatory anxiety, which is believed to be related to the limbic lobe, the center of basic human emotions; and phobic avoidance. During the anticipatory anxiety stage, generalized anxiety created by panic attacks produces a kindling phenomenon. The phobic avoidance stage involves conscious, cognitive activity to avoid the event, object, or situation that prompted the panic attack. The cognitive activity occurs in the prefrontal cortex. A multimodal therapy approach is best utilized to manage this complex and often debilitating disorder.

Potential complications

Undiagnosed medical reasons for phobic or panic symptoms can lead to physical deterioration. If left untreated, these disorders can lead to increasing social withdrawal and isolation, which may severely impair the client's social and work life. Individuals with panic disorder have committed suicide, so a suicide and lethality assessment needs to be incorporated into the care of these clients.

ASSESSMENT GUIDELINES

Nursing history (functional health pattern findings)
Health perception–health management pattern
- Extreme concern over general health
- Persistent fear of some object or situation that poses no actual danger
- Fear of "going crazy"
- Numerous somatic complaints, with or without diagnostic validation
- Inability to move, speak, or identify ways of decreasing anxiety
- Worry over medication compliance, follow-up visits, and inability to control feelings
- Inability to control feelings
- Overuse or underuse of health care system to ease panic symptoms

Nutritional-metabolic pattern
- Concern over eating behaviors, such as using food to suppress feelings
- Significant weight fluctuations

Elimination pattern
- Concern over GI system disturbances, such as nausea, pain, diarrhea, and vomiting
- Frequent urination
- Concern over increased sweating, cold and clammy skin, or both

Activity-exercise pattern
- Restlessness or trembling
- Fear of situations that consistently lead to panic attacks, helplessness, and humiliation
- Concern about inability to participate in and enjoy leisure activities
- Manipulation of environment and dependence on others to avoid confrontation with certain situations or objects
- Concern about limitations and self-imposed activity restrictions caused by inability to predict panic attacks
- Difficulty accomplishing normal daily activities

Sleep-rest pattern
- Concern about falling or staying asleep and nightmares
- Concern about use or abuse of sleep aids, such as alcohol, benzodiazepines, and hypnotics
- Feeling fatigued after sleep
- Fatigue and inability to function during the day

Cognitive-perceptual pattern
- Difficulty concentrating
- Worry over inability to think clearly
- Distorted thinking and inability to test reality

• Difficulty with understanding and reacting to external stimuli

Self-perception–self-concept pattern
• Perception of self as being highly anxious
• Dread and certainty that death is near
• Perception of self as being incompetent and powerless

Role-relationship pattern
• Concern over relationships with family or loved ones
• Concern over the lack of response to or support of lifestyle changes from family or loved ones

Sexual-reproductive pattern
• Dissatisfaction with sexual relations
• Difficulty with intimacy

Coping–stress tolerance pattern
• Pervasive muscle tension
• Constant irritability, feeling on edge or keyed up
• Shakiness, trembling, or twitching
• Feeling unreal or depersonalized
• Belief that significant lifestyle changes are contributing to feeling out of control

Value-belief pattern
• Feeling powerless to achieve life goals
• Disbelief about present situation
• Concern over inability to believe in anything or anyone

Physical findings
Cardiovascular
• Chest pain or discomfort
• Elevated blood pressure
• Hot and cold flashes or chills
• Increased heart rate
• Palpitations
• Sweating
• Syncope
• Tachycardia

Respiratory
• Choking sensation
• Dyspnea
• Hyperventilation
• Increased respiratory rate
• Shortness of breath
• Smothering sensation

Gastrointestinal
• Abdominal distress
• Diarrhea
• Difficulty swallowing
• Dry mouth
• Lump in throat
• Nausea
• Vomiting

Musculoskeletal
• Muscle aches
• Muscle tension
• Restlessness
• Shakiness
• Trembling

Neurologic
• Dilated pupils
• Dizziness or faintness
• Light-headedness
• Paresthesia
• Inability to fall asleep or difficulty staying asleep
• Vertigo or unsteadiness

Psychological
• Fear of losing control or dying
• Feeling keyed up or on edge
• Feeling unreal or depersonalized
• Inability to concentrate or focus
• Irritability
• Blank mind
• Perceptual field deficits

Anxiety disorders

NURSING DIAGNOSIS

Anxiety related to confrontation with feared object or situation

Nursing priority

Help the client become desensitized to the phobic object or situation.

Patient outcome criteria

As the treatment progresses, the client, family, or both should be able to:
• verbalize signs and symptoms of increasing anxiety
• identify current level of anxiety
• identify specific situations, events, activities, or objects that initiate the panic or phobic reaction.

Interventions

1. Collaborate with the client to identify the feared object or situation.

2. Teach assertiveness skills that reduce submissive and fearful responses.

3. Explore the client's anticipatory thinking about the feared object or situation.

4. Teach the client relaxation and thought-stopping techniques, such as progressive muscle relaxation and guided imagery. Provide time for practice sessions using role-playing scenarios.

5. Encourage the client to imagine encountering the feared situation or object and then taking steps to alleviate that fear. Encourage the client to describe the coping process step-by-step.

6. Collaborate with the client and multidisciplinary team to develop and implement a systematic desensitization program.

7. Collaborate with the client and multidisciplinary team to assess the need for pharmacologic intervention.

8. Administer antiphobic or antipanic agents, such as antianxiety agents (benzodiazepines: alprazolam [Xanax], clonazepam [Klonopin]), tricyclic antidepressants (amitriptyline [Elavil], doxepin [Sinequan]), monoamine oxidase inhibitors (isocarboxazid [Marplan], phenelzine [Nardil]), or SSRIs (paroxetine [Paxil], fluoxetine [Prozac], sertraline [Zoloft], fluvoxamine [Luvox]), as prescribed. Often these medications may be prescribed in combination to augment the effect, such as benzodiazepine and an SSRI along with cognitive-behavioral therapy. Monitor the client's response and observe for and educate the patient and family about adverse reactions and specific adverse effect management strategies.

Rationales

1. Identifying the phobic object or situation can enable the client to avoid or at least limit contact with it. This limited contact can be especially helpful initially when the nurse and client are developing a definitive treatment program.

2. Such strategies enable the client to experiment with new ways of coping (for example, making "I" statements, such as "I feel," "I want," or "I need") and discard old ways, which may be perpetuating the phobic response.

3. Anticipating a future or imminent phobic reaction can escalate the physiologic manifestations of fear. Identifying anticipatory thinking enables the client to make the necessary changes to stop it.

4. Relaxation techniques enable the client to alleviate anxiety's negative consequences. Thought-stopping techniques provide the client with a means of recognizing a negative feeling and its accompanying thought and then stopping that thought and replacing it with a positive one. By role playing, the client can rehearse ways to relax while confronting a feared object or situation.

5. Examining specific behaviors and coping strategies can increase the client's sense of control and strengthen skill mastery.

6. A well-developed desensitization program, one in which the client is systematically exposed to the feared object or situation in a controlled and supportive environment, may diminish the client's fear.

7. The appropriate use of antiphobic or antipanic agents can relieve the physical symptoms associated with phobic and panic disorders.

8. These agents have a significant calming effect and may facilitate the client's ability to change behavior by reducing anxiety during desensitization sessions. Educating the client about both positive effects and adverse reactions (including nausea, dry mouth, dizziness, and potential dependency) facilitates compliance.

Nursing diagnosis

Ineffective breathing pattern related to choking or smothering sensation, shortness of breath, or hyperventilation associated with panic

Nursing priority

Help the client restore a normal breathing pattern.

Patient outcome criteria

As the treatment progresses the client, family, or both should be able to:
• demonstrate the correct use of breathing techniques to decrease anxiety and increase oxygenation during an acute attack
• report an increased ability to breathe normally through an attack.

Interventions

1. Remain with the client while maintaining a calm, supportive but direct approach.

2. Assess the client's respiratory status by determining respiratory rate and ability to breathe and by noting the color of lips and nail beds.

3. Loosen all of the client's tight clothing, including ties, collars, and belts.

4. During an acute attack, demonstrate slow- and deep-breathing techniques and breathe along with the client.

5. If necessary, instruct the client to breathe into a paper bag to counteract hyperventilation during an acute attack.

Rationales

1. The client needs simple directions and reassurance that suffocation or death are not imminent.

2. Any sign of hyperventilation, difficulty breathing, or cyanosis indicates hypoxia, which requires immediate medical attention.

3. Decreasing bodily restrictions helps to decrease choking and suffocating sensations.

4. Active participation and role modeling can be effective when instructing a client with an impaired or restricted perceptual field.

5. This procedure maintains normal acid-base balance by normalizing CO_2 levels and preventing respiratory acidosis, which can cause depressed respirations.

Nursing diagnosis

Powerlessness related to a perceived inability to maintain control over a situation

Nursing priority

Help the client verbalize about the situation and exhibit more control in life.

Patient outcome criteria

As the treatment progresses, the client, family, or both should be able to:
• report a sense of being in control
• verbalize having a concrete plan to manage those times when feeling overwhelmed with anxiety.

Interventions

1. Encourage the client to assume responsibility for establishing and maintaining self-care practices.

Rationales

1. The client who can assume responsibility for self-care practices will probably feel more in control.

Anxiety disorders

2. Collaborate with the client to establish realistic, achievable goals.

2. Realistic goals should make the client more comfortable with the treatment. Achieving goals builds self-confidence.

3. Explore ways in which cultural values and religious beliefs might support helpless and dependent behavior.

3. A person's interpretation of cultural values and religious beliefs sometimes reinforces a sense of rigidity, shame, guilt, self-protection, and self-deprecation as well as a distorted sense of reality. By becoming aware of how these value systems can work negatively, the client may gain a better sense of self-control.

4. Continue to clarify the client's unmet goals (for example, the client's inability to assume responsibility for an increase in dependence).

4. The client should become more adept at modifying behavior as personal insight deepens.

5. Help the client to identify areas in life that are beyond personal control.

5. Recognizing such limitations promotes acceptance of what cannot be changed and allows the client to focus on resolvable issues.

6. Encourage the client to investigate and consider participation in self-help and support groups.

6. Incorporating additional outside support can reinforce the client's self-management and control.

NURSING DIAGNOSIS

Sensory-perceptual alteration related to diminished perceptual field during panic-level anxiety

Nursing priority

Ensure the client's safety during panic attacks.

Patient outcome criteria

As treatment progresses, the client, family, or both should be able to:
- verbalize the ability to remain focused on a concrete plan to manage high levels of anxiety
- demonstrate the ability to use relaxation skills
- report being able to obtain external support when need during panic attacks.

Interventions

1. Remain with and reassure the client that you are both safe, that you will remain, and that the attack will end.

2. Speak to the client in simple, one-step sentences.

3. Decrease environmental stimuli (for example, by dimming lights or closing doors). If necessary, move the client to a quieter, smaller area.

Rationales

1. During a panic attack, a client typically fears being abandoned. Remaining with the client and offering reassurance that the attack will end provides the first measure of security needed to decrease anxiety.

2. The client's severely restricted perceptual field limits the ability to comprehend complicated thoughts and sentences.

3. Exposure to environmental stimuli can escalate anxious behavior, especially in someone with an impaired ability to deal with such stimuli. A smaller, quieter area can make the client feel more secure.

Nursing diagnosis

Altered family processes related to the inability of family members to express feelings

Nursing priority

Help family members verbalize and demonstrate feelings of intimacy.

Patient outcome criteria

As the treatment progresses, the client, family, or both should be able to:
- recognize the need for support and follow up on referrals for community-based support networks
- verbalize increased feelings of intimacy and respect
- verbalize an understanding of the disease process, treatment, and need for treatment follow-up
- demonstrate increased responsibility for identifying and meeting needs within the family structure.

Interventions

1. Help individual family members to define and clarify their roles and relationships within the family.

2. Teach family members assertiveness techniques to express thoughts, feelings, and needs. Include the use of "I" statements, such as "I feel" and "I need."

3. Teach family members how to express what they need from each other to feel loved, cared for, and emotionally supported. For example, teach them to tell each other when they are frightened or when they need a hug. Demonstrate these behaviors and have family members practice them.

Rationales

1. Increasing the family's knowledge about family system dynamics can facilitate self-appraisal and restructuring of family functioning.

2. Encouraging open expression helps family members to identify their feelings and needs and address any built-up resentment. Open discussions also provide insight into how the client's illness has disrupted their family structure.

3. Although the family is traditionally viewed as the primary group in which feelings of intimacy and caring are nurtured and fostered, many families have difficulty recognizing the lack of support and do not know how to ask for help from one another.

Discharge criteria

Nursing documentation indicates that the client:
- has expressed an ability to recognize symptoms of phobia or panic
- can use newly learned skills to manage phobia- or panic-provoking situations
- understands the diagnosis, treatment, and expected outcomes
- is aware of available group, family, or marital support resources
- arranged for scheduled follow-up appointments.
Nursing documentation also indicates that the family:
- understands the client's diagnosis, treatment, and expected outcomes
- has been referred to appropriate group, family, or marital support resources
- can use alternative coping skills such as cognitive restructuring techniques
- has scheduled necessary follow-up appointments.

Selected references

Ballenger, J.C., et al. "Focus on Panic Disorder: Antidepressants in Practice," *Journal of Clinical Psychiatry* 59(8) supplement:3-54, 1998.

Boyd, M.A., and Nihart, M.A. *Psychiatric Nursing: Contemporary Practice.* Philadelphia: Lippincott-Raven Pubs., 1998.

Diagnostic and Statistical Manual of Mental Disorders, 4th ed. Washington, D.C.: American Psychiatric Association, 1994.

Grove, C., et al. "The Neuroanatomy of 5HT Dysregulation and Panic Disorder," *Journal of Neuropsychiatry and Clinical Neuroscience* 9(2):198-207, 1997.

Stahl, S.M. *Essential Psychopharmacology: Neuroscientific Basis and Practical Applications.* New York: Cambridge University Press, 1997.

Varcarolis, E.M. *Foundations of Psychiatric-Mental Health Nursing,* 3rd ed. Philadelphia: W.B. Saunders Co., 1998.

Wakefield, M., and Pallister, R. "Cognitive-Behavioral Approaches to Panic Disorder," *Journal of Psychosocial Nursing* 35:12, 1997.

Anxiety disorders

Obsessive-compulsive disorder

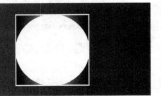

DSM-IV classification

300.30   Obsessive-compulsive disorder

INTRODUCTION

Description

Obsessive-compulsive disorder (OCD) is characterized by a compulsive response to an obsessive thought or impulse (obsession). The individual usually considers the obsession to be unacceptable or irrational but also feels powerless to control its persistent intrusion into consciousness. Fear that the obsession may actually be enacted generates considerable anxiety, and the compulsive acts are attempts to allay this anxiety.

Compulsive behaviors are as diverse as the people who display them. The individual may perform repetitive acts or engage in seemingly purposeless behavior to divert the conscious mind from its obsession. Such behaviors include frequent hand or body washing; constant counting, an overemphasis on cleanliness, checking and rechecking lights or gas stoves before leaving the house, and masturbation.

The estimated prevalence of obsessive-compulsive disorder is approximately 2% to 3% of the general population. It occurs most frequently in individuals in their early 20s, and about equally in adults of both sexes. In childhood, OCD is more common in boys. OCD appears to be less common among blacks than among whites. Individuals experiencing OCD are more likely to utilize general and psychiatric services than individuals with phobic disorder. (For more information, see *Common obsessions and compulsions.*)

Etiology and precipitating factors

Recent neuroimaging and neurochemical studies have revealed a prominent neurobiological basis for OCD, as well as a genetic vulnerability. Although neuroimaging studies, using computed tomography (CT) and magnetic resonance imaging (MRI) of individuals with OCD have been limited, findings suggest a link with abnormalities in the frontal cortex, limbic system, and basal ganglia. Positron emission tomography (PET) scans reveal differences in cerebral glucose metabolism between individuals with OCD and control groups. Presently, the most replicated results demonstrate increased glucose metabolism in the caudate nuclei, the orbitofrontal gyri, and cingulate gyri. The biochemical theories of causation are also being probed for a better understanding of the role that neurotransmitters play in the development of OCD.

Although it is unlikely that only one neurotransmitter is responsible for the development of OCD, the specific neurotransmitter that has been implicated so far is serotonin. Challenge testing with serotonin agonists showed that individuals with OCD responded with an increase of symptoms. The most compelling evidence for serotonin's contribution in OCD comes from the fact that antidepressants that act selectively on serotonin relieve the OCD symptoms in most of these individuals.

Psychological theories of causation provide a rich foundation for understanding the symptoms and behaviors related to OCD, although the psychological theories of OCD have not been scientifically tested. The behavioral treatments that have been developed from these hypotheses have become an important strategy in the multimodal approach to treating OCD, especially for individuals with severe compulsions and treatment-resistant OCD.

Potential complications

Untreated, obsessive-compulsive disorder can lead to aggressive behavior toward the self or others as well as depression, skin breakdown from obsessive washing, and infection caused by skin breakdown. There is increased risk of physical harm if the individual acts on a violent obsession.

ASSESSMENT GUIDELINES

Nursing history (functional health pattern findings)

Health perception–health management pattern
- Extreme concern about diet, germs, and disease
- Concern about or evidence of inadequate attention to health care needs
- Extreme concern over general health
- Exaggerated worry over daily life circumstances
- Worry over medication compliance, follow-up visits, and inability to follow through
- Fear of "going crazy"
- Inability to control feelings
- Numerous somatic complaints, with or without diagnostic validation
- Overuse or underuse of health care system to ease anxiety symptoms

Common obsessions and compulsions

Type of obsession	Example	Compulsion
Checking or doubt	Is worried about turning off an appliance or lights or about locking door.	Checks several times to see if appliance lights are off or door is locked. May return during the day when at work or school.
Germs or dirt	Believes everything is dirty or contaminated.	Avoids touching surfaces or people and will scrub hands if forced to touch objects.
Somatic obsessions, such as illness, death, and decay	Believes that teeth, mouth, insides are decaying and rotting or that he has bugs in his head.	Performs repetitive rituals of brushing, flossing, and gargling with antiseptic for several hours every day or trying to use remedies to rid the body of bugs.
Need for order and organization	Needs to have everything in its place.	Constantly arranges and rearranges items.
Sexual ideation or imagery	Has recurrent thought of touching a woman's breast when in the presence of a woman.	Avoids women and, when in presence of a woman, excuses self several times to wash hands.
Violence	Constantly thinks about cutting off red-headed women's heads.	Leaves a room when a red-headed woman enters.

Anxiety disorders

Nutritional-metabolic pattern
• Weight loss resulting from fear of contaminated food or ritualistic behaviors that interfere with meal time and eating ability
• Weight gain resulting from compulsive eating
• Worry over eating behaviors, such as using food to calm or soothe self
• Changes in appetite, including anorexia and binges

Elimination pattern
• Constipation resulting from fear of contacting excrement
• Concern over GI system disturbances, such as pain, flatulence, diarrhea, nausea, constipation, vomiting, and intestinal bleeding
• Frequent urination
• Concern over increased sweating, cold and clammy skin, or both

Activity-exercise pattern
• Concern about compulsive behavior interfering with personal, occupational, scholastic, and social functioning
• Restlessness or trembling
• Concern about being easily fatigued
• Difficulty in accomplishing normal daily activities
• Concern about inability to participate in and enjoy leisure activities
• Concern about any limitations and restrictions of activity caused by disease or condition
• Withdrawn or apathetic behavior

Sleep-rest pattern
• Decreased sleep resulting from obsessive thoughts or impulses
• Inability to relax because of constant activity resulting from an inability to prevent intrusive obsessive thoughts or impulses
• Concern about falling or staying asleep and nightmares
• Feeling fatigued after sleep
• Concern about use or abuse of sleep aids, such as alcohol, benzodiazepines, and hypnotics

Cognitive-perceptual pattern
• Concern about the disturbing nature of obsessions
• Awareness of illogical thoughts and behavior and of the inability to control them
• Self-destructive or aggressive ideas or impulses
• Difficulty concentrating
• Difficulty understanding and reacting to external stimuli
• Worry over inability to think clearly
• Distorted perceptions

Self-perception–self-concept pattern
• Low self-esteem and feelings of powerlessness resulting from the inability to control thoughts and behavior
• Feelings of worthlessness secondary to feeling unclean
• Concern over inability to meet expectations
• Concern over being indecisive and dependent
• Perception of self as being highly anxious
• Perception of self as being incompetent
• Concerns about body image

Role-relationship pattern

- Disturbance in interpersonal relationships
- Diminished ability to meet occupational, functional, interpersonal, or parental expectations
- Intense concern over relationships with family and friends
- Rumination over engaging in social situations with friends, fellow employees, or family
- Concern over the lack of response to or support of lifestyle changes from family and friends
- Concern about a distressful work situation
- Concern about how community members and neighbors may respond to the disease and associated behaviors

Sexual-reproductive pattern

- Fear of intimate contact with others resulting from fear of contamination and disease
- Sexual dysfunction
- Compulsive or ritualistic sexual activity, such as compulsive masturbation, excessive fascination with pornography, or use of others as sex objects
- Dissatisfaction with sexual relations
- Difficulty with intimacy
- Concern about involvement in high-risk sexual behavior, such as unprotected sex or promiscuity
- Concern about involvement with high-risk partners, including I.V. drug users, homosexual or bisexual partners, and strangers

Coping–stress tolerance pattern

- Feeling overwhelmed
- Avoiding social situations
- Concern over increasing frequency and duration of compulsive behaviors
- Pervasive muscle tension
- Constant irritability, feeling on edge or keyed up
- Constant shakiness, trembling, or twitching
- Concern over experiencing an exaggerated startle response (hypervigilance)
- Denial of clearly manifest anxiety
inability to identify those persons or measures that alleviate rather than exacerbate the condition
- Belief that significant lifestyle changes are contributing to feeling out of control

Value-belief pattern

- Fear of condemnation
- Feelings of powerlessness, hopelessness, or unworthiness
- Concern that the condition is punishment for sin or previous acts
- Overreliance on or identification with religious themes associated with ritualistic behavior
- Desire to increase or decrease involvement in spirituality or religion
- Concern over impaired ability to believe in anything or anyone
- Disbelief about present situation

Physical findings

Cardiovascular

- Cold, clammy skin
- Elevated blood pressure
- Hot and cold flashes
- Increased heart rate
- Palpitations
- Sweating
- Tingling

Respiratory

- Increased respiratory rate
- Shortness of breath
- Smothering sensation
- Choking sensation

Gastrointestinal

- Dry mouth
- Abdominal distress
- Nausea
- Vomiting
- Diarrhea
- Difficulty swallowing

Genitourinary

- Frequent urination

Integumentary

- Skin irritation from constant washing

Musculoskeletal

- Increased fatigue
- Muscle aches, pains, or soreness
- Muscle tension
- Restlessness
- Shakiness
- Trembling
- Twitching

Neurologic

- Dilated pupils
- Dizziness or faintness
- Light-headedness
- Paresthesia
- Restlessness
- Inability to sleep or to stay asleep

Psychological

- Feeling keyed up or on edge
- Inability to concentrate
- Irritability
- Blank mind

NURSING DIAGNOSIS

Ineffective individual coping related to checking and rechecking actions or other ritualistic behaviors

Nursing priority

Help the client gradually decrease ritualistic behavior and learn alternative strategies for coping with stress and anxiety.

Patient outcome criteria

As the treatment progresses, the client, family, or both should be able to:
- identify signs and symptoms of increasing anxiety
- report the level of anxiety being experienced
- demonstrate a slow but steady reduction in ritualistic behaviors
- demonstrate alternative coping strategies
- verbalize sense of self-control.

Interventions

1. Assess the degree of interference with daily functions by determining how much time the client spends on compulsive behaviors. Involvement of 1 hour or less a day on such behavior is considered mild interference; 1 to 3 hours per day, moderate; 3 to 5 hours per day, severe; and almost constant involvement, extreme.

2. As part of the structured care, provide the client with time for rituals and compulsive behaviors without focusing attention on them. As the client's anxiety abates, gradually decrease the time allowed for these behaviors.

3. Encourage the client to verbalize feelings and to discuss the maladaptive or disruptive nature of the behavior.

4. Have the client collaborate with team to develop the plan of care and set realistic goals and expectations.

5. Establish behavioral contracts in which the client agrees to refrain from certain behaviors in exchange for certain rewards. (For example, if the client decreases the number of hand washings after meals from 50 to 40 times, the client is rewarded with a predetermined reinforcement.)

6. Provide realistic, alternative coping methods, such as social interaction, occupational therapy, diversionary activities, relaxation, and self-help support groups.

7. Respond positively when the client makes productive behavioral adaptations to cope with anxiety.

Rationales

1. As the involvement level increases, the client typically has less time to devote to normal daily functions. A client exhibiting severe or extreme involvement is unable to use adaptive problem-solving skills.

2. Allowing time for the client's compulsive behaviors can decrease anxiety, thereby decreasing the need for rituals and compulsions. Furthermore, acknowledging the client's feelings and fears helps establish a trusting nurse-client relationship.

3. A frank discussion about the condition and feelings can help the client develop a more realistic perspective about the behavior. Such discussion also fosters trust between the nurse and client.

4. Such participation can increase the client's self-esteem and sense of control while decreasing anxiety and frustration.

5. Positive reinforcements for nonritualistic behaviors enhance the client's self-esteem and encourage the continuation of those behaviors.

6. Success with new behaviors and coping methods can increase self-esteem, decrease feelings of powerlessness, provide structure, and reinforce behavioral change. Self-help support groups provide both support and the opportunity for the client to talk about fears.

7. Reinforcing the successful use of new behaviors increases the client's self-esteem and feelings of control.

Anxiety disorders

8. Gradually begin to set limits on the frequency and duration of compulsive behaviors.

8. Reducing the time allowed for compulsive behaviors can give the client a sense that treatment is progressing. Furthermore, limiting such behaviors decreases the potential for client injury.

9. Encourage the client to talk about the cause of and need for the compulsive behavior. Also encourage the client to describe feelings just before and during such behavior.

9. As the client's understanding of the behavior, its causes, and personal feelings about it become clearer, the client will be better able to choose more appropriate adaptive behaviors.

10. Collaborate with the client to develop a set of positive coping cards to be kept for emergency use.

10. The client's ability to cope with OCD symptoms during a crisis may be enhanced with preset messages that are written and specific for the client. This can assist clients in refocusing on what they are able to do rather than on the OCD symptoms and feelings of inadequacy.

Nursing diagnosis

Potential for impaired skin integrity related to ritualistic behaviors involving cleaning, such as hand washing, scrubbing, teeth brushing, and showering

Nursing priority

Help the client maintain intact skin to prevent infection.

Patient outcome criteria

As the treatment progresses, the client, family or both should be able to:
• demonstrate evidence of skin integrity
• demonstrate evidence of being infection-free
• demonstrate use of less abrasive and antibacterial cleaning products.

Interventions

1. Assess the client's skin integrity and mucous membranes of the mouth (if compulsion involves teeth brushing).

2. Encourage the client to use only a mild soap and skin cream during ritualistic behaviors involving cleaning.

Rationales

1. Assessment is necessary to ensure that the client's behaviors are not compromising the integumentary system.

2. Using a mild soap and skin cream can prevent or minimize trauma to the integumentary system until the client can alter the compulsive behavior.

Nursing diagnosis

Altered family processes related to inability to express feelings and develop intimate relationships

Nursing priority

Facilitate the family's participation in a therapy program.

Patient outcome criteria

As the treatment progresses, the client, family, or both should be able to:
• recognize the need for support external to their family system
• report their understanding of the illness and corresponding treatment
• utilize community-based resources to develop a supportive network.

Interventions

1. Collaborate with family members to define and clarify their relationships with one another.

2. Help family members to identify their feelings and to understand the importance of sharing those feelings with each other.

3. Teach family members assertiveness techniques, and rehearse these techniques with them.

4. Teach the family about obsessive-compulsive behavior and ways they can assist the client, such as through use of relaxation and behavioral modification. Instruct the family about psychopharmacologic interventions utilized to treat individuals with OCD.

Rationales

1. Making the client and family more aware of how families function can enable them to continually evaluate and, if necessary, redefine their relationships.

2. Families that are aware of and able to openly exchanges emotions function more positively. Clearly expressing and communicating feelings also enhances family functioning.

3. Family members need to assume responsibility for their own thoughts, feelings, and actions rather than blame others.

4. Adequate information about OCD enables the family to better understand the client's condition and behavior. By reinforcing client relaxation, using behavioral contracts, helping the client recognize anxious behavior, and praising appropriate coping strategies, family members can enhance the client's self-esteem and feelings of control.

Anxiety disorders

DISCHARGE CRITERIA

Nursing documentation indicates that the client:
• has demonstrated an increased ability to recognize obsessive-compulsive symptoms
• uses alternative coping methods
• reports a reduction or an absence of intrusive thoughts
• displays an increased ability to use social skills
• reports a positive mood change
• is aware of aftercare options and plans
• has improved sleep and elimination patterns
• can maintain skin integrity.
Nursing documentation also indicates that the family:
• understands the client's condition and needs, including medication management
• has planned for the client's aftercare
• reports improvements in family relationships
• reports improved sleep patterns
• reports a decrease in or absence of suicidal or homicidal impulses.

SELECTED REFERENCES

Boyd, M.A., and Nihart, M.A. *Psychiatric Nursing: Contemporary Practice.* Philadelphia: Lippincott-Raven Pubs., 1998.
Bystritsky, A., et al. "A Preliminary Study of Partial Hospital Management of Severe OCD," *Psychiatric Services* 47:170, 1996.
Diagnostic and Statistical Manual of Mental Disorders, 4th ed. Washington, D.C.: American Psychiatric Association, 1994.
Mavissakalian, M., and Prien, R. *Long-Term Treatment of Anxiety.* Washington, D.C.: American Psychiatric Association, 1996.
McCloskey, J.C., and Bulechek, G.M. *Nursing Interventions Classification (NIC),* 2nd ed. St. Louis: Mosby–Year Book, Inc., 1996.
New Developments in the Biology of Mental Disorders. Piscataway, N.J.: Research and Education Association, 1997.
Osborn, I. *Tormenting Thoughts and Secret Rituals: The Hidden Epidemic of Obsessive Compulsive Disorder.* New York: Pantheon Press, 1998.
Schwartz, J.M., et al. "Systematic Changes in Cerebral Glucose Metabolic Rate after Successful Behavior Modification Treatment of OCD," *Archives of General Psychiatry* 53(2):109, 1996.
Stahl, S.M. *Essential Psychopharmacology: Neuroscientific Basis and Practical Applications.* New York: Cambridge University Press, 1997.
Varcarolis, E.M. *Foundations of Psychiatric-Mental Health Nursing,* 3rd ed. Philadelphia: W.B. Saunders Co., 1998.

Stress-related anxiety disorders

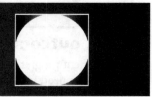

DSM-IV classifications
308.3   Acute stress disorder
309.81   Posttraumatic stress disorder

INTRODUCTION

Description

Acute stress disorder (ASD) is a relatively new diagnosis presented in the *DSM-IV* based on much review of traumatic stress literature and research. ASD occurs within one month after exposure to a traumatic event. The individual is typically exposed to or experiences an event that involves actual or threatened harm or death to the self, significant others, or other persons nearby, and responds with fear, helplessness, or horror. The individual must exhibit three dissociative symptoms during or after the traumatic event: a sense of numbing, detachment, or an absence of emotional response; reduced awareness of surroundings (dazed state); and derealization, depersonalization, and amnesia for important aspects of the traumatic event.

Posttraumatic stress disorder (PTSD) affects individuals who have experienced traumatic events in a similar manner as the individual with ASD, including military combat, hostage situations, natural disasters, rape, criminal assaults, and interpersonal abuse or violence. Rescue workers and health care providers who have daily or frequent exposure to traumatic and emotionally charged events may develop ASD or PTSD.

After the traumatic event, the individual typically experiences anxiety characterized by elevated autonomic responses (rapid pulse, increased blood pressure, and increased respiratory rate), cognitive impairment, and altered memory function. The individual persistently reexperiences the traumatic event through intrusive and unwanted thoughts or nightmares and tries to cope by suppressing emotional responsiveness. These behaviors are characteristic symptoms of PTSD.

Etiology and precipitating factors

Recent research shows that severe psychological and physical trauma can cause alterations in the neurobiological response to stress, even several years after the original exposure or insult. These long-standing alterations may contribute to a number of complaints and symptoms that are commonly experienced by individuals with ASD or PTSD.

Neurobiological studies provide evidence for at least two relatively consistent neurobiological alterations in chronic PTSD. Findings from psychophysiologic, hormonal, receptor-binding, and intravenous challenge studies have demonstrated repeatedly that reminders of the original trauma provoke hyperresponsiveness of the sympathetic nervous system in individuals with PTSD.

Additionally, findings of HPA (hypothyroid-pituitary-adrenal) axis alterations in PTSD suggest increased responsiveness of this system. Low baseline cortisol, along with heightened response to exogenous dexamethasone, is consistent with an HPA axis that is extremely sensitive to the stress-mediated hormones. These neurobiological findings are consistent with a behavioral sensitization model of PTSD. Behavioral sensitization produces an increased magnitude of response following repeated presentation of a particular stimulus such as a traumatic event.

Potential complications

Undiagnosed or untreated ASD can and probably will progress to PTSD. Undiagnosed or untreated PTSD can lead to substance abuse or dependence, engaging in high-risk behaviors, social isolation and withdrawal from the family, violent behavior, and suicide.

ASSESSMENT GUIDELINES

Nursing history (functional health pattern findings)

Health perception–health management pattern
• Extreme concern about "going crazy"
• Fear of being confined in a hospital
• Extreme concern over general health
• Exaggerated worry over daily life circumstances
• Worry over medication compliance, follow-up visits, and inability to follow through
• Inability to control feelings
• Numerous somatic complaints, with or without diagnostic validation
• Overuse or underuse of health care system to ease anxiety symptoms

Nutritional-metabolic pattern
• Concern over eating behaviors, such as using food to suppress feelings
• Concern over weight fluctuations
• Inattentiveness to dental problems
• Changes in appetite, including anorexia and binges

Elimination pattern
- Concern over GI system disturbances, such as pain, flatulence, diarrhea, nausea, constipation, vomiting, and intestinal bleeding
- Frequent urination
- Concern over increased sweating, cold and clammy skin, or both

Activity-exercise pattern
- Agitation and restlessness
- Concern about fluctuations in energy and activity level
- Decreasing interest and participation in leisure or social activities
- Trembling
- Concern about being easily fatigued
- Difficulty accomplishing normal daily activities
- Concern about any limitations and restrictions of activity caused by disease or condition
- Withdrawn or apathetic behavior

Sleep-rest pattern
- Feeling fatigued after sleep
- Dreams or nightmares of traumatic event
- Sleep disturbances, such as falling asleep but not staying asleep or awakening early in the morning
- Use or dependence on sleep aids, such as alcohol, benzodiazepines, or hypnotics
- Concern about use or abuse of sleep aids

Cognitive-perceptual pattern
- Memory impairment
- Difficulty concentrating
- Acute or chronic pain
- Difficulty learning
- Difficulty understanding and reacting to external stimuli
- Worry over inability to think clearly
- Distorted perceptions

Self-perception–self-concept pattern
- Anxiety or feelings of inadequacy
- Feeling detached or estranged from others
- Feelings of having no control over life
- Concern over being indecisive and dependent
- Perception of self as being highly anxious
- Perception of self as being incompetent and powerless
- Concerns about body image, self-esteem, and self-worth

Role-relationship pattern
- Concern over inability to maintain relationships with loved ones
- Inability to maintain consistent or rewarding employment
- Concern about feeling alone and not being involved in the community
- Intense concern over relationships with family and friends
- Rumination over engaging in social situations with friends, fellow employees, or family
- Concern over the lack of response to or support of lifestyle changes from family and friends
- Concern about a distressful work situation
- Concern about how community members and neighbors may respond to the disease or condition

Sexual-reproductive pattern
- Decrease in sexual desire
- Difficulties with sexual performance or satisfaction
- Dissatisfaction with sexual relations
- Difficulty with intimacy
- Concern about involvement in high-risk sexual behavior, such as unprotected sex or promiscuity
- Concern about involvement with high-risk partners, including I.V. drug users, homosexual or bisexual partners, and strangers

Coping–stress tolerance pattern
- Feeling tense most of the time
- Flashbacks or recurrences of traumatic event can progress to illusions and hallucinations (in severe presentation)
- Significant number of stressful events during the last year
- Inability to cope
- Feelings of "going crazy"
- Pervasive muscle tension
- Constant irritability, feeling on edge or keyed up
- Constant shakiness, trembling, or twitching
- Concern over experiencing an exaggerated startle response (hypervigilance)
- Denial of clearly manifested anxiety
- Inability to identify persons or measures that alleviate rather than exacerbate the condition
- Belief that significant lifestyle changes are contributing to feeling out of control

Value-belief pattern
- Inability to achieve goals in life
- Desire to increase or decrease involvement in spirituality or religion
- Concern over impaired ability to believe in anything or anyone
- Disbelief about present situation

Physical findings
Cardiovascular
- Excessive perspiration
- Increased heart rate
- Cold, clammy skin
- Elevated blood pressure
- Hot and cold flashes
- Palpitations
- Tingling sensation

Respiratory
- Hyperventilation

- Increased respiratory rate
- Shortness of breath
- Smothering sensation
- Choking sensation

Gastrointestinal
- Abdominal distress
- Diarrhea
- Nausea
- Gastric ulcers
- Dry mouth
- Vomiting
- Difficulty swallowing

Genitourinary
- Frequent urination

Musculoskeletal
- Muscle aches, pains, or soreness
- Muscle tension
- Restlessness
- Trembling
- Fatigue
- Shakiness
- Twitching

Neurologic
- Headaches
- Hyperalertness
- Hypervigilance
- Memory impairment
- Inability to sleep or to remain asleep
- Startle reactions
- Tremors or tics
- Dilated pupils
- Dizziness or faintness
- Light-headedness
- Paresthesia
- Restlessness

Psychological
- Anger to rage
- Anxiety at or around the time of year that the traumatic event occurred
- Feeling constricted
- Diminished interest in life activities or work
- Feeling detached or estranged
- Sleep-induced hypnagogic hallucinations (such as might occur when a war veteran falls asleep and reexperiences a bombing incident)
- Hypnopompic hallucinations, or dreams that continue after waking (such as those that make an exhostage continue to feel as if he is being held hostage after awaking from a dream about the experience)
- Nightmares
- Recurrent dreams about the traumatic event
- Illusions of being back in the traumatic situation (such as might occur when a veteran hears a car backfire and thinks he is back in combat)
- Intrusive thoughts of the traumatic event
- General numbing of emotional responsiveness
- Self-hatred
- Significant irritability
- Social withdrawal
- Substance abuse or dependence
- Sudden acting or feeling as if the traumatic event were recurring
- Survivor guilt
- Feeling keyed up or on edge
- Inability to concentrate
- Blank mind

NURSING DIAGNOSIS

Post-trauma syndrome related to the subjective experience of an overwhelming traumatic event, such as disaster, war, rape, torture, catastrophic illness, injury, assault, or being held hostage, or of vicarious traumatization (secondary traumatization)

Nursing priority

Assess the traumatic event and degree of client anxiety to determine the seriousness of the perceived threat.

Patient outcome criteria

As the treatment progresses, the client, family, or both should be able to:
- report that intrusive thoughts and memories produce less anxiety
- demonstrate an ability to manage emotional reactions
- demonstrate appropriate lifestyle changes
- report ability to pursue support from family members.

Interventions

1. Observe for and identify any physical injury to the client.

2. Identify the client's symptoms (such as numbness, headache, nausea, palpitations, or chest tightness) and ensure that they are anxiety-related and not the products of a physiologic condition.

3. Identify any physical effects of the traumatic event on the client. Such effects might include disfigurement, chronic physical conditions, and disabilities.

4. Identify and document the client's psychological responses (such as shock, anger, panic, bewilderment, and confusion) and emotional changes. Observe for emotional instability evidenced by crying, alternating calm and agitation, hysteria, and statements of self-blame or disbelief concerning the event.

5. Identify the client's cultural beliefs and ethnic background.

6. Determine the degree of disorganization in the client's thinking and coping.

7. Observe for verbal and nonverbal expressions of survivor guilt (self-blame or guilt over having survived the traumatic event) and for signs of increasing anxiety.

Rationales

1. Physical injuries can occur during a traumatic event as well as during a recurrence of that event.

2. Anxiety-related symptoms must be differentiated from medical symptoms so that appropriate treatment can be instituted.

3. Sequelae from the traumatic event may significantly interfere with normal daily functioning. They also may serve as constant reminders of the event.

4. The behavioral range following a traumatic event is naturally broad; however, such responses must be managed or they will become repetitive and chronic.

5. Knowing the client's cultural beliefs and ethnic background can help the nurse better understand responses to both the event and treatment. For example, a male client whose culture emphasizes macho behavior may have particular difficulty coping with a frightening experience that caused him to run away or hide for self-protection and survival.

6. Evaluating the client's thinking and coping abilities helps the nurse determine the degree of intervention necessary during hospitalization, crises, follow-up care, and support group therapy.

7. Self-blame, guilt, and increasing anxiety indicate a decreased coping ability. Should these symptoms occur and escalate during the initial interview, the nurse should assess the client's suicide potential and institute suicide precautions if necessary.

NURSING DIAGNOSIS

Powerlessness related to feelings of helplessness, inadequate problem-solving and coping skills, and overwhelming anxiety

Nursing priority

Help the client regain control over feelings and behaviors.

Patient outcome criteria

As treatment progresses, the client, family, or both should be able to:
• express a sense of control over the present situation
• acknowledge that the present situation has increased anxiety related to the traumatic event
• become actively involved in the decision-making processes concerning present and future treatment.

Interventions

1. Assess the client's pre-event coping abilities and degree of success with these skills and abilities.

2. Explore cultural and religious beliefs that may support helpless behavior as well as those that might be used to support the client.

3. Collaborate with the client to establish realistic, achievable goals for an effective plan of care.

4. Collaborate with the client to identify feelings of powerlessness as well as factors that contribute to these feelings.

5. Teach the client strategies to diffuse intense stress and escalating anxiety. Rehearse the strategies with the client.

6. Encourage the client to participate in group psychotherapy and self-help support groups; possibly consider a therapist educated in Eye Movement Desensitization Reprocessing techniques.

Rationales

1. Acknowledging any past success that the client has had in dealing with the condition fosters self-confidence and self-control. It also reminds the client that other behavior exists.

2. Cultural and religious beliefs need to be examined in terms of the rigidity, shame, guilt, and sense of powerlessness they can instill. Understanding the influence of such beliefs can enable the client to see that feelings have certain foundations and that they are not beyond control. Positive cultural and religious beliefs, such as those that promote self-control and self-determination, can help the client regain a sense of control.

3. Involvement in the plan of care can enhance the client's sense of control.

4. Identifying stressors that contribute to or trigger feelings of powerlessness can enhance client self-confidence and self-control.

5. Strategies such as deep breathing, using thought-stopping techniques to interrupt irrational thinking, counting to refocus energy, and reviewing the situation with a staff or family member or friend provide alternative coping methods for feelings of powerlessness and can increase the client's sense of self-management.

6. Participating in such groups enables the client to learn and share new coping strategies with peers who have experienced similar traumatic events and reactions.

Nursing diagnosis

Sleep pattern disturbance related to recurrent nightmares, dreams of personal death, or fear of reexperiencing the traumatic event

Nursing priority

Help the client establish a restful environment to increase hours of refreshing sleep.

Patient outcome criteria

As treatment progresses, the client, family, or both should be able to:
• verbalize an understanding of any sleep disturbance
• identify and utilize focused sleep hygiene measures to reduce sleep pattern disturbance
• report improved sleep pattern.

Interventions

1. Gather information from the client, loved ones, or family members to assess the client's usual sleep pattern and any changes in that pattern that have occurred since the traumatic event.

Rationales

1. Both subjective and objective information can help the nurse assess the client's specific sleep disturbance and focus interventions.

2. Assess the client's usual sleep-related behaviors, such as time of retiring and rising, bedtime rituals, alcohol and sleep aid use, and caffeine intake before bedtime.

2. Knowing when the client goes to bed and arises and usual bedtime rituals can help the nurse evaluate potential difficulties. For example, alcohol and sleep aids interfere with the rapid-eye-movement (REM) sleep cycle, thereby preventing refreshing sleep. Coffee, exercise, or animated conversations before bed can cause restlessness and interfere with the normal sleep cycle.

3. Teach the client effective sleep measures, such as retiring and rising at regular times, avoiding naps, and avoiding caffeine and alcohol in the evening. Encourage the client to remain fairly active during the early evening and not to spend most of the night on the couch resting or watching television.

3. Taking measures to modify behaviors and promote sleep can help decrease the client's anxiety about sleeplessness.

4. Arrange a quiet, restful environment that is not too warm and that has no direct light.

4. These measures can facilitate a sleep-inducing environment.

5. Encourage the client to install a dim night-light in the bedroom.

5. Should the client awake quickly from a nightmare, a night-light promotes orientation, thereby reducing overwhelming fear.

6. Help the client to develop an individualized relaxation program. Demonstrate and rehearse such techniques as self-hypnosis, imagery, and muscle relaxation.

6. These strategies can produce both physical and mental relaxation, which may decrease the client's anxiety and induce sleep. Relaxation can reduce the incidence of nightmares.

7. Refer the client to a support group concerned with similar traumatic events.

7. Exploring trauma-related nightmares and fears in a supportive and understanding environment can help diminish the client's feelings of isolation and loneliness.

8. In collaboration with the client and doctor, select, administer, and monitor psychopharmacologic medications to manage ASD or PTSD symptoms that are interfering with client's sleep-wake cycle.

8. The client may require short-term psychopharmacotherapy to decrease exhaustion, fatigue, or fear and to alleviate the symptoms that are interring with their ability to sleep. Frequent assessments are necessary to determine the therapeutic response to the medication and assist in adverse effect management.

NURSING DIAGNOSIS

Self-esteem disturbance related to the traumatic experience

Nursing priority

Help enhance the client's self-esteem.

Patient outcome criteria

As treatment progresses, the client, family, or both should be able to:
• identify effective coping strategies to alleviate negative self-perception
• verbalize positive statements about successes when coping with increase level of anxiety.

Anxiety disorders

Interventions

1. Discuss with the client any experiences related to community response to the traumatic event. (For example, a Vietnam veteran might recall his reception upon returning home or complain of a perceived lack of recognition on Veterans Day; a plane crash victim may recall the sights, smells, and sounds of the crash when listening to the news of the event.)

2. Explore cultural and social values that might contribute to the client's emotional response and potential for lowered self-esteem.

Rationales

1. Relating these experiences can give the client an opportunity to explore specific events of prejudicial behavior.

2. Cultural and social values can instill a sense of shame related to certain traumatic events, such as rape. Helping the client to differentiate these views from personal feelings may enhance self-esteem.

NURSING DIAGNOSIS

Risk for violence, self-directed or directed toward others, related to inability to verbalize feelings

Nursing priority

Ensure the safety of the client and others.

Patient outcome criteria

As treatment progresses, the client, family, or both should be able to:
• identify factors that lead to violence
• demonstrate increased self-control.

Interventions

1. Teach the client to recognize early warning signs of impending violence. Verbal signs include the content of remarks and tone of voice. Nonverbal signs include trembling, sweating, pacing, hypervigilance, rapid startle reaction, pounding of clenched fists, and angry facial expressions.

2. Explore with the client the relation between high anxiety and hostile, possibly aggressive behaviors.

3. Help the client to identify and remove the causes of escalating anxiety.

4. Collaborate with the client to understand and verbalize the reasons for angry, vengeful, retaliatory feelings.

5. Collaborate with the client to discover and rehearse different methods for expressing feelings.

6. Remain calm and nonthreatening during a client crisis.

Rationales

1. Early identification can help de-escalate the violence cycle and prevent loss of control.

2. High anxiety can increase underlying hostility and lead to a loss of control.

3. Preventing anxiety escalation can help halt the aggression to violence cycle.

4. Verbal expression of anger can diminish the need for physical outbursts, which in turn can decrease the incidence of rejection or disapproval by others.

5. The client needs to find rational, acceptable ways to manage feelings rather than resort to destructive, violent behavior.

6. During any interaction with an angry, hostile, or threatening client, the nurse must remember to control personal anxieties. If the healthcare providers become fearful or avoid the client, the situation can escalate. Loss of objectivity can result in a nurse-client power struggle, which increases anxiety and worsens the crisis.

7. Provide for and monitor the client's use of immediate, safe outlets for the physical expression of tension. Such outlets might include a punching bag and gloves, walking, aerobic exercising, or weight lifting.

8. Determine the probability of impending violence while removing potential weapons or dangerous objects.

9. Ensure clear access to the client and a safe exit route for the staff when managing a potentially violent episode.

7. The client needs to discharge the physical energy that high-level anxiety produces; however, the nurse must be present to prevent self-injury, property damage, or injury to others.

8. The nurse must limit the possibility of harm or injury to the client and to others in the area.

9. The nurse and health care team must collaborate to ensure a safe, injury-free intervention during a violent episode. An effective strategy is for one member to talk to the client while other team members prepare for specific tasks should restraints be necessary. This approach reinforces that the client is in a safe, controlled environment.

NURSING DIAGNOSIS

Spiritual distress related to the client's perception of the world as threatening after the traumatic event

Nursing priority

Help the client manage personal fears.

Patient outcome criteria

As treatment progresses, the client, family, or both should be able to:
• report believing that they will again be safe in their life
• verbalize an understanding that they are not to blame for this traumatic event.

Interventions

1. Encourage the client, loved ones, and family to express feelings about the traumatic event.

2. Collaborate with the client, family members, and a religious counselor to discover the reasons for the traumatic event.

3. Discuss support systems available to both the client and family members.

4. Determine whether the client's spiritual practices are adversely affecting treatment.

Rationales

1. Doing so prevents suppression or denial of feelings.

2. Understanding that such events occur for specific reasons can help the client accept that he was not a random victim, which in turn can give the client a more positive outlook on life.

3. Knowing that support is available can make the client and family feel more connected to others and diminish feelings of isolation.

4. Understanding the client's spiritual or religious beliefs can help the nurse determine any conflict between such beliefs and treatment.

DISCHARGE CRITERIA

Nursing documentation indicates that the client:
• has demonstrated an increased ability to recognize the impact of intrusive thoughts or memories and to use strategies that diminish that impact
• can effectively use strategies that diminish feelings of powerlessness
• has demonstrated a willingness to participate in the plan of care and decision making
• can effectively use methods that facilitate sleep
• can use alternative coping skills
• is aware of available group, family, or marital support resources
• understands the importance of and participates in an ongoing therapy program
• understands the prescribed drug regimen
• understands how to obtain emergency help.
Nursing documentation also indicates that the family:
• can cope with the client's illness
• is aware of community organizations that can help them meet legal or financial needs
• has been referred to appropriate family, group, or marital support resources
• can administer the client's prescribed drug regimen if necessary
• can identify client behaviors that indicate the client's need for immediate assistance.

SELECTED REFERENCES

Acute Stress Disorder
Blanchard, E.B., and Hickling, E.J. *After the Crash: Assessment and Treatment of MVA Survivors*. Washington, D.C.: American Psychiatric Press, 1997.
Bryant, R.A., and Harvey, A.G. "Initial Post-Traumatic Stress Response Following Motor Vehicle Accidents," *Journal of Traumatic Stress* 9(2): 223-234, 1996.
Diagnostic and Statistical Manual of Mental Disorders, 4th ed. Washington, D.C.: American Psychiatric Association, 1994.
Stuber, M.L., et al. "Appraisal of Life Threat and Acute Trauma Responses in Pediatric Bone Marrow Transplant Patients," *Journal of Traumatic Stress* 9(4):673-86, 1996.
Ursano, R.J., et al. *Individual and Community Responses to Trauma and Disaster: The Structure of Chaos*. London: Cambridge University Press, 1996.
Van der Kolk, B.A., et al. *Traumatic Stress: The Effect of Overwhelming Experiences on Mind, Body and Society*. New York: Guilford Press, 1996.
Posttraumatic Stress Disorder
Bremner, J.D., et al. "Magnetic Resonance Imaging-Based Measurement of Hippocampal Volume in Post Traumatic Stress Disorder Related to Childhood Sexual Abuse," *Biological Psychiatry* 41(1): 23-32, 1997.
Ford, N. "The Use of Anticonvulsants in PTSD," *Journal of Traumatic Stress* 9(4):857-63, 1996.
Fullerton, C.S., and Ursano, R.J. *Post-Traumatic Stress Disorder: Acute and Long-Term Responses to Trauma and Disaster*. Washington, D.C.: American Psychiatric Association, 1997.
Holden, G.W., et al. *Children Exposed to Marital Violence: Theory, Research and Applied Issues*. Washington, D.C.: American Psychological Association, 1998.
Hossack, A., and Bentall, R.P. "Elimination of Post-Traumatic Symptomatology by Relaxation and Visual-Kinesthetic Dissociation," *Journal of Traumatic Stress* 9(1):99-110, 1996.
Noyes, F. "Oklahoma City Bombing: Evaluation of Symptoms in Veterans with PTSD," *Archives of Psychiatric Nursing* 10(1):55, 1996.
Shapiro, F., and Forrest, M.S. *EMDR: The Breakthrough Therapy for Overcoming Anxiety, Stress and Trauma*. New York: Basic Books, 1997.
Snell, F., and Padin-Rivera, E. "Group Treatment for Older Veterans with PTSD," *Journal of Psychosocial Nursing* 35:10, 1997.

General anxiety disorders

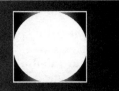

DSM-IV classifications

300.00	Anxiety disorder not otherwise specified
300.02	Generalized anxiety disorder

INTRODUCTION

Description

Generalized anxiety disorder (GAD) is characterized by unrealistic or excessive worry about life circumstances. This disorder lasts at least 6 months. It is associated with sustained and pervasive feelings of distress and physiologic changes that contribute to the discomfort. Onset of GAD is gradual, and many patients report being nervous all their life. GAD affects individuals across the life span; although onset is most common after age 20, it often occurs in childhood and adolescence. Many individuals diagnosed with GAD suffer with other psychiatric disorders and have a history of major depression.

GAD is one of the most common psychiatric disorders in the United States. Approximately 10% of the population will experience symptoms meeting the diagnostic criteria for GAD during some point in their life. Women are approximately twice as likely as men to experience GAD.

The residual classification *anxiety disorders not otherwise specified* covers those disorders that do not conform to the classification criteria for any other specific anxiety disorder (generalized anxiety disorder, phobic and panic disorders, obsessive-compulsive disorder, acute stress disorder, posttraumatic stress disorder, anxiety disorder due to a medical condition, substance-induced anxiety disorder). Management for the two anxiety disorder classifications covered in this plan of care is the same.

Etiology and precipitating factors

Currently, no single etiology thoroughly explains the psychophysiologic manifestations of anxiety as it relates to generalized anxiety disorder and anxiety disorders not otherwise specified. There have been fewer biological theories of causation researched for GAD than for panic disorder. However, the physical syptomatology of GAD and responsiveness of these symptoms to psychopharmacologic agents have led investigators to focus their research on several biological possibilities. There has been only limited research evidence of norepinephrin system dysregulation in GAD. Investigators followed the postitive effects of the SSRIs and GAD and this led to more promising investigations of serotonin dysfunction related to GAD. There has been some research evidence that implicates a down-regulation of benzodiazepine receptors, which does normalize after treatment.

Only a few studies have examined genetic and familial factors in the etiology of GAD. Some studies have indicated a familial tendency toward GAD may be related more to genetic factors than to effects of a shared familial environment; this seemed to be particularly true for females.

Cognitive-behavioral theory postulates that the disorder results from an inaccurate appraisal of perceived environmental threat. This results from a selective focus on negative details, distorted information processing, and an overly pessimistic view of one's own coping ability. Psychoanalytic theory, on the other hand, proposes that anxiety represents unresolved unconscious conflicts, such as loss of or separation from a loved one or loss of self-esteem. These sources of anxiety change as the individual passes through different developmental stages.

Currently, there is no focused sociocultural research related to the development of GAD. However, it appears that high-stress lifestyles and multiple, simultaneous stressors in one's life can contribute to the development of GAD. Individuals with GAD have a hypersensitivity to stress and anxiety-provoking events.

Potential complications

Undiagnosed medical reasons for anxiety could lead to physical deterioration and a delay in obtaining appropriate treatment.

ASSESSMENT GUIDELINES

Nursing history (functional health pattern findings)

Health perception–health management pattern

- Extreme concern over general health
- Exaggerated worry over daily life circumstances
- Worry over medication compliance, follow-up visits, and inability to follow through
- Fear of "going crazy"
- Inability to control feelings
- Numerous somatic complaints, with or without diagnostic validation

• Overuse or underuse of health care system to ease anxiety symptoms

Nutritional-metabolic pattern
• Worry over eating behaviors, such as using food to calm or soothe self
• Weight gain or loss
• Changes in appetite, including anorexia and binges

Elimination pattern
• Concern over GI system disturbances, such as pain, flatulence, diarrhea, nausea, constipation, vomiting, and intestinal bleeding
• Frequent urination
• Concern over increased sweating, cold and clammy skin, or both

Activity-exercise pattern
• Restlessness or trembling
• Concern about being easily fatigued
• Difficulty in accomplishing normal daily activities
• Concern about inability to participate in and enjoy leisure activities
• Concern about any limitations and restrictions of activity caused by disease or condition
• Withdrawn or apathetic behavior

Sleep-rest pattern
• Concern about falling asleep or staying asleep and nightmares
• Feeling fatigued after sleep
• Concern about use or abuse of sleep aids, such as alcohol, benzodiazepines, and hypnotics

Cognitive-perceptual pattern
• Difficulty concentrating
• Difficulty with understanding and reacting to external stimuli
• Worry over inability to think clearly
• Distorted perceptions

Self-perception–self-concept pattern
• Concern over being indecisive and dependent
• Perception of self as being highly anxious
• Perception of self as being incompetent and powerless
• Concerns about body image, self-esteem, and self-worth

Role-relationship pattern
• Intense concern over relationships with family and friends
• Rumination over engaging in social situations with friends, fellow employees, or family
• Concern over the lack of response to or support of lifestyle changes from family and friends
• Concern about a distressful work situation
• Concern about how community members and neighbors may respond to the disease or condition

Sexual-reproductive pattern
• Dissatisfaction with sexual relations
• Difficulty with intimacy

• Concern about involvement in high-risk sexual behavior, such as unprotected sex or promiscuity
• Concern about involvement with high-risk partners, including I.V. drug users, homosexual or bisexual partners, and strangers

Coping–stress tolerance pattern
• Pervasive muscle tension
• Constant irritability, feeling on edge or keyed up
• Constant shakiness, trembling, or twitching
• Concern over experiencing an exaggerated startle response (hypervigilance)
• Denial of clearly manifest anxiety
• Inability to identify those persons or measures that alleviate rather than exacerbate the condition
• Belief that significant lifestyle changes are contributing to feeling out of control

Value-belief pattern
• Feeling powerless to achieve life goals
• Desire to increase or decrease involvement in spirituality or religion
• Concern over impaired ability to believe in anything or anyone
• Disbelief about present situation

Physical findings
Cardiovascular
• Cold, clammy skin
• Elevated blood pressure
• Hot and cold flashes
• Increased heart rate
• Palpitations
• Sweating
• Tingling sensation

Respiratory
• Increased respiratory rate
• Shortness of breath
• Smothering sensation
• Choking sensation

Gastrointestinal
• Dry mouth
• Abdominal distress
• Nausea
• Vomiting
• Diarrhea
• Difficulty swallowing

Genitourinary
• Frequent urination

Musculoskeletal
• Increased fatigue
• Muscle aches, pains, or soreness
• Muscle tension
• Restlessness
• Shakiness
• Trembling
• Twitching

Neurologic
• Dilated pupils
• Dizziness or faintness
• Light-headedness
• Paresthesia
• Restlessness
• Insomnia

Psychological
• Feeling keyed up or on edge
• Inability to concentrate
• Irritability
• Blank mind

NURSING DIAGNOSIS

Anxiety related to real or perceived threat to physical integrity or self-concept

Nursing priority

Help the client recognize the anxiety and use effective coping strategies.

Patient outcome criteria

As treatment progresses, the client, family, or both should be able to:
• verbalize awareness of signs and symptoms of anxiety
• identify current level of anxiety
• identify effective and healthy coping strategies to manage anxiety-provoking situations.

Interventions

1. Establish and maintain trust with the client while using active listening and showing empathy and respect.

2. Recognize and manage your own anxiety or negative feelings that may occur in response to the client's resistance to recommended changes. (See *Autonomic responses to anxiety,* page 54.)

3. Identify client behaviors that produce anxiety in others. Explore these behaviors with the client as the therapy progresses.

4. Encourage the client to keep a daily journal and to make entries recording feelings, behaviors, stressors, coping strategies, and degrees of anxiety relief achieved. Help the client to describe any anxiety associated with specific activities or events, such as work, relationships, holidays, and social activities.

5. Identify the types and significance of stressors in the client's life.

Rationales

1. These strategies may alleviate any perceived threats that the client feels, thereby decreasing the client's anxiety level.

2. Anxiety and negative feelings in response to the client's resistance to recommended changes can inhibit the nurse's problem-solving abilities, thereby blocking effective interventions.

3. Identifying and exploring such behaviors can facilitate client growth and change and may help the client to recognize how such negative behavior affects others.

4. Developing effective coping strategies requires that the client recognize anxiety and its attendant feelings and overcome resistance to change. Recording thoughts, feelings, and actions (in a thought-feeling-and-action [T-F-A] journal) may facilitate self-awareness, help to clarify the client's resistance patterns, and identify what actions are successful in reducing the client's anxiety. Describing anxiety in specific situations can help the client to identify its causes and prevent free-floating anxiety (anxiety without an identifiable cause), which, if untreated, can cause progressive dysfunction.

5. Identifying stressors and determining their significance helps the client understand which stressors play a positive and a negative role.

Autonomic responses to anxiety

Anxiety can be contagious. When interacting with an anxious client, you may become aware that you are experiencing similar feelings as your client. Nurses need to learn and recognize physical signs and symptoms of anxiety in themselves. Awareness of these feelings and learning and utilizing self-regulation strategies assists the nurse in attaining a healthier balance while taking care of individuals who are experiencing varying levels of anxiety. This chart identifies how the autonomic nervous system, divided into the sympathetic (accelerator) and parasympathetic (decelerator) branches, responds to anxiety.

Body system	Sympathetic response	Parasympathetic response
Cardiovascular	• Accelerates heart rate • Increases blood pressure	• Slows heart rate • Decreases blood pressure
Respiratory	• Dilates bronchi • Causes rapid, shallow breathing	• Constricts bronchi • Slows respiratory rate
Gastrointestinal (alimentary system)	• Inhibits peristalsis • Inhibits secretin	• Stimulates peristalsis • Stimulates secretin • Stimulates release of bile
Genitourinary	• Stimulates conversion of glycogen to glucose • Causes secretion of adrenaline and noradrenaline • Inhibits flow of saliva in oral cavity • Inhibits bladder contraction	• Stimulates flow of saliva • Contracts bladder
Vision	• Dilates pupil	• Constricts pupil

6. Help the client to develop new, adaptive coping strategies by first exploring past methods used to reduce anxiety. Identify both effective and ineffective strategies as well as destructive or overused and ineffective ones. Explore the negative consequences of the ineffective strategies and work with the client to suggest new, effective strategies.

6. Learning new, adaptive coping strategies enables the client to use available resources and to accept personal responsibility for making and maintaining positive changes.

7. Encourage the client to participate in an exercise or physical activity program, within any functional status limitations.

7. Exercise is a healthy and effective means of decreasing the physical manifestations of anxiety and improving effective problem solving.

8. Encourage proper nutrition and direct the client to record dietary intake in daily journal entries.

8. Food, stimulants (such as nicotine and caffeine), and depressants (such as alcohol) may initially help to suppress the client's anxiety. However, if overused, they can cause additional problems (compulsive overeating, nicotine or caffeine addiction, and alcoholism) that may require treatment. Journal records can provide evidence of how the client uses food, alcohol, and nicotine to cope with anxiety.

9. If appropriate, use role playing in a supervised, safe environment.

9. Role playing allows the client to rehearse new coping strategies. Many coping skills require practice, feedback, and rehearsals before the client feels comfortable and skillful using them.

10. Teach the client relaxation techniques, such as guided imagery (recalling a pleasant, serene scene to induce relaxation), meditation, muscle relaxation (conscious tensing and relaxing of each muscle group), biofeedback (monitoring the reduction of tension that occurs during relaxation techniques), and hypnosis.

10. These techniques can help alleviate the emotional distress that accompanies anxiety and may decrease anxiety-related symptoms.

11. Administer medication, as ordered. Monitor drug levels and report any signs of adverse reactions.

12. Provide instruction about the medication regimen. Monitor the client's self-administration and provide written instructions for managing any adverse reactions, indicating when to call the primary care provider, psychiatrist, or prescribing advanced practice psychiatric nurse.

11. Antianxiety (anxiolytic) medications can relieve the physical symptoms of anxiety; however, they can cause significant adverse reactions, such as dizziness, drowsiness, insomnia, and dependency.

12. Adequate information about prescribed anxiolytic medication enables the client and family to take appropriate action should adverse reactions occur.

NURSING DIAGNOSIS

Ineffective individual coping related to inadequate coping strategies, inadequate support systems, high anxiety level, personal vulnerability or fragility, or multiple stressors

Nursing priority

Help the client identify ineffective coping behavior and negative consequences of this behavior.

Patient outcome criteria

As treatment progresses, the client, family, or both should be able to:
• identify ineffective coping strategies, unhealthy (risky) behaviors and their consequences
• demonstrate problem-solving and decision-making skills to manage increased anxiety levels.

Interventions

1. Assess the client's stressors and any factors that may cause stress, including negative self-concept, disapproval by others, inadequate problem-solving skills, loss or grief, inadequate support system, sudden lifestyle changes, a recent change in health status, and moral or ethical conflict.

2. Assess the client's developmental level and functional capacity to determine ability to cope with anxiety.

3. Identify any chemical substances (such as alcohol or drugs) and potentially compulsive behaviors (involving eating, gambling, sexual behaviors, smoking, spending, or working) that the client might be using to suppress anxiety.

4. Observe and monitor the client's behavior. Describe and clarify your observations for the client in clear, objective terms. Monitor complaints of physical disturbances. Clarify discrepancies among behavioral, cognitive, and physical manifestations of anxiety.

Rationales

1. Identifying the degree and impact of stressors and contributing factors can guide the nurse in developing appropriate treatment, especially for a client with multiple stressors or a high stress level. Such a client may become physically or emotionally ill, and coping abilities may regress.

2. Developmental and functional levels determine how a client can cope with stress. For example, a young boy might cry and run to his mother when anxious, whereas an adolescent might turn to peers or drugs. In addition, how well a person copes is affected by current events in the person's life. A client working full time while going to school may not have time to continue activities or sports that in the past helped to decrease anxiety.

3. Drugs and compulsive behaviors are commonly used to suppress anxiety; however, overuse can interfere with the client's ability to manage anxiety. Chemical substances or compulsive behaviors then become stressors rather than effective methods of reducing stress.

4. This procedure can help the nurse avoid making judgmental evaluations while increasing the client's awareness. Anxiety-ridden clients typically have more somatic complaints that need assessment, such as headaches, stomachaches, and nonspecific complaints of pain.

5. Provide the client with information and instructions for problem-solving techniques that can decrease negative and automatic responses to anxiety-provoking situations. For example, instruct the client to record events that precede anxiety attacks and then avoid those events or develop focused strategies to manage the situation in a less threatening manner.

5. This method gives the client an opportunity to learn and practice new coping skills.

6. Help the client to evaluate daily routines and stressors in family, work, and social relationships and situations.

6. Examining relationships and situations that may be contributing to the client's anxiety allows the client to make informed, conscious changes rather than impulsive, automatic, and often hurtful decisions that further contribute to their anxiety.

7. Collaborate with treatment team members on providing the client with referrals for group, family, or marital therapy as well as information about support groups, spiritual resources, and financial assistance.

7. The client and family may need various types of support to continue improvement.

Nursing diagnosis

Self-esteem disturbance related to perceived inability to cope

Nursing priority

Collaborate with the client develop and maintain an enhanced self-esteem.

Patient outcome criteria

As the treatment progresses, the client, family, or both should be able to:
• demonstrate enhanced ability to cope with anxiety-provoking situations
• verbalize and acknowledge successful anxiety management
• verbalize positive comments about their ability to achieve these successes.

Interventions

1. Establish a trusting, supportive relationship with the client.

2. Set up opportunities for the client to interact socially with others. Although you want to avoid overprotecting the client, take care not to make too many demands or overestimate their ability and readiness to take on new challenges.

3. Collaborate with the client to describe self-image and identify any factors that threaten that self-image.

4. Through a discussion of past incidents, collaborate with the client to recognize personal strengths and capabilities in coping with previous anxiety-provoking situations.

5. Use role playing to help the client discover and rehearse coping strategies that can be used in threatening or anxiety-provoking situations.

Rationales

1. A trusting relationship between the nurse and client can put the client at ease, which in turn may help the client establish a positive sense of self.

2. Structured interactions can develop the client's ability to socialize. They also can help the client to realize that others have similar social needs.

3. This self-examination may give the client a better sense of reality, which may have been distorted by increased anxiety.

4. These discussions should acknowledge the client's previous successes and abilities to cope with anxiety.

5. Allowing the patient to act out situations and practice well-defined coping strategies can diminish anticipatory anxiety and improve self-esteem.

NURSING DIAGNOSIS

Impaired social interaction and social isolation related to altered mental status, altered sensory and perceptual status, inadequate personal resources, lack of social support, self-esteem disturbance, or unsuccessful social interactions

Nursing priority

Collborate with the client to recognize anxiety and identify factors that lead to impaired social interaction and social isolation.

Patient outcome criterion

As the treatment progresses, the client, family, or both should be able to:
• participate in activities that enhance interactions and decrease social isolation.

Interventions

1. Encourage the client to discuss and analyze reasons for and feelings about social isolation.

2. Encourage the client to identify what causes the anxiety that inhibits social interaction.

3. Express a positive regard for the client.

4. Assess the client's use of coping skills and defense mechanisms.

5. Assess the client's communication skills.

6. Recommend that the client participate in psychoeducational programs directed at conflict areas or skill deficiencies. Such programs may address assertiveness skills, body awareness, debt recovery and financial planning, managing multiple commitments, and stress-management strategies.

Rationales

1. Discussing reasons for and feelings about being alone can help the client differentiate between choosing to be alone for enjoyment and purposefully isolating oneself from society.

2. Identifying specific causes can guide the client in adapting strategies to deal with anxiety in social situations.

3. Doing so communicates a belief in the client and establishes a safe, secure environment in which the client can feel comfortable about disclosing thoughts, fears, and feelings.

4. Identifying when and to what degree defense mechanisms are used allows the client to make informed choices when changing behavior. This allows the client to develop adaptive social interaction skills.

5. Teaching effective communication skills can increase self-esteem and decrease anxiety.

6. Participating in psychoeducational programs can instill in the client a sense that an anxiety-related disorder is a manageable condition and not something that need be suffered in isolation or forever.

NURSING DIAGNOSIS

Sleep pattern disturbance related to physiologic disturbance, psychological stress, or thought intrusion

Nursing priority

Help the client recognize the relationship between anxiety and sleep disturbance and identify appropriate interventions that restore and maintain normal sleep patterns.

Anxiety disorders

Patient outcome criteria

As treatment progresses, the client, family, or both should be able to:
• identify and use appropriate sleep hygiene interventions to facilitate an effective and restorative sleep pattern
• report improvement in sleep (decreased sleep latency with an increase in sleep efficiency and feeling refreshed after sleep cycle).

Interventions

1. Identify the sleep pattern disturbance and assess the client's usual sleep rituals (sleep hygiene regimen).

2. Encourage the client to restrict stimulant and depressant intake before bedtime (especially nicotine and caffeine-containing beverages and foods).

3. Teach the client relaxation techniques to use at bedtime.

4. Teach the client methods to decrease the amount of waking time spent in bed.

5. Encourage the client to increase daytime activities, participate in an exercise program, and avoid exercise 2 hours before bedtime.

6. Teach the client about prescribed sedative or hypnotic medications. Encourage the client to use the medication only as directed. Encourage the client to keep a journal describing responses to the medication and to behavioral interventions regarding their sleep time and feeling refreshed and restored after sleeping.

Rationales

1. Identifying usual sleep rituals in clients with sleep pattern disturbances can help determine specific sleep-inducing strategies. For example, the client may find that drinking a glass of warm milk before retiring promotes relaxation and sleepiness.

2. Stimulants (such as caffeine and nicotine) and depressants (such as alcohol) interfere with the normal sleep cycle and can contribute to a sleep pattern disturbance.

3. Relaxation techniques can reduce anxious feelings and muscle tension, thereby improving the ability to sleep.

4. Having a concrete plan to manage sleep disturbance can alleviate any immediate anxiety the client has about falling asleep and staying asleep.

5. Regular, moderate exercise increases body fatigue and the desire to rest and sleep without stimulating the client too much before going to bed.

6. Sedatives and hypnotic agents interfere with non-rapid eye movement (NREM) and rapid eye movement (REM) sleep and alter the quality of rest. A significant problem of rebound insomnia can develop, characterized by intense dreaming, nightmares, and increased sleep disruption. Therefore, sedative-hypnotic medications need to be monitored closely by the prescriber for the risk-benefit outcome.

NURSING DIAGNOSIS

Ineffective family coping related to misinformation or lack of knowledge about the client's condition, resulting in transient family disorganization and role disruptions

Nursing priority

Help the client's family recognize their own needs for support and identify and use resources effectively.

Patient outcome criteria

As the treatment progresses, the client, family, or both should be able to:
• recognize their needs for support related to family functioning
• follow up with recommendations for building a support network
• use these resources to decrease sense of isolation, resentment, and lack of knowledge.

Interventions

1. Assess the learning needs of the client's family members.

2. Identify the client's role in the family, and determine how the condition has altered the family function and organization.

3. Explain to the family the client's needs and behaviors.

4. Clarify with the family which members are experiencing problems and which need to be involved in solving the problems.

5. Encourage the family to develop problem-solving and decision-making skills.

6. Refer family members to appropriate resources, including support groups, financial counseling and support, family therapy, and spiritual counseling.

Rationales

1. Lack of knowledge or misunderstanding of the client's behavior can disrupt the way the family normally interacts. This disruption may escalate anxiety in family members.

2. Family organization and function may be influenced significantly by a member who is unable to contribute positively or fulfill usual roles.

3. Understanding the client's needs and behaviors as well as the nature of the condition or disease can help other family members to cope with the situation.

4. Understanding who needs help and why enables family members to understand their responsibilities better. It also encourages family members to ask for and offer help in a mutually beneficial manner.

5. Doing so allows the family to learn and use new strategies for coping with conflicts and for preventing anxiety-provoking situations.

6. The family may require additional assistance and support to maintain family integrity and functioning.

DISCHARGE CRITERIA

Nursing documentation indicates that the client:
• has demonstrated an increased ability to recognize anxiety symptoms
• can use newly learned skills to manage anxiety-provoking situations
• understands the diagnosis, treatment, and expected outcomes
• is aware of available group, family, or marital support resources and their referrals
• can use alternative coping skills (for example, anxiety reduction, cognitive restructuring, learning new behavior)
• has scheduled follow-up appointments.
Nursing documentation also indicates that the family:
• understands the client's diagnosis, treatment, and expected outcome
• has been referred to appropriate group, family, and other support services and knows how to contact these referrals
• can use alternative coping skills
• has scheduled necessary follow-up appointments.

SELECTED REFERENCES

Boyd, M.A., and Nihart, M.A. *Psychiatric Nursing: Contemporary Practice.* Philadelphia: Lippincott-Raven Pubs., 1998.

Diagnostic and Statistical Manual of Mental Disorders, 4th ed. Washington, D.C.: American Psychiatric Association, 1994.

Gorman, L.M., et al. *Davis's Manual of Psychosocial Nursing for General Patient Care.* Philadelphia: F.A. Davis Co., 1996.

Haber, J., et al. *Comprehensive Psychiatric Nursing,* 5th ed. St. Louis: Mosby–Year Book, Inc., 1997.

Howell, T. "Anxiety Disorders," in *Psychiatric Care in the Nursing Home.* Edited by Reichman, W.E., and Katz, P.R. New York: Oxford University Press, 1996.

Krupnick, S. "Antianxiety and Hypnosedative Medications," in *Psychiatric Nursing: A Comprehensive Reference,* 2nd ed. Edited by Lego, S. Philadelphia: Lippincott-Raven Pubs., 1996.

Mavissakalian, M., and Prien, R. *Long-Term Treatments of Anxiety Disorders.* Washington, D.C.: American Psychiatric Association, 1996.

Stuart, G.W., and Laraia, M.T. *Principles and Practice of Psychiatric Nursing,* 6th ed. St. Louis: Mosby–Year Book, Inc., 1997.

Varcarolis, E.M. *Foundations of Psychiatric-Mental Health Nursing,* 3rd ed. Philadelphia: W.B. Saunders Co., 1998.

Anxiety disorders

Part 3

Mood disorders

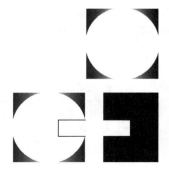

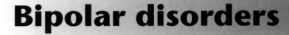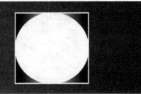

Bipolar disorders

DSM-IV classifications

296.0x	Bipolar I disorder
296.40	Bipolar I disorder, most recent episode hypomanic
296.4x	Bipolar I disorder, most recent episode manic
296.6x	Bipolar I disorder, most recent episode mixed
296.5x	Bipolar I disorder, most recent episode depressed
296. 7	Bipolar I disorder, most recent episode unspecified
296.89	Bipolar II disorder
296.80	Bipolar disorder not otherwise specified
301.13	Cyclothymia

INTRODUCTION

Description

Bipolar disorder is a chronic neurobiological illness. The course and chronicity are variable with the multiple treatment options that are currently available. Primary bipolar disorder has a prevalence from 0.4% to 1.6% in the general population. The estimated mean age at onset is between 21 and 30 years. It has been determined that approximately 10% to 15% of adolescents with a recurrent major depressive disorder will develop bipolar I disorder.

Bipolar disorder is further classified as bipolar I (and its variations), bipolar II, and bipolar disorder not otherwise specified. Cyclothymic is a chronic fluctuating mood disturbance. There is a risk that the person will develop bipolar I or II disorder.

Bipolar I disorder is a recurrent disorder. Approximately 90% of individuals who have a single manic episode will experience future episodes. There is some evidence that indicates a mean number of affective (depression and manic) episodes in a bipolar patient as nine. Some patients have been known to have more rapid mood shifts in short periods of time, known as rapid cycling.

Although the majority of individuals with bipolar I disease return to a fully functional level between episodes, approximately 20% to 30% continue to exhibit mood instability and interpersonal or occupational difficulties. Psychotic symptoms may develop after days or weeks. When an individual has manic episodes with psychotic features, subsequent manic episodes are more likely to develop psychotic features.

Bipolar II disorder is characterized by the occurrence of one or more major depressive episodes accompanied by at least one hypomanic episode. Individuals with bipolar II may not perceive the hypomanic episode as pathological, although others may be concerned by the individual's erratic behavior.

Bipolar II disorder may be more common in women than men. Incidence in the general population is 0.5%. Some studies have indicated that first-degree biological relatives of individuals with bipolar II have increased rates of bipolar II, bipolar I, and major depressive disorder when compared with the general population.

Bipolar disorder not otherwise specified includes disorders with bipolar features that do not meet criteria for any specific bipolar disorder. Some examples include very rapid alteration (over several days) between manic symptoms and depressive symptoms that do not meet minimal duration criteria for a manic episode or a major depressive episode, recurrent hypomanic episodes without intercurrent depressive episodes, and situations in which there is a bipolar disorder present but it is unclear if it is a primary (due to a general medical condition) or secondary (substance induced) condition.

Cyclothymic disorder is characterized by a chronic, fluctuating mood disturbance involving numerous periods of hypomanic symptoms as well as numerous periods of depressive symptoms. Although some individuals may function well during some of the periods of hypomania, they usually experience clinically significant distress or impairment in social, occupational, or other functions as a result of this mood disturbance. The impairment may develop as a result of prolonged periods of cyclical, sometimes unpredictable mood changes. Cyclothymic disorder usually begins early in life and is sometimes considered to reflect a temperamental disposition to other mood disorders. It is equally common in males and females. The lifetime prevalence is 0.4% to 1%; however, prevalence of this disorder in mood disorder clinics is from 3% to 5%.

Etiology and precipitating factors

Current research on biological factors in major depression and bipolar disorders often overlaps and may reflect the fact that they are closely linked. Some studies have shown that patients with bipolar disorder have decreased norepinephrine metabolites during depression and increased amounts during mania, which supports the norepinephrine imbalance hypothesis. There is also evidence that suggests that an increased activity of the norepinephrine-dopamine component tends to promote mania. Additionally, it has been proposed that an imbalance between acetylcholine and norepinephrine is associated with mania.

The National Institutes of Mental Health reports that bipolar disorder has demonstrated a significant genetic predisposition. First-degree biological relatives of individuals with bipolar disorder have elevated rates of bipolar I disorder (4% to 24%) and bipolar II disorder (1% to 5%). However, the mode of transmission and its genetic relationship to other affective disorders have not been identified.

The role of psychosocial or physical stress in precipitating episodes of bipolar illness has been studied, but current research indicates that environmental conditions contribute more to the timing of an episode than the actual causes of the disorder. Finally, many research scientists believe sleep deprivation is connected to the pathophysiology of mania. An individual with primary bipolar disorder often moves from depression to mania after experiencing sleep loss from only one sleep cycle.

Potential complications

If left untreated, bipolar disorder can lead to fatigue, exhaustion, and poor judgment, which in turn can lead to financial problems, unrealistic decisions, and alcohol or drug abuse. Violence, including child or spouse abuse, may occur during a manic episode. If the individual has a coexisting chronic medical condition, the mania could exacerbate that condition and require emergency medical treatment. Completed (successful) suicide occurs in 10% to 15% of individuals with bipolar I and II disorder. School and occupational failure may occur.

ASSESSMENT GUIDELINES

Nursing history (functional health pattern findings)

Health perception–health management pattern
- Euphoria over being in the best health ever
- Overconfidence in managing health-related issues
- Denial of need for health care attention
- Noncompliance with medication regimen
- Excessive drug or alcohol use
- Exaggerated lack of concern over health-related issues

Nutritional-metabolic pattern
- Inadequate or irregular food and fluid intake
- Significant weight loss
- Appetite loss
- Short attention span during meals

Elimination pattern
- Abdominal distress, including pain, flatulence, indigestion, and nausea
- Excessive, frequent urination
- Increased perspiration

Activity-exercise pattern
- Restlessness and boundless energy
- Excessive time spent exercising
- Denial of fatigue
- Sexual promiscuity, excessive spending, irresponsible enterprises, or other activities that have a high potential for painful or unpleasant consequences
- Psychomotor agitation
- Poor personal hygiene

Sleep-rest pattern
- Decreased need for sleep
- Feeling rested after only 2 or 3 hours of sleep
- Drug or alcohol use to aid sleep
- Disrupted sleep with initial, middle, or late insomnia
- Nightmares, illusions, or hallucinations during the night

Cognitive-perceptual pattern
- Confusion
- Racing thoughts
- Being easily distracted
- Decreased short-term memory
- Difficulty concentrating
- Illusions or hallucinations
- Disorganized, incoherent, and accelerated speech
- Poor impulse control
- Poor judgment
- Grandiose, unrealistic ambitions
- Denial of feeling painful stimuli
- Slowed reactions

Self-perception–self-concept pattern
- Perception of self as being magically omnipotent
- Intolerance of criticism
- Lack of shame or guilt
- History of angry or aggressive outbursts

Role-relationship pattern
- Grandiose delusions about special relationships with political, religious, entertainment figures or with God
- Inappropriate enthusiasm during social interactions and an increased involvement in social groups
- Concern over the lack of support shown by family and loved ones concerning lifestyle or behavioral changes
- Intrusive, demanding, or domineering behaviors
- Isolated, stressful living circumstances
- Frequent, angry outbursts directed at loved ones
- Manipulative and limit-testing behaviors

Sexual-reproductive pattern
- Involvement in multiple sexual encounters
- Concern about involvement in high-risk sexual behavior, such as promiscuity
- Concern about involvement with high-risk partners, including bisexual or homosexual partners and I.V. drug users

Mood disorders

- Irregular menstrual periods or other menstrual cycle changes
- Disrupted relations with spouse or loved one
- Difficulty with issues of dependence and independence
- Difficulty with intimacy
- Difficulty doing things for others
- Fear of social isolation

Coping–stress tolerance pattern
- Increased irritability and tension
- Drug or alcohol use
- Loss of control
- Exaggerated startle response (hypervigilance)
- Engagement in significant, stressful situations before symptom exacerbation
- Inability to identify what may be helpful

Value-belief pattern
- Grandiose delusions involving religious themes
- Exaggerated feelings of power
- Denial of illness and nonparticipation in care
- Inability to trust anyone
- Inability to control situation
- Feelings of hopelessness about the condition
- Concern about real or perceived personal failures

Physical findings
Cardiovascular
- Hypotension or hypertension
- Palpitations
- Sweating
- Rapid heart rate
- Irregular rhythm

Respiratory
- Increased respiratory rate
- Shortness of breath

Gastrointestinal
- Abdominal pain
- Diarrhea
- Dry mouth
- Flatulence
- Heartburn
- Indigestion
- Nausea
- Vomiting

Genitourinary
- Menstrual irregularities
- Increased sex drive
- Sexually transmitted diseases
- Frequent urination

Integumentary
- Changes in hair amount, texture, and distribution
- Changes in nail growth and texture
- Rashes or scales
- Pigmentation and skin temperature changes

Musculoskeletal
- Aches or pains
- Cramping
- Fractures
- Muscle weakness
- Numbness
- Tingling
- Tremors
- Twitching

Neurologic
- Agitation
- Dizziness

Psychological
- Alternating euphoria and irritability
- Delusions
- Decreased ability to concentrate
- Extreme self-confidence
- Impaired judgment
- Lack of insight

NURSING DIAGNOSIS

Risk for violence, self-directed or directed at others, related to poor impulse control or cognitive and perceptual changes

Nursing priority

Maintain the client's safety.

Patient outcome criteria

As the treatment progresses, the client, family, or both should be able to:
• verbalize and demonstrate a sense of personal control
• remain free from harm
• refrain from verbal outbursts
• refrain from interpersonal violence and violence against animals or objects
• report and demonstrate increasing mood stability

Interventions

1. Provide a safe environment for the client by removing potentially dangerous items, such as sharp objects and belts, and rearranging furniture as needed.

2. Intervene at the beginning stages of agitation, and frequently assess the client's agitation level.

3. Communicate in simple, direct sentences.

4. Allow the client to resume interactions with other clients gradually as behavior improves.

5. When feasible, encourage the client to participate in decision making. Avoid arguing with the client.

6. When feasible, develop with the client written behavioral plans that clearly state limits on undesirable or destructive behavior as well as rewards for appropriate, positive behavior.

7. Address the client's needs promptly.

8. Administer antimanic medications as ordered. (See *Overview of mood-stabilizing medications,* page 66.) Monitor the client's response, and assess for any adverse reactions.

9. Encourage the client to identify and discuss conditions that cause anger and agitation.

Rationales

1. The client whose thinking is impaired and who is behaving in a psychotic manner can be a physical threat to self and others. Removing potentially destructive implements can help prevent violent incidents.

2. Intervening when agitation begins can help prevent the situation from escalating and can allow the nurse to treat the client in a less restrictive manner. Such intervention may include speaking in a calm, reassuring voice; decreasing stimulation by having the client limit interactions with others; and restricting the client to one room if necessary.

3. The impulsive, agitated, and easily distracted client cannot process complex messages. Simple, clear directions can help ease client agitation.

4. Gradually resuming interactions with others promotes, reinforces, and enhances the client's self-esteem and sense of self-control.

5. Participating in treatment can increase the client's sense of control. Arguing can escalate an agitated client's behavior and may increase the sense of powerlessness.

6. Plans that clearly spell out behavioral limits discourage nurse-client power struggles, limit manipulative client behaviors, and enhance continuity of care. A plan that provides positive reinforcement for desirable behavior increases the client's desire to repeat that behavior.

7. The agitated and impulsive client cannot tolerate waiting. Unnecessary delays and delayed gratification can provoke client violence.

8. Neuroleptics, benzodiazepines, lithium, and anticonvulsants — all indicated for mania — have different actions and potential adverse effects. Careful monitoring of the client's response and of blood levels decreases the risk of adverse effects or toxic reactions and allows for more accurate titration.

9. Knowing the conditions and factors that cause agitation can enable the client to recognize when such episodes might occur, which in turn allows the client to implement alternative coping methods.

Mood disorders

Overview of mood-stabilizing medications

Medications	Pretreatment tests
Lithium lithium carbonate (Eskalith, Lithane, Lithotabs, Lithonate, Eskalith CR, and Lithobid sustained-release) lithium citrate (Cibilith)	**Before starting any mood-stabilizing agent** • Comprehensive medical history • Physical examination • Pregnancy test
Anticonvulsant agents carbamazepine (Tegretol) divalproex (Depakote) (combination of valproate and valproic acid) gabapentin (Neurontin)	**Before starting lithium** • Complete blood count • Electrocardiogram • Electrolyte levels • Renal function studies (renal panel); blood urea nitrogen, creatinine, routine urinalysis • Thyroid panel
	Before starting valproate (divalproex) • Hepatic function tests • Hematologic function tests
	Before starting carbamazepine • Blood and platelet counts • Hepatic function tests • Renal function tests • Urinalysis

10. Monitor rapid mood shifts and behavioral changes, paying special attention to depressive thoughts and feelings.

10. Emotional instability and impulsive behavior may lead to suicidal gestures or aggressive outbursts. Monitoring mood swings and related behavioral changes can protect the client and others in the area from danger.

NURSING DIAGNOSIS

Sleep pattern disturbance related to hyperactivity and perceived lack of need for sleep

Nursing priority

Help the client reestablish a regular and restful sleep pattern.

Patient outcome criteria

As the treatment progresses, the client, family, or both should be able to:
• establish an efficient and effective sleep pattern
• report feeling rested after a sleep cycle.

Interventions

1. Establish a distraction-free environment at bedtime.

2. Restrict the client's caffeine and nicotine intake.

3. Establish a daily morning and afternoon exercise routine. Discourage strenuous evening activity 2 hours before bedtime.

Rationales

1. A quiet, comfortable environment induces relaxation and decreases the client's attention to stimuli.

2. Stimulants can interfere with normal sleep and exacerbate the client's manic symptoms.

3. Daily exercise induces fatigue and promotes sleep. Strenuous evening activity may energize the client and interfere with sleep.

4. Administer prescribed medications as ordered, and monitor the client's response.

5. Establish with the client a bedtime routine to manage any sleep disturbance.

6. Offer warm milk and a snack at bedtime.

4. Medications may assist in reestablishing a normal sleep pattern and reduce the client's restlessness.

5. Establishing a planned bedtime routine helps to alleviate client anxiety, frustration, and irritability associated with a sleep disturbance.

6. A bedtime snack can help the client to relax. Warm milk contains tryptophan, a natural substance that can induce sleep.

Nursing diagnosis

Altered nutrition: less than body requirements related to increased metabolic rate, distractibility, and poor attention span

Nursing priority

Help the client establish better eating habits and maintain proper nutrition.

Patient outcome criteria

As the treatment progresses, the client, family, or both should be able to:
• reestablish an adequate fluid and electrolyte balance
• demonstrate a stable weight
• verbalize a need to eat.

Interventions

1. Monitor the client's serum electrolyte and albumin levels, weight, and fluid intake and output status daily.

2. Offer small, frequent meals of high-calorie foods. Include foods that the client likes as well as those that can be eaten while moving about.

3. Serve the client meals in an area with few distractions.

Rationales

1. This enables the nurse to determine the client's fluid and electrolyte status, ongoing nutritional needs, and hydration status.

2. The manic client has a generally high metabolic rate and may be too distracted to eat complete meals. Foods that can be eaten while moving around may be indicated for the client who is too agitated to sit long enough to eat a meal.

3. Reducing mealtime distractions encourages the client to focus attention on eating.

Nursing diagnosis

Impaired social interaction related to impulsive behavior, distractibility, impaired judgment, cognitive or perceptual changes, and paranoid ideation

Nursing priority

Protect the client from harmful consequences of poor and diffuse personal and social boundaries and enhance the establishment and maintenance of interpersonal relationships.

Mood disorders

Patient outcome criteria

As the treatment progresses, the client, family, or both will be able to:
• recognize and control intrusive, demanding behavior in social situations
• interact effectively and appropriately using assertive communication strategies
• recognize how interaction styles affect communication within the family
• identify constructive ways to interact.

Interventions

1. Intervene as needed to protect the client from harmful social interactions.

2. Approach the client in a nondefensive, casual manner, and explain any refusals of irrational or inappropriate requests.

3. Discuss the impact the client's behaviors and verbal messages have on others, and encourage the use of more appropriate interaction styles.

Rationales

1. The manic client typically does not recognize the intrusive, demanding nature of personal interactions. The nurse can diffuse potentially violent outbursts by intervening during such interactions.

2. The manic client is highly sensitive to communication styles, which inadvertently may trigger impulsive, angry responses. By providing rationales for refusing irrational requests, the nurse can discourage such responses.

3. The nurse may be able to encourage the manic client to use a heightened sensitivity to nonverbal behavior and verbal messages to explore the impact of behavior on others. As concentration and attention span improve, the client should be better able to accept feedback regarding interaction styles.

NURSING DIAGNOSIS

Sensory-perceptual alterations related to decreased ability to concentrate, racing thoughts, distractibility, flight of ideas, hallucinations, delusions, sleep deprivation, or anxiety

Nursing priority

Orient the client to reality, maintain a safe environment for the client and others, and encourage realistic, goal-directed thinking.

Patient outcome criteria

As the treatment progresses, the client, family, or both should be able to:
• report and demonstrate increasing mood stability
• identify early signs and symptoms of decompensation
• verbalize and appropriate plan for relapse management

Interventions

1. Frequently orient the client to reality, speaking in a clear, simple, nonargumentative manner.

2. Provide the client with a relaxing area with decreased environmental stimulation.

Rationales

1. Frequently orientating the client to reality helps reduce potential agitation resulting from confused perceptions and thoughts.

2. An environment free from distractions decreases anxiety and reduces the potential for agitation or hyperactivity.

3. Gradually integrate the client into a social environment while observing for changes in tolerance of such activity.

4. Design a daily schedule appropriate to the client's mental status. Reevaluate the schedule and add activities as the client's ability to process and tolerate stimuli improves.

5. Be sensitive to the client's physical and psychological boundaries during interaction; for example, use physical contact cautiously and clearly distinguish your own experiences from the client's in conversation.

3. Interacting with others can decrease the client's feelings of isolation and allow for nonpressured participation in a social environment.

4. An established daily schedule defines both client and staff expectations of behavior and guides daily planning. It also keeps client choices to a minimum, which in turn avoids agitation.

5. Clearly separating the client from others, including the nurse, decreases client confusion, reduces paranoia and anxiety, and shows respect for the client's territorial space.

Nursing diagnosis

Self-esteem disturbance related to delusions and grandiosity

Nursing priority

Collaborate with the client to plan for recovery and develop a realistic perception of abilities and self-esteem.

Patient outcome criteria

As the treatment progresses, the client, family, or both should be able to:
- verbalize self-acceptance
- recognize and verbalize self-limitations
- verbalize pride in self
- demonstrate ability to accept constructive feedback from others.

Interventions

1. Establish expectations of self-care and provide guidance, assistance, and support as needed. Reevaluate and revise expectations as the client's functioning level increases.

2. Address the client in a respectful, dignified manner while helping to maintain personal privacy.

3. Offer the client choices related to treatment, and encourage participation in the treatment plan.

4. Reinforce the client's successes and gains made toward achieving personal goals.

Rationales

1. Establishing standards encourages the client to assume personal responsibility, promotes independent functioning, and enhances self-worth.

2. By behaving respectfully, the nurse can enhance the client's sense of self-worth.

3. The client who participates in treatment should develop an increased sense of control and value.

4. Acknowledging accomplishments and efforts toward achieving goals reinforces the client's sense of self-worth.

Nursing diagnosis

Powerlessness related to feelings of hopelessness and perceived lack of control over life situations and illness

Nursing priority

Collaborate with the client to regain a sense of self-control and mastery over life situations and illness.

Mood disorders

Patient outcome criteria

As the treatment progresses, the client, family, or both will be able to:
• verbalize realistic, goal-directed thinking related to abilities, recovery and maintenance of bipolar disorder
• discuss the bipolar disorder as a neurobiological condition that can be triggered by sleep deprivation and psychosocial stressors
• recognize the need for and benefit of support systems
• utilize support systems to enhance feelings of being empowered.

Interventions

1. Collaborate with the client to develop and implement the treatment plan.

2. Discuss with the client early signs and symptoms, such as increased activity, little appetite, or decreased need for sleep, that may indicate a recurrence of the illness. Collaborate with the client to develop early intervention strategies.

3. Provide the hospitalized client with opportunities to demonstrate self-control. For example, instruct the client to ask for quiet time when becoming overstimulated.

4. Explore the client's feelings of hopelessness and identify misperceptions, distortions, and irrational beliefs.

5. Collaborate with the client to set realistic, attainable goals for the present and future.

Rationales

1. Helping to make treatment-related decisions can enhance the client's sense of self-control and mastery within their chronic illness.

2. Making the client aware of early symptoms of the illness and developing steps to minimize its recurrence can help to avoid or minimize future hospitalization resulting from an acute episode.

3. Opportunities to rehearse self-control can foster confidence and mastery in personal abilities.

4. Doing so helps the client differentiate between irrational and real concerns. It also enables the client to examine the accuracy of perceptions and helps to increase positive thinking.

5. Setting realistic goals can increase the client's sense of self-control while eliminating distorted, unattainable objectives that could promote being unsuccessful and foster feelings of demoralization.

NURSING DIAGNOSIS

Altered family processes related to role changes, economic crisis, or lack of knowledge about the client's illness

Nursing priority

Teach family members about bipolar disorder while encouraging discussion of thoughts and feelings about how the client's and the family's behaviors affect one another.

Patient outcome criteria

As treatment progresses, the client, family, or both should be able to:
• verbalize their concerns and needs to the treatment team
• verbalize feelings of anger, resentfulness, frustration, and guilt and be validated for these feelings
• demonstrate decrease intensity of these feelings
• verbalize understanding of bipolar disorder as a genetically transmitted, neurobiological, chronic mental disorder
• recognize the importance and benefit to family member well-being of utilizing outside support systems.

Interventions

1. Assess the family's external support network and encourage participation in family therapy and support groups.

2. Assess communication patterns and boundaries within the family.

3. Observe interaction patterns within the family and discuss their influence on the client and family functioning.

4. Provide the family with information regarding bipolar disorder and the client's treatment and prognosis.

Rationales

1. External support networks can provide a safe, nurturing environment for the expression of fears and concerns. Such groups encourage the formation of friendships based on common interests.

2. Knowing basic information about the family's functioning, the ability of family members to resolve problems, and the family's impact on the client can help the nurse develop a more effective treatment plan.

3. Both the client and family need to be aware of how the client's behaviors affect family relationships in order to adapt to necessary changes.

4. Such knowledge may relieve guilt, encourage discussion of issues, and increase the family's ability to detect early signs of the disorder's degeneration.

DISCHARGE CRITERIA

Nursing documentation indicates that the client:
• has demonstrated stable mood, thoughts, perceptions, and behavior
• can interact appropriately with others and care for self
• can recognize early signs of illness recurrence and implement an appropriate plan of action
• can use effective coping methods
• understands the need for follow-up care and is willing to comply with recommended treatment
• knows when and how to use emergency services
• is aware of appropriate community resources.
Nursing documentation also indicates that the family:
• is maintaining a stable sleep cycle and nutritional status
• has scheduled necessary follow-up appointments
• has been referred to the appropriate community resources
• understands the potential problems that can develop during the transition from inpatient to outpatient care.

SELECTED REFERENCES

Bauer, M., and McBride, L. *Structured Group Psychotherapy for Bipolar Disorder: The Life Goals Program.* New York: Springer Publishing Co., 1996.

Diagnostic and Statistical Manual of Mental Disorders, 4th ed. Washington, D.C.: American Psychiatric Association, 1994.

Ginns, E.L., et al. "A Genome-Wide Search for Chromosomal Loci Linked to Bipolar Affective Disorder in the Old Order Amish," *National Genetics* 12(4):431, 1996.

Johnson, M., and Maas, M. *Nursing Outcomes Classification (NOC).* St. Louis: Mosby–Year Book, Inc., 1997.

McCloskey, J.C., and Bulechek, G.M. *Nursing Interventions Classification (NIC),* 2nd ed. St. Louis: Mosby–Year Book, Inc., 1996.

Nathan, P.E., and Gorman, J.M. *A Guide to Treatments That Work.* New York: Oxford University Press, 1998.

New Developments in the Biology of Mental Disorders. Piscataway, N.J.: Research and Education Association, 1997.

Ramirez Basco, M., and Rush, A.J. *Cognitive-Behavioral Therapy for Bipolar Disorder.* New York: Guilford Press, 1996.

Tohen, M., et al. "Risperdone in the Treatment of Mania," *Journal of Clinical Psychiatry* 57:249-253, 1996.

Torrey, E.F., et al. *Schizophrenia and Manic-Depressive Disorder: The Biological Roots of Mental Illness as Revealed by the Landmark Study of Identical Twins.* New York: Basic Books, 1994.

Whybrow, P.C. *A Mood Apart: Depression and Mania and Other Afflictions of the Self.* New York: Basic Books, 1997.

Wise, M.G., and Rundell, J.R. *Text of Consultation Liaison Psychiatry.* Washington, D.C.: American Psychiatric Association, 1996.

Mood disorders

Depressive disorders

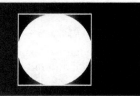

DSM-IV classifications

296.2x	Major depression, single episode
296.3x	Major depression, recurrent
300.4	Dysthymic disorder
311	Depressive Disorder Not Otherwise Specified

INTRODUCTION

Description

Major depression is a mood disorder in which the major symptoms — depressed mood and loss of interest or pleasure in all or almost all activities (anhedonia) — occur daily for at least 2 weeks. Related symptoms include appetite disturbance, sleep disturbance, weight changes, psychomotor agitation or retardation, low energy, decreased libido, feelings of worthlessness, difficulty concentrating, recurrent thoughts of death, and suicidal ideation or suicide attempts. Major depression can occur during infancy, represented by failure-to-thrive syndrome, and throughout adulthood.

Major depression may be classified as a single episode (one occurrence) or as recurrent (two or more depressive episodes separated by at least 2 months). The symptoms are not related to bereavement or due to the direct physiologic effects of a substance or a general medical condition. Approximately 17% of the general population will experience a depressive episode at some time in their lives.

Dysthymic disorder is a chronic mood disorder characterized by a depressed mood during most of the day and lasting at least 2 years (1 year for children and adolescents). The symptoms are not as severe or disabling as a major depressive disorder. Dysthymic disorder can be associated with impairment in functional capacity and typically has an early onset (childhood, adolescence, or early adulthood).

Depressive disorder not otherwise specified (DDNOS) includes disorders with depressive features that do not meet the criteria for major depressive disorder, dysthymic disorder, adjustment disorder with depressed mood, or adjustment disorder with mixed anxiety and depressed mood. Examples of DDNOS include premenstrual dysphoric disorder, minor depressive disorder, recurrent brief depressive disorder, or postpsychotic depressive disorder of schizophrenia.

Etiology and precipitating factors

The explosion of biological research in mood disorders has provided significant data in the areas of psychoneuroendocrinology, psychoneuroimmunology, and neurotransmitter receptors and genetics. The research in these areas has advanced the biological theories of causation as well as the focused treatment of depressive disorders.

Studies of major depression in families, twins, and adopted children demonstrate that genetic influences have a substantial role in the etiology of depressive disorders. Major depressive disorder (MDD) is 1.5 to 3 times more prevalent among first-degree biological relatives of individuals with this disorder than in the general population. Current research is focusing on developing a more thorough understanding of how genetic factors contribute to the development of major depression.

Several biological theories of causation have been investigated. Currently, the focus of biological research is on neurotransmitters and receptor sites — two areas that have advanced our knowledge and pharmacologic treatment of individuals suffering with depressive disorders. There is considerable evidence indicating that the secretion of hypothalamic hypophysiotropic hormones is controlled by several neurotransmitters; including serotonin, acetylcholine, norepinephrine, dopamine, and gamma aminobutyric acid. Additional neurotransmitter research is focused on the receptors and transporters of these molecules, in conjunction with the enzymes that control their metabolism. The neuroendocrine and neuropeptide hypothesis of major depression is associated with multiple alterations in the neuroendocrine and neuropeptide systems. Specifically, the hypothalamic-pituitary adrenal axis, hypothalamic-pituitary-thyroid axis, hypothalamic-pituitary-gonadal axis, and hypothalamic-growth hormone axis. Additionally, there is increasing evidence that neuromodulating peptides (that is, corticotropin releasing factor) contributes to the symptoms of depression.

Psychoneuroimmunologic studies examine interactions among behavioral, neural, endocrine, and immune processes, each serving a regulatory and homeostatic function. The relation between immune dysfunction and specific psychiatric disease genesis is not yet delineated, but is a growing area of research.

Cognitive factors may contribute to the development of depression. The cognitive approach proposes that irrational beliefs and distorted attitudes toward the individual, his environment, and his future perpetuate depressive feelings. There is support for the impact of developmental factors on an individual. Developmental factors, such as the premature or permanent loss of a parent or loved one by death or separation, significantly contribute to the development of depression as does inadequate emotional parenting. There is some evidence that significant losses in life can change the brain's neurochemistry and thereby produce depression.

Behavioral theory holds that depression is caused primarily by a severe reduction of pleasant experiences or an increase in unpleasant experiences in the individual's life. As depression develops, the unpleasant experiences multiply, thus feeding a downward and increasingly restrictive cycle, which intensifies the mood disturbance.

Social and family system theories emphasize the individual's role within the family system. According to these theories, interpersonal difficulties, dysfunctional family communication, and abusive lifestyle patterns cause depression. Major depression is often found to correlate with an intensely adverse life event, especially if it involved the loss of an important human relationship or role in life. Social isolation places individuals, especially those who are elderly or economically disadvantaged, at greater risk for depression.

Potential complications
An undiagnosed or undertreated (primary) depressive disorder can lead to significant impairments in functional status, and activities of daily living may become drastically curtailed. This can put the individual at risk for dehydration, infection, and an exacerbation of a concurrent medical condition. Unrelenting depression can lead to suicidal feelings and possible action; potential for a successful suicide does exist. MDD is diagnosed in 20% to 25% of clients with general medical conditions. If MDD is not detected or is undertreated, clients with a coexisting medical condition may begin to fail in their responses to treatment and their overall condition and functional ability worsen.

ASSESSMENT GUIDELINES

Nursing history (functional health pattern findings)
Health perception–health maintenance pattern
• Concern over somatic complaints
• Increased irritability
Nutritional-metabolic pattern
• Decreased or increased appetite
• Weight loss or gain
Elimination pattern
• Decreased motility
• Constipation
Activity-exercise pattern
• Increased fatigue

• Decreased libido
• Psychomotor retardation
• Withdrawal from daily life activities
• Decreased ability to enjoy life or to function at work
Sleep-rest pattern
• Early morning awakening and depression
• Difficulty falling asleep
• Hypersomnia as a method of withdrawal
• Alcohol or drug use to induce sleep
Cognitive-perceptual pattern
• Difficulty concentrating
• Difficulty making decisions
• Ruminating thoughts
• Impoverished thinking
• Distorted perceptions
Self-perception–self-concept pattern
• Preoccupation with self
• Low self-esteem
• Feelings of inadequacy or guilt
• Increased irritability
• Perception of self as being worthless or incompetent
Role-relationship pattern
• Perception of self as a burden to spouse or loved one
• Feelings of worthlessness at work
Sexual-reproductive pattern
• Decreased libido
• Difficulty with intimacy
• Fertility, reproductive, or menstrual disturbances
Coping–stress tolerance pattern
• Considering suicide as coping mechanism
• Suicidal ideation or gestures
• Difficulty coping
• Inability to reach reasonable solutions to problems
Value-belief pattern
• Feelings of powerlessness or hopelessness in achieving life goals

Physical findings
Cardiovascular
• Elevated blood pressure
Respiratory
• Increased respiratory rate
• Increased sighing
• Shortness of breath
Gastrointestinal
• Abdominal distress
• Anorexia
• Constipation
• Diarrhea
• Increased appetite
• Weight gain or loss
Musculoskeletal
• Fatigue
• Lethargy
• Muscle tension, aches, pains

(Text continues on page 76.)

Mood disorders

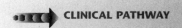

CLINICAL PATHWAY

Major depression

	Day 1	**Day 2**	**Day 3**
Admission and consultations	• History and physical • Vital signs • Nursing assessment • Medical consultation, if indicated • Weigh patient • Assess suicidality (+ or −)	• Reassess or confirm diagnosis • Review test results • Medical-surgical or neurologic consults if indicated • Assess suicidality (+ or −)	• Assess suicidality (+ or −)
Tests	• Complete blood count • Thyroid-stimulating hormone, thyroxine, urinalysis, rapid plasma reagin • Pregnancy test if indicated • Chest X-Ray • Electrocardiogram	• Repeat abnormal tests • List quantity and quality of sleep	
Treatments	• Milieu • Verbal group • Activities • Psychotherapy	• Same as Day 1	• Treatment plan completed and signed by patient • Family assessment and therapy
Medications	• Antipsychotic medications • Antidepressants • Hypnotics • Antianxiety medications • Medications for preexisting condition	• Adjust medications as indicated	• Same as Day 2
Teaching	• Medications • Psychiatric condition • Tests • Procedures • Health maintenance • Family	• Continue to reinforce teaching of patient and significant other.	• Same as Day 2
Discharge planning and social services	• Expected length of stay • Contact with family members for information • Initiate Social Services assessment	• Daily morning meeting • Discharge planning in progress	• Same as Day 2
Outcomes	• Baseline • Beck Depression Inventory	• Assess daily: – sleep – mood – psychotic symptoms – appetite – change observation status – suicidal Ideation.	• Same as Day 2

Day 4	Day 5	Day 6	Day 7 (Day of discharge)
• Assess suicidality (+ or −)	• Assess suicidality (+ or −)	• Assess suicidality (+ or −)	• Weigh patient • Assess suicidality (+ or −)
			• Quantity and quality of sleep
• Same as Day 1	• Same as Day 1	• Same as Day 1	• Same as Day 1
• Same as Day 2	• Same as Day 2	• Same as Day 2	• Same as Day 2
• Same as Day 2	• Same as Day 2	• Same as Day 2	• Discharge instructions • Wrap-up session • Review medication
• Same as Day 2	• Same as Day 2 • Social Services assessment on chart	• Same as Day 2	• Review discharge plan with patient and family or significant other • Review with community staff as indicated
• Same as Day 2	• Same as Day 2	• Same as Day 2	• Same as Day 2 • Repeat Beck Depression Inventory

Adapted with permission from Doylestown (Pa.) Hospital

Mood disorders

Neurologic
- Agitation
- Memory difficulties
- Restlessness
- Sleep disturbance
- Slowed thinking

Psychological
- Anhedonia
- Crying or fearfulness
- Delusions
- Difficulty concentrating
- Restlessness
- Excessive concern with physical health
- Feelings of inadequacy
- Feelings of worthlessness, shame, or guilt
- Indecisiveness
- Loss of interest in environment
- Preoccupation with certain thoughts
- Social withdrawal
- Suicidal thoughts

NURSING DIAGNOSIS

Ineffective individual coping related to depression in response to identifiable stressors

Nursing priority

Help the client develop positive coping mechanisms and understand how stress affects the condition.

Patient outcome criteria

As the treatment progresses, the client, family, or both should be able to:
- identify ineffective coping behaviors and consequences
- express feelings and thoughts more clearly and directly
- report decreases signs and symptoms of depression.

Interventions

1. Encourage the client to identify events that cause unpleasant emotional responses. Help the client to distinguish between extraneous issues and relevant stressors.

2. Assess real, significant losses that the client has experienced. Also identify cultural and social factors that may have determined how the client coped with these losses.

3. Assess the client's support network.

4. Assess the client's alcohol and drug use as well as suicide potential.

5. Help improve the client's self-esteem by suggesting simple, success-oriented tasks.

Rationales

1. Gaining insight about how certain events can affect feelings is an important step in developing self-control. Organizing and ranking stressors can enhance the client's sense of control.

2. Cultural and social values can negatively affect how people cope with grief and loss. For example, a person may feel that crying over or mourning the death of a loved one is socially unacceptable; such suppression and denial of feelings can lead to depression.

3. A support network including family and friends can help the client recover from depression.

4. Alcohol or drug use is an ineffective coping method. Alcohol, a depressant, can increase depression. Other drugs may mask the client's feelings but do not remove the depression's cause. A depressed client is at higher risk for suicide, especially one who sees no way out of the situation. Alcohol or drug use increases the risk for suicide in such clients.

5. Low self-esteem commonly accompanies depression. Giving the client simple, success-oriented tasks can increase feelings of self-worth.

6. Collaborate with the multidisciplinary team to determine and monitor appropriate pharmacologic and other somatic therapies, such as electroconvulsive therapy or phototherapy. Concomitant use of monoamine oxidase (MAO) inhibitors and serotonergic drugs can lead to serotonin syndrome (See *Identifying and treating serotonin syndrome*.) Make sure the client and family receive clear guidelines for using tricyclic antidepressants or MAO inhibitors before the client is discharged from the unit. (See *Food and drug interactions with monoamine oxidase inhibitors,* page 78.)

6. The client may require a combination of therapies to relieve depression. Some forms of depression respond well to medication, whereas others may need electroconvulsive therapy or other treatments.

Identifying and treating serotonin syndrome

Early phase characteristics	Middle phase characteristics	Late phase characteristics	Treatment
• Agitation • Confusion • Diaphoresis • Diarrhea • Flushing • Lethargy • Myoclonic jerks • Restlessness • Tremors	• Hypertension • Hypertonicity • Increased myoclonus • Rigor	• Acidosis • Disseminated intravascular coagulation • Respiratory failure • Renal failure • Rhabdomyolysis	• Discontinuation of serotonergic medications • Emergency medical treatment in middle to late phase to support physiologic recovery • Cooling blankets for hyperthermia • Clonazepam for myoclonus • Chlorpromazine I.M. for hyperthermia and sedation • Nifedipine for hypertension • Serotonin antagonists and beta blockers

NURSING DIAGNOSIS

Risk for self-directed violence related to suicidal ideation

Nursing priority

Ensure the client's safety, paying specific attention to suicide prevention.

Patient outcome criteria

As the treatment progresses, the client, family, or both should be able to:
• comply voluntarily with signing and adhering to a safety contract
• control self-harm impulses and actions.

Mood disorders

Food and drug interactions with monoamine oxidase inhibitors

Monoamine oxidase (MAO) inhibitors interact with certain foods and drugs to produce a significant increase in blood pressure. Some interactions can cause severe and even life-threatening complications. Generally, foods that can cause a reaction have been aged, fermented, pickled, or smoked.

Foods and beverages to avoid completely

Dairy products
Most cheeses (especially if aged)
Yogurt
Meats and fish
Caviar
Dried fish
Fermented sausage (bologna, pepperoni, salami, summer
  sausage)
Marinated meats
Pickled herring
Unrefrigerated fermented fish
Sauces and seasonings
Chocolate
Hoisin (fermented oyster sauce used in Oriental dishes)
Soy sauce
Yeast (all yeast products, extracts, and preparations such as
  Marmite and brewer's yeast)
Vegetables
Chinese pea pods
English broad beans
Fava beans
Sauerkraut
Combination foods
Caesar salad
Eggplant parmesan
Lasagna
Macaroni and cheese
Pate (liver)
Pizza
Quiche
Soufflés
Beverages
Imported, aged beers
Chianti, aged red wines

Foods and beverages to avoid in large amounts

Caffeine products
Chocolate
Coffee
Colas
Dairy products
Processed American cheese
Fruits
Avocados
Bananas
Canned figs
Plums
Prunes
Raisins
Beverages
Domestic (jug) red wines
Domestic beers, ales, and stouts
Sherry

Foods and beverages that cause no reactions

Dairy products
Cottage cheese
Cream cheese
Cream
Ice cream
Milk
Beverages
White wines

Drugs to avoid

Amphetamines, such as dexedrine, methylamphetamine
  (Desoxyn), and methylphenidate (Ritalin)
Anesthesia, general and local
Antiasthmatic agents
Antidepressants (cyclics, especially clomipramine, Anafranil,
  and possibly fluoxetine; Prozac; nonselective serotonin reup-
  take inhibitors: venlafaxine, Effexor)
Antihistamines
Antihypertensive drugs
Antiparkinson drugs
Barbiturates
Cocaine
Cold remedies and antiallergy medications:
Over-the-counter (OTC) medications containing pseu-
  doephedrine: Actifed, Sudafed, Contac, CoTylenol,
  Dimetapp, Vicks Formula products, Sine-tab, Sine-Aid, Tylenol
  Maximum Strength Sinus Medication
OTC medications containing phenylephrine: Dimetane
  Decongestant, Dristan Advanced formula, Neosynephrine,
  Nostril, Vicks Sinex, Robitussin Night Relief
OTC medications containing phenylpropanolamine: Coricidin,
  Dimetapp, Dimetane-DC cough, Vicks Formula-44
  Decongestant Cough mixture, CoTylenol, Acutrim, Dexatrim,
  Allerest, Alka-Seltzer Plus Cold Medicine, Sine-Off, Triaminic
MAO (another MAO, selegiline)
meperidine (Demerol)
metrizamide (Amipaque)
Narcotics

Interventions

1. Periodically evaluate the client's risk for suicide.

2. Assess the suicide potential if the client suddenly appears in a better mood.

3. Implement suicide precautions, including a written contract with the client, to focus on safety measures.

4. If in an inpatient psychiatric setting, check the client's condition every 15 minutes. Be alert to potentially lethal items, administer medications in liquid or injectable form, and check packages brought to the client; if in a nonpsychiatric (medical-surgical, long-term care, subacute care) unit, consult with a psychiatric clinical nurse specialist and employ all of the safety precautions listed above.

Rationales

1. Suicide methods vary with the seriousness of the intent; for example, taking an overdose of medication near the presence of others is a less lethal attempt than driving a car into a highway barrier at high speed. Suicide clues include making vague references to others as being "better off without me," giving away objects, feelings of hopelessness, withdrawn behavior, and impulsive self-harming actions.

2. A depressed client may be at greater risk for suicide when the depression begins to lift because there is more energy to carry out the self-destructive activity.

3. A written contract with the client can represent concrete commitments to self-preservation.

4. Suicidal clients typically are hospitalized when they are no longer capable of maintaining their own safety. During the hospital stay, the nurse is responsible for ensuring the client's safety.

NURSING DIAGNOSIS

Decisional conflict related to an inability to concentrate and a need for perfection

Nursing priority

Help the client recognize and use the ability to make logical decisions.

Patient outcome criteria

As the treatment progresses, the client, family, or both should be able to:
• demonstrate decision-making ability
• report satisfaction with their decisions
• acknowledge feelings of anxiety and emotional upheaval related to decision making
• report decrease in the level of anxiety and emotional upheaval related to decision making.

Interventions

1. Assess the client's impairment level.

2. Help the client to identify one decision that has to be made.

3. Help the client develop and rehearse problem-solving skills.

4. Implement safe, structured activities involving limited demands on the client such as occupational therapy.

Rationales

1. The nurse must determine the degree of impairment before planning appropriate interventions.

2. Focusing on one decision at a time can decrease the client's feelings of being overwhelmed and helpless.

3. Developing new skills presents the client with alternative behavior and can help point out the inadequacies of old behaviors.

4. Directed activities can facilitate initial decision-making as the client develops these skills. Such activities increase self-confidence and self-esteem.

Mood disorders

5. Encourage the client to delay making major life decisions until the depressive disorder has improved. Help the client to set reasonable time tables for such decisions.

5. Making rational major life decisions requires optimal psychophysiologic functioning.

NURSING DIAGNOSIS

Diversional activity deficit related to inability to be gratified because of overwhelming depressive feelings

Nursing priority

Promote the client's engagement in satisfying diversional activities within the scope of any functional status limitations.

Patient outcome criterion

As the treatment progresses, the client, family, or both should be able to:
• engage in satisfying activities within their functional status limitations.

Interventions

1. Determine the client's ability and interest to participate in available activities such as helping to plan a unit party.

2. Motivate the client to participate in activities by jointly selecting personally meaningful activities that provide immediate gratification and ensure success.

3. Encourage the client to assist in scheduling required as well as optional activities. Encourage the client to gradually assume more responsibility for the daily schedule.

4. Do not make changes in the daily schedule without first conferring and negotiating with the client.

Rationales

1. A severely depressed or physically impaired client may not have the psychic or physical energy to initiate and participate in activities.

2. Helping the client to select and participate in such activities can decrease feelings of inadequacy and incompetence.

3. Client involvement reestablishes feelings of control and self-reliance.

4. The nurse and other staff members must adhere to their commitments and thereby serve as role models for responsible behavior.

DISCHARGE CRITERIA

Nursing documentation indicates that the client:
• no longer indulges in suicidal ideation or self-harm behaviors
• has demonstrated improved coping mechanisms, relaxation techniques, and direct communication skills
• has demonstrated a willingness to enlist family involvement in ongoing treatment
• is aware of available support resources
• understands the potential adverse effects associated with drug therapy, electroconvulsive therapy, phototherapy, and sleep deprivation therapy.
Nursing documentation also indicates that the family:
• has demonstrated a willingness to involve themselves in the client's treatment

• has been referred to the appropriate group or family support resources in the community
• understands when, how, and why to contact the health care provider in an emergency.

SELECTED REFERENCES

Akiskal, H.S., and Cassano, G.B. *Dysthymia and the Spectrum of Chronic Depressions.* New York: Guilford Press, 1997.
American Psychiatric Association. *Practice Guidelines.* Washington, D.C.: American Psychiatric Association, 1996.
Boyd, M.A., and Nihart, M.A. *Psychiatric Nursing: Contemporary Practice.* Philadelphia: Lippincott-Raven Pubs., 1998.
Diagnostic and Statistical Manual of Mental Disorders, 4th ed. Washington, D.C.: American Psychiatric Association, 1994.
Fava, M., and Rosenbaum, M.A. "Treatment-Emergent Side Effects of the Newer Antidepressants," *Psychiatric Clinics of North America* 3:13-29, 1996.

Krupnick, J.L., et al. "The Role of the Therapeutic Alliance in Psychotherapy Outcome: Findings in the National Institute of Mental Health Treatment of Depression." Collaborative Research Program. *Journal of Consulting and Clinical Psychology* 64(3):532-39, 1996.

Nathan, P.E., and Gorman, J.M. *A Guide to Treatments that Work.* New York: Oxford University Press, 1998.

Pollack, M.H., et al., eds. *Challenges in Clinical Practice: Pharmacologic and Psychosocial Strategies.* New York: Guilford Press, 1996.

Shuchter, S.R., et al. *Biologically Informed Psychotherapy for Depression.* New York: Guilford Press, 1996.

Thompson, L.W. "Cognitive-Behavioral Therapy and Treatment for Late-Life Depression," *Journal of Clinical Psychiatry* 57(supplement 5):29-37, 1996.

Varcarolis, E.M. *Foundations of Psychiatric-Mental Health Nursing,* 3rd ed. Philadelphia: W.B. Saunders Co., 1998.

Winokur, G. *The Natural History of Mania, Depression and Schizophrenia.* Washington, D.C.: American Psychiatric Association, 1996.

Worthington, J., et al. "Consumption of Alcohol, Nicotine, and Caffeine among Depressed Outpatients: Relationship with Response to Treatment," *Psychosomatics* 37(6):518-22, 1996.

Yudofsky, S.C., and Hales, R.E. *Textbook of Neuropsychiatry.* Washington, D.C.: American Psychiatric Association, 1997.

Mood disorders

Organic-related mood disorders

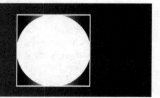

DSM-IV classifications

293.83 Mood disorder due to a general medical condition

292.84 Substance-induced mood disorder (specify type of substance)
Cocaine-induced mood disorder
Hallucinogen-induced mood disorder
Inhalant-induced mood disorder
Phencyclidine-induced mood disorder
Sedative-hypnotic or anxiolytic-induced mood disorder

291.8 Alcohol-induced mood disorder

INTRODUCTION

Description

Mood disorder due to a general medical condition is often referred to as *secondary depression* or *secondary mania* because these disorders are not primary psychiatric disorders. In this disorder, clinically significant depression or mania are caused by the direct physiologic effects of one or more general medical conditions.

Secondary depression presents as depressed mood accompanied by vegetative symptoms. The individual manifests depressed, irritable, or dysphoric mood, along with loss of interest and appetite and sleep disturbances. An individual with secondary mania has an elated, expansive, or euphoric mood that is accompanied by actions that increase the risk of exacerbating the individual's medical condition.

The age and mode of onset are determined by the underlying disease and the progression of that condition. The history, physical assessment, and laboratory findings must provide evidence that the depression or mania is the direct physiologic consequence of a general medical condition.

Substance-induced mood disorder is characterized by symptoms of depression or mania that are caused by the direct physiologic effects of a substance, such as prescribed medications, over-the-counter (OTC) medications, or illicit substances. The clinical presentation depends on the effects of the substance and the context (intoxication or withdrawal) in which the signs and symptoms occur. A variety of medications have been implicated.

Etiology and precipitating factors

The etiologic factors of secondary depression and secondary mania are summarized in the charts related to underlying medical conditions and medications or illicit drugs. (See *Disorders that cause depression*, *Drugs that cause depression,* page 84, and *Disorders and drugs that cause mania*, page 85, for more details.)

Potential complications

An undiagnosed, untreated, or incorrectly treated underlying medical condition can lead to further psychophysiologic deterioration, leading to increased fatigue and exhaustion. This could lead to emergency hospitalization if the individual is being treated in the home care environment, or transfer to a medical or critical care environment. Additionally, the individual might become agitated or violent, or successfully commit suicide or homicide.

ASSESSMENT GUIDELINES

Nursing history (functional health pattern findings)

Health perception–health management pattern

With depression
- Concern over somatic complaints
- Increased irritability
- Trouble following treatment regimen

With mania
- Denial of feeling ill
- Euphoria
- Overconfidence in managing health care issues

Nutritional-metabolic pattern

With depression
- Appetite decreased or increased
- Weight loss or gain

With mania
- Appetite loss
- Hyperphagia (with steroid use)
- Inadequate or irregular food and fluid intake
- Short attention span during meals
- Weight loss

Elimination pattern

With depression
- Constipation
- Decreased motility

Disorders that cause depression

Cardiovascular-pulmonary disorders
• Arrhythmias (especially life-threatening ventricular tachycardia)
• Chronic obstructive pulmonary disease (End-stage lung disease)
• Heart failure (End-stage heart disease)
• Myocardial infarction

Endocrine disorders
• Adrenal insufficiency
• Cushing's disease
• Diabetes
• Hyperparathyroidism or hypoparathyroidism
• Hyperprolactinemia
• Hypothyroidism or hyperthyroidism
• Menopause

Gastrointestinal disorders
• Chronic abdominal pain
• Colitis
• Islet cell adenoma
• Hepatitis

Infectious and inflammatory disorders
• Acquired immunodeficiency syndrome
• Chronic fatigue syndrome
• Mononucleosis
• Pneumonia (bacterial and viral)
• Rheumatoid arthritis
• Sjögren's arteritis
• Systemic lupus erythematosus
• Temporal arteritis
• Tuberculosis

Metabolic disorders
• Electrolyte imbalance
• Gout
• Hypercalcemia
• Pernicious anemia
• Porphyria
• Uremia (and other renal diseases)

Neurologic disorders
• Cerebrovascular disease
• Chronic pain
• Central nervous system tumors
• Dementias (including Alzheimer's disease)
• Hydrocephalus
• Migraine headache
• Multiple sclerosis
• Narcolepsy
• Parkinson's disease
• Progressive supranuclear palsy
• Seizure disorders
• Sleep apnea

Nutritional disorders
• Dehydration
• Iron deficiency
• Obesity
• Vitamin deficiencies (Vitamin B_{12}, vitamin C, folate, niacin)

Miscellaneous disorders
• Alcoholism
• Bilateral cataracts
• Cancer (especially pancreatic and other GI cancers)
• Hypertension
• Influenza

Mood disorders

With mania
• Abdominal distress (nausea, pain, vomiting)
• Excessive urination
• Increased perspiration
Activity-exercise pattern
With depression
• Anhedonia (no pleasure in activities)
• Decreased functional status
• Decreased libido
• Increased fatigue
• Inattention to personal hygiene
With mania
• Denial of fatigue

• Excessive time spent exercising
• Inattention to personal hygiene
• Psychomotor agitation
• Restlessness, pacing
Sleep-rest pattern
With depression
• Difficulty falling asleep
• Drug or alcohol use to induce sleep
• Early morning awakening
• Hypersomnia
With mania
• Decreased need for sleep
• Drug or alcohol use to induce sleep

Drugs that cause depression

Analgesics
- ibuprofen
- indomethacin
- Opioids

Antibacterials and antifungals
- ampicillin
- cycloserine
- ethionamide
- griseofulvin
- metronidazole
- nitrofurantoin
- streptomycin
- sulfamethoxazole
- Sulfonamides
- Tetracyclines

Antihypertensives
- beta blockers: propranolol (Inderal)
- clonidine (Catapres)
- Digitalis glycosides
- guanethidine (Ismelin)
- hydralazine (Apresoline)
- lidocaine
- methyldopa (Aldomet)
- propranolol (Inderal)
- reserpine (Serpasil)

Antiparkinsonians
- amantadine
- levodopa

Cancer chemotherapeutics
- amphotericin B
- bleomycin
- interferon
- L-asparaginase

- procarbazine
- trimethoprim
- vinblastine, vincristine
- zidovudine

Hormones
- Contraceptives (oral)
- estrogen (Premarin)
- progesterone (Gesterol)

Psychoactives
- Antipsychotics (butyrophenones, phenothiazines, oxyindoles)
- bromocriptine
- carbamazepine (Tegretol)
- Sedative-hypnotics (barbiturates, benzodiazepines, chloral hydrate)

Steroids
- Corticosteroids (including corticotropin)
- dexamethasone (Decadron)
- prednisone

Stimulants
- Amphetamines (flenfluramine)
- cocaine
- methylphenidate (Ritalin)

Miscellaneous drugs
- acetazolamide
- choline
- cimetidine (Tagamet)
- cyproheptadine
- diphenoxylate
- disulfiram
- methylsergide

- Nightmares
- Sleep disturbance
- Vivid, colorful dreams (with steroid use)

Cognitive-perceptual pattern

With depression
- Difficulty concentrating
- Difficulty making decisions
- Distorted perceptions (everyone hates me)
- Impoverished thinking
- Ruminating thoughts

With mania
- Confusion
- Decreased short-term memory
- Difficulty concentrating
- Disorganized, incoherent, and accelerated speech
- Tendency to be easily distracted
- Grandiose, unrealistic ideas
- Illusions, hallucinations
- Poor impulse control
- Poor judgment

Disorders and drugs that cause mania

Endocrine disorders
- Cushing's syndrome
- Hyperthyroidism

Immune-mediated disorders
- Systemic lupus erythematosus

Infectious disorders
- Acquired immunodeficiency syndrome
- Neurosyphilis

Metabolic disorders
- Hepatic encephalopathy

Neurologic disorders
- Epilepsy
- Fahr's disease

- Multiple sclerosis
- Neoplasms (central nervous system)
- Sydenham's chorea
- Trauma
- Wilson's disease

Pharmacologic agents
- Anabolic steroids
- bromocriptine
- Bromides
- chloroquine
- Corticosteroids
- isoniazid
- procarbazine

Self-perception–self-concept pattern
With depression
- Feelings of inadequacy or guilt
- Increased irritability
- Low self-esteem

With mania
- Intolerance of criticism
- History of angry outbursts
- Perception of self as being omnipotent and indestructible

Role-relationship pattern
With depression
- Dependence on support systems
- Feelings of worthlessness
- Perception of self as a burden to others

With mania
- Grandiose delusions about special relationships with God or with political, religious, or entertainment figures
- Inappropriate enthusiasm during social interactions
- Isolated, stressful living circumstance
- Intrusive, demanding, or domineering behaviors

Sexual-reproductive pattern
With depression
- Decreased libido
- Difficulty with intimacy
- Fertility and reproductive disturbances
- Menstrual disturbances

With mania
- Concern about involvement in high-risk sexual behavior
- Disrupted relationships with spouse or significant other

Coping–stress tolerance pattern
With depression
- Consideration of suicide
- Difficulty coping
- Inability to reach reasonable solutions to problems
- Suicidal ideation, plan, and "practice"
- Suicide attempt

With mania
- Increased alcohol or drug use
- Exaggerated startle response (hypervigilance)
- Inability to identify what would be helpful
- Loss of control
- Several stressful events before symptom exacerbation

Value-belief pattern
With depression
- Feelings of hopelessness
- Feelings of powerlessness
- Inability to master illness and treatment regimen

With mania
- Exaggerated feelings of power
- Grandiose religious delusions
- Hopelessness about condition
- Inability to control illness or situation

Physical findings
Cardiovascular
- Chest discomfort, pain
- Elevated blood pressure

Respiratory
- Increased respiratory rate
- Increased sighing
- Shortness of breath

(Text continues on page 88.)

Mood disorders

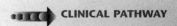

Mood disorders

	Day 1	Day 2
Clinical assessment	• Suicide risk • Multidisciplinary assessment initiated • Physical examination initiated • Initial family meeting scheduled • Appetite deficit • Sleep deficit • Activities of daily living (ADLs) deficit	• Suicide risk • Assessments completed: – care level – nursing – multidisciplinary –physical examination –psychiatric
Tests	• SMA-6, complete blood count (CBC), liver function tests (LFT) • Urinalysis and urine toxocology (if applicable • Thyroid-stimulating hormone (TSH) • Other: _____	• Laboratory results: Normal Abnormal – SMA-6, CBC, LFT? __ __ – TSH __ __ – Other: _____ __ __
Treatments	• Initiate contact with outpatient • Orient to level system • Evaluate group appropriateness	• Increase participation in programs and groups • 1:1 support
Patient and family education and patient rights	• Orient to unit • Patient rights, consent, and confidentiality • Release of information • Relaxation techniques	• Patient discusses: – diagnosis – treatment options – discharge planning
Discharge planning	• Initiate discharge plan	• Home or resource assessment • Discharge plan presented to team, patient, and significant other • Liaison with outpatient care providers
Psychosocial supports	• Psychosocial assessment • Assessment of stressors • Assessment of coping skills • Discuss outside resources patient can utilize when feeling suicidal	• Assessment of illness progression
Medications	• Assessment of: – current medications – symptoms – history • Continue or start medication and teaching	• Continue teaching related to medication and its adverse effects
Nutrition, hydration, and elimination	• Assess bowel and bladder functions • Monitor intake t.i.d. • Regular diet • Nutritional assessment • Vital signs • Weight	• Assess bowel and bladder functions • Monitor intake t.i.d. • Regular diet • Nutritional assessment • Vital signs • Weight
Activity	• Level 2	• Assess for level advance • Full engagement in unit activities

Day 3	Day 4 (Discharge)	Discharge outcomes

• Suicide risk
• Assessments completed:
  – social work
  – occupation therapy
	• Suicide risk
	• Biopsychological summary completed
	• Adequate sleep, appetite, and ADLs
		• Assessment for discharge readiness:
		  – affect appropriate
		  – mood stabilized
		  – no evidence of thought disorder
		  – denies suicidal ideation

• As indicated	• As indicated	• Laboratory values within normal limits
• Continue to increase participation in programs and groups	• Outpatient transition begun	• Verbalizes importance of compliance with outpatient follow-up
• Teaching protocol completed	• Continue to reinforce teaching	• Identifies reportable signs and symptoms of relapse • Verbalizes understanding of teaching
• Continue to discuss and finalize discharge plans	• Continue to discuss and initialize discharge plans	• Patient or family verbalize discharge plan • Patient is discharged • Follow-up referrals
• Focus on post-hospital plans and support system	• Engage post-hospital support system	• Patient sets realistic goals and demonstrates willing attempt to reach them • Identifies resources outside of the hospital to utilize when feeling depressed or suicidal
• Continue teaching related to medication and its adverse effects • Monitor response to medication	• Continue teaching related to medication • Monitor response to medication	• Discharge preparation • Prescriptions • Instructions • Verbalizes knowledge of schedule, desired effects, and adverse effects for each medication
• Assess bowel and bladder functions • Monitor intake t.i.d. • Regular diet • Nutritional assessment • Vital signs • Weight	• Assess bowel and bladder functions • Monitor intake t.i.d. • Regular diet • Nutritional assessment • Vital signs • Weight	• Verbalizes relevant dietary restrictions • Adequate intake • Demonstrates willingness to interact with others around treatment issues
• Assess for level advance	• Assess for level advance	

Adapted with permission from Danbury (Conn.) Hospital

Mood disorders

- Wheezing
Gastrointestinal
- Abdominal distress
- Anorexia or hyperphagia
- Conception
- Diarrhea
- Dry mouth
- Pain
- Weight gain or loss
Musculoskeletal
- Fatigue
- Lethargy
- Muscle tension, aches, pains
Neurologic
- Agitation
- Memory difficulties
- Restlessness
- Sleep disturbances

- Slowed thinking
Psychological
- Anhedonia
- Crying or tearfulness
- Delusions
- Difficulty concentrating
- Excessive concern with physical health
- Feelings of being a burden
- Feelings of inadequacy
- Feelings of worthlessness, shame, or guilt
- Indecisiveness
- Loss of interest in the world or environment
- Preoccupation with certain thoughts
- Social withdrawal
- Suicidal thoughts
- Violence (homicidal thoughts, violence against property, animals, or caregivers)

NURSING DIAGNOSIS

Sleep pattern disturbance related to effects of medical condition, medical treatments, or medications or substances

Nursing priority

Help the client reestablish a regular and restful sleep pattern.

Patient outcome criteria

As the treatment progress, the client, family, or both should be able to:
- report an increase in the amount of hours of sleep
- demonstrate improved sleep pattern
- report more uninterrupted sleep time (less sleep time awakenings)
- report feeling refreshed and restored after sleep cycle.

Interventions

1. Identify the sleep pattern disturbance and assess the client's usual sleep rituals.

2. Establish a distraction-free sleep environment.

3. Encourage the client to restrict stimulant and depressant intake before bedtime.

Rationales

1. Identifying a client's usual sleep rituals can assist in determining the causative factors and selection of focused interventions to manage sleep disturbances. For example, the client may be taking medications that are stimulating them in the evening or awakening them to urinate at night.

2. A quiet, comfortable, and safe environment induces relaxation and decreases the client's attention to stimuli.

3. Stimulants (such as caffeine, nicotine, psychostimulants, some selective serotonin reuptake inhibitors [SSRIs]) and depressants (such as alcohol) interfere with the normal sleep cycle and can exaggerate a preexisting one.

4. Establish a daily exercise routine (within functional limitations) and avoid exercise 2 hours before bedtime. Teach the client specific sleep hygiene methods to enhance their sleep pattern.

5. Reschedule medications that interfere with sleep cycle (such as activating antidepressants, steroids, psychostimulants, and diuretics) for the early part of the day.

6. Teach the client about sedative-hypnotic medications that might be added to their medication regimen to promote and reestablish their sleep pattern.

4. Regular, light to moderate exercise (within the individual's functional limitations) increases body fatigue and the desire to rest and sleep without overstimulating the client before going to bed.

5. Rescheduling the timing of medications and treatments can decrease the stimulating effects or awakenings that the medication can produce. Often a simple rescheduling of medications can reduce the activating effects of psychostimulants or SSRIs or the need to get up to urinate in the middle of the night.

6. Sedative-hypnotic medications can interfere with the non-rapid eye movement (NREM) part of the sleep cycle as well as the rapid eye movement (REM) part of the sleep cycle and alter the quality of the sleep. A significant problem of rebound insomnia, characterized by intense dreaming, nightmares, and increased sleep disruption, can occur. Also, these medications can further cloud the assessment of secondary mania and depression and need to be used cautiously.

NURSING DIAGNOSIS

Sensory-perceptual alterations related to decreased ability to concentrate, racing thoughts, distractibility, flight of ideas, hallucinations, delusions, sleep deprivations, or depression

Nursing priority

Orient the client to reality, maintain a safe environment for the client and others in their proximity, and encourage realistic, focused, and goal-directed thinking.

Patient outcome criteria

As the treatment progresses, the client, family, or both should be able to:
• demonstrate increasing mood stability
• report feeling more focused
• report improved concentration
• demonstrate less distractibility.

Interventions

1. Gently orient the client to reality and his current situation (home, hospital, office of primary provider).

2. Provide the client with a calm environment with decreased stimulation.

3. Collaborate with the primary care provider and other treating health care providers to determine the effects of the client's medical condition or medications on his behavior and mental well-being.

Rationales

1. Frequently and gently orienting and reassuring the client helps to reduce potential escalation of agitation resulting from confused thoughts.

2. An environment free from distractions and high levels of stimulation can reduce the potential for agitation and hyperactivity.

3. Effective and focused treatment of the individual with a secondary mania or depression must begin with collaboration from all the prescribing and treating health care providers. This collaboration will provide the most complete view of the individual to help determine if this is a primary disorder (major depression) or truly a secondary disorder due to a medical or substance-induced condition.

Mood disorders

4. Administer prescribed psychotropic medications and monitor client response.

4. Monitoring the effects of prescribed medications is imperative to ensure that the individual is responding to the treatment and not worsening. Also, the client and family must have an understanding of the goal of medication, especially if medications caused the behavioral health problem.

5. Teach the client and family about the physical basis for their behavioral changes and about the treatment plan and expected outcomes.

5. Individuals who have an understanding of their illness and expected outcomes can identify a relapse situation earlier and seek treatment sooner. Psychoeducation for both the client and family can reduce their fears that they or the client is "going crazy" and is going to be considered mentally ill or unbalanced.

Nursing diagnosis

Powerlessness related to feelings of hopelessness and perceived lack of control over the client's life due to a medical condition, medical treatments, or both

Nursing priority

Assist the client to regain a sense of self-control and mastery related to his medical condition and corresponding treatment regimen.

Patient outcome criteria

As the treatment progresses, the client, family, or both will be able to:
• verbalize realistic, goal-directed, and focused thinking
• demonstrate ability to master illness and corresponding treatments.

Interventions

1. Discuss with the client early signs and symptoms, such as significant changes in activity level, sleep, or appetite or use of alcohol, nicotine, or other substances.

2. Explore the client's feelings of hopelessness and identify misperceptions, distortions, and irrational thoughts

3. Collaborate with the client to establish realistic goals for the present and future.

4. Recommend and refer the client and family to resources to assist them in achieving their goals.

Rationales

1. Informing the client and family of the early symptoms of the behavioral manifestations and developing concrete steps to manage their recurrence can help avoid future hospitalization or exacerbation of underlying medical conditions.

2. This helps the client to differentiate between irrational and real concerns. It also enables the client to examine accuracy of perceptions and helps to validate his concerns.

3. Setting realistic goals that are attainable can increase the client's sense of self-control and enhance his feelings of mastery over his illness. It also helps him become future-oriented and have something on which to focus in his future.

4. Both the family and client will benefit from social support in the community that can help decrease their sense of isolation (for example, "I am the only one who has ever had this problem with this medication or treatment").

DISCHARGE CRITERIA

Nursing documentation indicates that the client:
• has demonstrated stable mood, thoughts and perceptions, and behavior
• recognizes early signs and symptoms of relapse
• implements a concrete plan to manage symptoms
• understands the need for treatment and follow-up with primary care provider and psychiatric services
• has made a connection with community resources
• has scheduled necessary follow-up appointments
• maintains a more regular sleep cycle pattern
• maintains an improved nutritional status.
Nursing documentation also indicates that the family:
• has been referred to appropriate community resources
• understands the potential problems that can develop during the initial recovery phase.

SELECTED REFERENCES

Barry, P.D. *Psychosocial Nursing: Care of Physically Ill Patients and Their Families.* Philadelphia: Lippincott-Raven Pubs., 1996.

Boyd, M.A., and Nihart, M.A. *Psychiatric Nursing: Contemporary Practice.* Philadelphia: Lippincott-Raven Pubs., 1998.

Diagnostic and Statistical Manual of Mental Disorders 4th ed. Washington, D.C.: American Psychiatric Association, 1994.

Lang, D., and Territo, J. *Coping with Lyme Disease,* 2nd ed. New York: Henry Holt and Company, 1997.

Lishman, W.A. *Organic Psychiatry: The Psychological Consequences of Cerebral Disease,* 3rd ed. London: Blackwell Science, 1998.

McEnamy, G.W., et al. "Depression and HIV: A Nursing Perspective on a Complex Relationship," *Nursing Clinics of North America* 31:57, 1996.

Moore, D.P., and Jefferson, J.W. *Handbook of Medical Psychiatry.* St. Louis: Mosby–Year Book, Inc., 1996.

Moran, M.G. "Psychiatric Aspects of Rheumatology," *Psychiatric Clinics of North America* 19(3):575-87, 1996.

Morris, N.J. "Depression and HIV Disease: A Critical Review," *Journal of American Psychiatric Nurses Association* 2:154, 1996.

Reichman, W.E., and Katz, P.R. *Psychiatric Care in the Nursing Home.* New York: Oxford University Press, 1996.

Shapiro, M. "Chronic Fatigue Syndrome," *Psychiatric Clinics of North America* 19(3):549-73, 1996.

Shapiro, P. "Psychiatric Aspects of Cardiovascular Disease," *Psychiatric Clinics of North America* 19(3):613-29, 1996.

Stuart, G.W., and Laraia, M. *Principles and Practice of Psychiatric Nursing.* St. Louis: Mosby–Year Book, Inc., 1998.

Varcarolis, E.M. *Foundations of Psychiatric Mental Health Nursing,* 3rd ed. Philadelphia: W.B. Saunders Co., 1998.

Wyszynski, A.A., and Wyszynski, B. *A Case Approach to Medical-Psychiatric Practice.* Washington, D.C.: American Psychiatric Association, 1996.

Zukerman, E., and Inglefinger, J.R. *Coping with Prednisone and Other Cortisone-Related Medications.* New York: St. Martin's Press, 1997.

Mood disorders

Part 4

Psychotic disorders

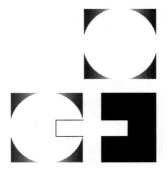

Schizophrenic disorders

DSM-IV classifications

295.10	Schizophrenia, disorganized type
295.20	Schizophrenia, catatonic type
295.30	Schizophrenia, paranoid type
295.60	Schizophrenia, residual type
295.90	Schizophrenia, undifferentiated type

INTRODUCTION

Description

Schizophrenia is a severe, persistent mental disorder that consists of two different categories of symptoms. The symptoms present for at least 1 month but usually persist for at least 6 months and are classified as positive and negative. (See *Positive and negative symptoms of schizophrenia.*) Positive symptoms reflect an excess of normal function, such as bizarre thinking, while negative symptoms reflect a lessening or loss of normal function, such as restricted or flattening in the range and intensity of emotion, thought, and speech.

Several subtypes of schizophrenia have been identified and are recognized by their clinical presentation. The subtypes include catatonic, disorganized, paranoid, undifferentiated, and residual. (See *Diagnostic characteristics of schizophrenia subtypes.*) These subtypes have some implications for the clinical course and the response to treatment. The clinical course of schizophrenia is variable due to the complex interactions of positive and negative symptoms from one individual to the next and even from one episode to the next. Onset usu-ally occurs in late adolescence and early adulthood. Many individuals are diagnosed with late-onset schizophrenia after age 45. Estimates of prevalence of schizophrenia in the general population range from 0.5% to 1%, to as high as 2%.

Schizophrenia is a clinically complex disorder for several reasons. The symptoms can combine in several different constellations, and an individual's symptoms differ from another's and, sometimes, from one episode to the next. The illness seems to have three distinct phases, including:

Phase 1. Initial diagnosis and early schizophrenia

Phase 2. Relative calm between episodes of overt signs and symptoms

Phase 3. Relapse, which includes those recurring periods of exacerbation or relapse.

Etiology and precipitating factors

Current biological research supports a link between one or more likely several genes and schizophrenic disorders. Generally, researchers believe that individuals inherit a predisposition to the disorder, which may be exacerbated by environmental factors. First-degree relatives of schizophrenics are 10 times more likely to develop a form of the disorder than the general population.

Some workers have suggested that infectious agents or autoimmune responses may contribute to developing schizophrenia. Possible causative agents include active infections, viral proteins that interfere with brain function, reactivation of latent viruses, retroviral sequences

Positive and negative symptoms of schizophrenia

Positive symptoms

Positive symptoms appear early in the first phase of the illness. These symptoms typically "get attention" and often precipitate a hospitalization and usually respond to antipsychotic medication.

- Catatonic behavior
- Delusions
- Disorganized or bizarre thinking
- Hallucinations
- Inappropriate affect
- Thought disorder

Negative symptoms

Negative symptoms develop over a period of time and interfere with the individual's adjustment and ability to survive and think.

- Anhedonia (loss of pleasure)
- Avolition (apathy)
- Blunted affect
- Loss of interest
- Loss of motivation
- Poor attention and concentration
- Poor attention to social tasks
- Poverty of speech

Diagnostic characteristics of schizophrenia subtypes

Catatonic type: *DSM-IV* 295.20
Echolalia
Echopraxia
Excessive purposeless motor activity
Extreme negativism
Motor immobility or stupor
Posturing, stereotypic movements, prominent mannerisms, or prominent grimacing
Resistance toward instructions

Disorganized type: *DSM-IV* 295.10
Disorganized behavior
Disorganized thought
Flat affect
Inappropriate affect
Chronic and disabling course
Medication management may be only moderately effective

Paranoid type: *DSM-IV* 295.30
Auditory hallucinations
Negative symptoms are less severe (blunted affect)
Preoccupied with delusions
Medication management may significantly reduce symptoms

Residual type: *DSM-IV* 295.60
Absence of prominent delusions
Absence of disorganized speech or grossly disorganized or catatonic behavior
Negative symptoms persist or two or more positive symptoms are present

Undifferentiated type: *DSM-IV* 295.90
Characteristic symptoms are present, but does not meet criteria of other subtypes

---

integrated in host cell DNA, and autoimmune responses against central nervous system (CNS) tissue. There is little evidence to support these ideas at present.

Neuroanatomic studies of brain tissue from individuals who had schizophrenia have shown three consistent structural changes: enlarged lateral ventricles, enlarged third ventricles, and enlarged sulci. Ventricular changes are indicative of brain atrophy, which is localized in the amygdala, hippocampus and parahippocampal gyrus. Enlarged sulci suggest cortical loss, particularly in the frontal lobe. Such neuroanatomic changes have diagnostic as well as treatment implications. There is evidence that individuals with enlarged ventricles have had a prominent prodromal period, had increased cognitive impairment, and were less responsive to treatment.

The dopamine hypothesis of schizophrenia was developed from observations that antipsychotic medications act primarily by blocking postsynaptic dopamine receptors in the brain. The dopamine hypothesis continues to receive intense research attention with further understanding of dopaminergic function. A recent change in the dopamine hypothesis suggests that there is relative hypodopaminergic function in the limbic system, prefrontal and neocortex. This evolution of the dopamine hypothesis is supported by positron emission tomography studies demonstrating hypofrontality, a reduced cerebral blood flow and glucose metabolism in the prefrontal cortex of persons with schizophrenia. The next few years of neurobiological research into the understanding and treatment of schizophrenia are very

promising and offer hope to those clients and families experiencing this often devastating, chronic mental illness.

Potential complications
If left untreated, schizophrenia can lead to aggressive, violent behavior toward the self or others as well as to catatonic behavior, profound depression, and suicide. Although uncommon, neuroleptic malignant syndrome, a severe and life-threatening condition, can develop and must be identified in the early stage. Tardive dyskinesia can develop from chronic use of antipsychotic agents, and the client must be regularly assessed for this syndrome using an objective rating tool. (See "Assessment of extrapyramidal effects," page 278.) Also, the individual's use of self-medication with alcohol or drugs rather than taking his prescribed medications may cause complications.

ASSESSMENT GUIDELINES

Nursing history (functional health pattern findings)
Health perception–health management pattern
• Presence or severity of symptoms
• Need for treatment
• Poor physical health secondary to psychotic symptoms and disorganized thoughts
• Weight loss
• Poor hygiene and grooming

Nutritional-metabolic pattern
• Fear that food is being tampered with

Elimination pattern
• Constipation secondary to poor nutritional status or medication use

Activity-exercise pattern
• Pacing to relieve anxiety
• Hypervigilance
• Decreased motivation and interest in activities
• Psychomotor retardation
• Restlessness secondary to adverse effects of medication or psychotic symptoms
• Disorganized or bizarre behavior and posturing

Sleep-rest pattern
• Insomnia secondary to hallucinations or delusions
• Sedation secondary to medication

Cognitive-perceptual pattern
• Hallucinations
• Delusions
• Decreased attention span
• Difficulty concentrating
• Disturbed thought processes (manifested as blocking, loose associations, flight of ideas, tangentiality, or ideas of reference)
• Lack of insight or denial of illness

Self-perception–self-concept pattern
• Low or exaggerated self-esteem
• Feelings of persecution

Role-relationship pattern
• Disturbed interpersonal relationships
• Inability to assume responsibilities for parenting, employment, or relationships
• Inability to trust others
• Feelings of loneliness

Sexual-reproductive pattern
• Sexual dysfunction secondary to medication effects

Coping–stress tolerance pattern
• Symptom escalation following exposure to stressors

Value-belief pattern
• Paranoia or grandiose delusions
• Delusions of possessing special powers or a different identity
• Overreliance on or identification with religion or religious figures

Physical findings

Cardiovascular
• Excessive perspiration
• Increased heart rate
• Increased or decreased blood pressure
• Orthostatic changes secondary to psychotropic medications

Gastrointestinal
• Constipation secondary to psychotropic medications
• Dry mouth secondary to psychotropic medications

Genitourinary
• Amenorrhea
• Difficulty achieving or maintaining erection
• Retarded ejaculation
• Diminished sex drive

Musculoskeletal
• Body posture alterations
• Balance disturbance
• Gait disturbances
• Muscle tension
• Restlessness related to anticholineigic medications

Neurologic
• Catatonia
• Dilated pupils
• Hyperreflexia
• Parkinsonian movements (such as tremors and pill-rolling finger movements)
• Sensory abnormalities (such as hyperesthesia, hypoesthesia, or paresthesia)
• Sleep disturbances (such as inability to sleep or difficulty staying asleep)

Psychological
• Ambivalence
• Anger
• Anxiety
• Apathy
• Argumentativeness
• Delusions
• Emotional lability
• Lack of facial expression
• Hallucinations
• Paranoia

NURSING DIAGNOSIS

Altered thought processes related to psychosis and evidenced by disruptions in thought flow, form, or content

Nursing priority

Help the client differentiate between delusions and reality.

Patient outcome criteria

As treatment progresses, the client, family, or both will be able to:
• demonstrate decreased suspiciousness
• verbalize or demonstrate improved reality orientation by recognizing and clarifying possible misinterpretations
• demonstrate an improved attention span and concentration ability.

Interventions

1. Provide the client with honest and consistent feedback.

2. Avoid challenging the content of the client's disturbed thoughts.

3. Focus interactions on the client's behavior.

4. Communicate with the client clearly, concisely, and honestly, avoiding slang and figures of speech.

5. Point out when you cannot understand the client's thoughts.

6. Maintain objectivity when listening to the client. Do not take personally any ethnic slurs or judgmental statements.

7. Be aware of the client's personal space, and use gestures and touch judiciously.

8. Administer medications as ordered and monitor the client's response.

9. Teach the client and family about the uses, actions, and adverse effects of any prescribed medication.

10. Do not minimize the client's subjective experience of an adverse reaction to a prescribed neuroleptic medication. (See "Assessment of extrapyramidal effects," page 278, and appendix D, Managing adverse effects of psychotropic medications, page 316.)

11. Teach the client and family how to recognize and cope with relapse symptoms, such as increased hallucinations and agitation.

Rationales

1. By being consistently honest, the nurse reinforces the client's orientation to reality and fosters trust.

2. The client believes that such thoughts are accurate. Challenging this perceived accuracy can only increase mistrust and conflict between the nurse and client.

3. By focusing on present behavior, the nurse minimizes the potential for conflict and misunderstanding.

4. Complex words and sentences as well as slang and idiomatic speech can increase client frustration and miscommunication. By speaking clearly, the nurse can prevent these problems and help the client to concentrate and communicate without anxiety.

5. Doing so demonstrates that the nurse is listening carefully and helps to establish trust between the nurse and client.

6. The client may frequently use these types of statements to create emotional and psychological barriers toward others because closeness increases anxiety. By not taking such statements personally, the nurse can gain the client's trust.

7. Invading the client's personal space can increase anxiety. The anxious client may misinterpret gestures as aggressive moves.

8. Medication can reduce psychotic symptoms and promote more organized thought processes.

9. Knowing about the prescribed medication and how to manage adverse reactions enhances compliance.

10. Acknowledging the potentially distressing adverse reactions to neuroleptic medications can foster client trust and compliance. Adverse reactions include drowsiness or sedation, dry mouth, blurred vision, photosensitivity (especially with phenothiazines), constipation or urine retention, orthostatic hypotension, general hypotension, weight gain, and altered sexual functioning. Extrapyramidal effects include parkinsonian symptoms, restlessness, acute muscle spasms, and tardive dyskinesia symptoms (including tongue protrusion, lip smacking, and grimacing).

11. Providing the client and family with effective coping strategies will increase their sense of control in coping with the disorder.

NURSING DIAGNOSIS

Altered thought processes related to psychosis-induced hallucinations

Nursing priority

Orient the client to reality and help alleviate hallucinations.

Patient outcome criteria

As treatment progresses, the client, family, or both should be able to:
• report or demonstrate a decrease in hallucinations
• report improved ability to socialize and communicate
• report or demonstrate an improved judgment and insight.

Interventions

1. Observe the client for signs of hallucinations, such as a listening pose, laughing or talking to self, and halting in mid-sentence.

2. Ask if the client hears or sees things that others do not.

3. If possible, determine the content of hallucinations.

4. Assess the client's response to hallucinations.

5. Acknowledge the client's feelings about any disturbing hallucinations.

6. Provide reality-based, supportive feedback.

7. Monitor the client's responses to the environment and make any appropriate changes.

8. Provide appropriate measures to ensure client safety and explain to the client why you are doing so.

Rationales

1. Early recognition of hallucinations and subsequent intervention may help the nurse prevent an aggressive client response to command hallucinations.

2. By doing so, the nurse acknowledges the validity of the client's perceptions without challenging them and promotes trust.

3. Knowing the content of the hallucinations can help the nurse determine the level of observation required for client safety. A client who hears deprecatory or hostile voices may become increasingly agitated or violent. Command hallucinations commonly contain suicidal or violent directives, which the client may act on impulsively.

4. Hallucinations may frighten and confuse the client, who may consequently require closer supervision.

5. Supportive, empathetic responses foster trust and enhance the client's sense of safety and reality. Acknowledging the client's feelings also can help prevent unnecessary agitation.

6. Acknowledging the client's perceptions and feelings related to the hallucination can help the client begin to distinguish real from unreal. Supportive feedback could include statements such as "I know you see that, and it is scaring you. We will keep you safe."

7. An overresponsiveness to environmental stimuli can increase client misperceptions, thereby increasing anxiety and, consequently, hallucinations. Changes to the environment might include reducing visual and auditory stimuli. This could require time out of the environment in his room or a seclusion room or a walk in a quiet area of the unit.

8. Implementing and explaining safety measures can promote trust and decrease anxiety while increasing the client's sense of security.

9. During any interaction, encourage the client to focus on you and your voice.

9. Doing so can help the client to distinguish the real from the unreal. It also can help prevent misunderstandings between the nurse and client.

10. Administer antipsychotic medications as ordered and monitor the client's response.

10. Antipsychotics can decrease hallucinations, thereby alleviating the client's subjective discomfort and agitation.

11. Encourage the client to participate in recreational and diversionary activities.

11. Such activities can reduce the client's preoccupation with internal stimuli. They also provide opportunities for improving self-esteem and self-confidence.

12. Encourage the client to identify situations or experiences that increase or decrease hallucinations.

12. Understanding the relationship between anxiety-producing experiences and hallucinations can enhance the client's feelings of self-control. For example, the client can learn to avoid situations (sleep deprivation, illicit drug use) that are stimulating and promote hallucinations, thus enhancing self-control.

13. Help the client and family to assess their communication patterns and emotional styles and to identify those that might be related to symptom development.

13. Research shows a relationship between certain styles of emotional expression and symptom escalation. Identifying aggravating behaviors is necessary before adjustments in those behaviors can be made.

14. Provide opportunities for the client to learn adaptive social skills in a nonthreatening environment.

14. Learning new social skills can enhance the client's adjustment after discharge.

NURSING DIAGNOSIS

Risk for violence, directed at self or others, related to delusional thinking

Nursing priority

Ensure that the client does not harm self, others, or the environment while in the hospital.

Patient outcome criteria

As treatment progresses, the client, family, or both will be able to:
• remain injury-free from self-directed violence
• demonstrate a decrease in agitation, aggressive behavior, and violent outbursts
• remain in control and seek out assistance when experiencing increased feelings of wanting to destroy property, hurt self, or someone else.

Interventions

Agitation
Early interventions at the initial signs of agitation can prevent symptom escalation.

1. Monitor the client for behaviors that indicate increased anxiety. Assess the client using the Overt Agitation Severity Scale (OASS) to determine degree of agitation and response to intervention (see "Overt Agitation Severity Scale," page 293).

2. Collaborate with the client to identify anxious behaviors as well as their probable causes.

Rationales

1. Early intervention can help prevent escalating anxiety, which usually precedes agitation and aggressive behavior.

2. Involving the client in self-examination of behavior can increase the client's sense of self-control.

3. Inform the client of available alternatives for dealing with anxiety and agitation.

3. Alternatives such as moving to a less stimulating environment, engaging in diversionary activities, talking with the nurse, and taking prescribed medications can enable the client to channel energy in more adaptive ways. Anxiolytics can be effective at this time because they provide fast relief of anxiety symptoms. Neuroleptics take longer to produce therapeutic effects, although their sedative effects can be beneficial at this point.

4. In an accepting, nonthreatening manner, encourage the client to verbalize feelings and perceptions.

4. By encouraging the client to express unacceptable feelings, the nurse can help put those feelings into perspective.

5. Tell the client that you will help him maintain control and that you are aware of his concern about losing control.

5. By acknowledging the client's possible fear of losing control, the nurse provides reassurance and fosters trust.

6. In a supportive, nonjudgmental, yet clear and firm manner, set limits on the client's behavior.

6. Setting limits for behavior helps the client identify boundaries and provides structure.

7. Remove all other clients and unnecessary spectators from the environment.

7. The client is more likely to cooperate with the nurse without an audience.

Escalation
If the client does not respond to early interventions and the anxiety continues to escalate, the nurse must assume more control through focused interactions.

8. Speak in a quiet, slow, self-assured manner, using clear, concise language.

8. By speaking quietly and slowly, the nurse might prevent the interaction from escalating out of control. A self-assured manner communicates a sense of control to the client.

9. To prepare for possible continued escalation, form a care team and designate one member to maintain client interaction.

9. Planning ahead gives everyone involved a sense of control and ensures teamwork. Having only one person interact with the client prevents confusion and provides the client with a single external stimulus on which to focus.

10. Give the client focused, realistic options; however, be sure you know and distinguish for the client what is optional and what is not.

10. Providing options allows the client to maintain self-esteem and can foster a sense of self-control. For example, if you have decided that the client needs medication, this need is no longer an option. However, the client could choose the administration route. You might say, "You need medication. Would you prefer to have it by mouth or by injection?"

11. Follow through with the options you provide.

11. The client usually will respond positively to structure and a sense of control. This can make the situation safer and more predictable. For example, you might say to the client, "I am going to ask you to go to the seclusion room; you can walk with me, or we can take you there." If the client chooses not to walk, make sure you have enough help.

12. Provide the client with adequate interpersonal space, taking care not to enter that space without warning.

12. As anxiety and agitation increase, the client may feel the need for increased interpersonal space. If crowded or threatened, the client might assault someone.

13. Maintain eye contact, but do not stare; be aware of the client's position and posture.

13. The client might perceive staring as intrusive or challenging. If preparing to strike out, the client will glance quickly to check for a clear path. The client also may be scanning the environment for a weapon.

14. Ensure that only one person maintains verbal interaction with the client. Do not have anyone rush to or move suddenly toward the client.

14. Restricted verbal interaction can keep the client focused and promotes a sense of being cared for and supported.

Aggression
If escalation continues, the nurse must take control and make decisions for the safety of the client and others.

15. Make sure that all potential weapons and obstacles are removed from the environment.

15. Removing potential weapons decreases the chance of injury and communicates to the client that everyone will be safe.

16. Inform the care team of your plan, and define each member's responsibility.

16. Doing so fosters confidence among team members and helps to ensure effective teamwork.

17. Determine the need for external controls, including seclusion or restraints. Communicate your decisions to the client.

17. This communicates to the client that the nurse is in control.

18. Once you have initiated a plan, follow through with it.

18. Interrupting a plan can create confusion and increase anxiety for all involved. If the client perceives that the nurse or other care team members are not in control, anxiety may escalate to violence, resulting in injury.

19. When agitation decreases, establish with the client a behavioral contract that identifies specific behaviors that indicate regained self-control.

19. Such a contract provides both the staff and client with criteria that indicate the client is ready and able to maintain control and tolerate frustration.

Nursing diagnosis

Risk for activity intolerance related to adverse reactions to medications

Nursing priority

Establish an activity routine for the client.

Patient outcome criteria

As treatment progresses, the client, family, or both should be able to:
• demonstrate an improved functional status as the client acclimates to medication
• report decreased impact of adverse effects and use of medication management strategies to minimize the impact of adverse effects
• report and demonstrate participation in light exercise activity to enhance functional status.

Interventions

1. Assess the client's response to any prescribed antipsychotic. (See *Understanding neuroleptic malignant syndrome,* page 102.)

2. Teach the client and family about therapeutic effects of and adverse reactions to antipsychotic medications.

Rationales

1. Assessment data helps the nurse to plan and implement appropriate interventions.

2. Client and family knowledge of the prescribed medication helps to ensure compliance.

Psychotic disorders

Understanding neuroleptic malignant syndrome

Neuroleptic malignant syndrome is a potentially fatal, idiosyncratic reaction to the use of dopamine-blocking or dopamine-depleting drugs or to the withdrawal of dopamine agonists.

Symptoms	Complications	Treatment
Early • Fever • Mild to moderate rigidity *Middle* • Catatonia (mute to stupor) • Delirium • High fever (>102° F [38.9° C]) • Marked and generalized rigidity • Tremor (coarse) *Late* • Autonomic instability • Blood pressure labile • Diaphoresis • Tachycardia • Tachypnea • Chest wall rigidity • Increased creatine kinase level (> 15,000 U/L) • Increased white blood cell count (> 15,000 µl) • Increased lactate dehydrogenase, aspartate aminotransferase, alkaline phosphatase levels • Pallor	• Acute renal failure from myoglobinuria • Disseminated intravascular coagulation • Respiratory failure • Rhabdomyolysis	• Administer dantrolene, as ordered. Repeat if necessary. • Administer bromocriptine orally or via nasogastric tube, as ordered. • Use a cooling blanket for temperature reduction. • Provide hydration as needed. • Provide ventilatory support.

3. Encourage the client to report any adverse reactions to the prescribed antipsychotic medications.

4. Teach the client strategies that decrease adverse reactions to antipsychotic medications. Monitor for signs of orthostatic hypotension, including a drop in blood pressure with a position change, increased heart rate when arising from a prone or sitting position, dizziness, light-headedness, and falls.

5. Assess the client's ability to perform activities of daily living. Take into consideration their identified deficits in the following areas: cognitive, coping, psychophysiologic, and social skills. (See *Identifying deficits and impairments that promote vulnerability in a client with schizophrenia.*) Collaborate with the client to establish a daily routine within physical limitations.

3. By knowing the client's response to prescribed medications, the nurse can help promote optimal functioning.

4. Strategies, such as gradually increasing activity, rising slowly from a prone or sitting position, and dangling the feet while sitting, can help decrease the dizziness caused by orthostatic hypotension and prevent accidental falls.

5. A realistic daily routine can help the client overcome adverse reactions to antipsychotic medications. For example, the nurse can avoid scheduling activities that require alertness when the client's sedative medication achieves its peak effect.

NURSING DIAGNOSIS

Risk for anxiety related to extrapyramidal effects of antipsychotic medications

Nursing priority

Decrease the client's anxiety over the extrapyramidal effects of antipsychotic medications.

Identifying deficits and impairments that promote vulnerability in a client with schizophrenia

Cognitive deficits
- Deficits in maintaining a steady focus of attention
- Deficits in processing complex information
- Difficulty forming consistent abstractions
- Impaired memory
- Inability to distinguish between relevant and irrelevant stimuli

Coping skills deficits
- Overassessment of threat
- Overuse of denial
- Underassessment of personal resources

Psychophysiologic deficits
- Deficits in sensory inhibition
- Poor control of autonomic responsiveness

Social skills deficits
- Deficits in conversational ability
- Deficits in experiencing pleasure
- Deficits in initiating and participating in activities
- Impairments in processing interpersonal stimuli (assertiveness, eye contact)

Adapted with permission from McGlashan, T.H. "Psychosocial Treatments of Schizophrenia: The Potential Relationships," in *Schizophrenia: From Mind to Molecule.* Edited by Andreasen, N.C. Washington, D.C.: American Psychiatric Association, 1994.

Patient outcome criteria

As treatment progresses, the client, family, or both should be able to:
- report a decrease in anxiety related to adverse effects
- demonstrate early recognition of these adverse effects
- report to the health care provider the beginning of the extrapyramidal effect to obtain early treatment.

Interventions

1. Assess the client for extrapyramidal effects. (See "Assessment of extrapyramidal effects," page 278).

2. Reassure the client that the extrapyramidal effects are reversible.

3. Teach the client about the extrapyramidal effects of antipsychotic medications.

4. Administer medications as ordered to alleviate extrapyramidal symptoms.

Rationales

1. Early identification of extrapyramidal effects can help diminish or eliminate the client's anxiety related to these symptoms. Signs and symptoms include abnormal posturing; continual hand, mouth, or body movements; drooling; fatigue; mandibular movements; masklike facial expression; opisthotonos; tongue protrusion; restlessness; tremors; and arm and leg weakness.

2. Knowing that the effects are reversible can reduce anxiety caused by these frightening symptoms.

3. Knowing about these effects, including the signs and symptoms of akathisia, dyskinesia, dystonias, and pseudoparkinsonism, can decrease the client's anxiety, help ensure early identification and treatment, and promote compliance.

4. Antiparkinsonian agents can reverse extrapyramidal symptoms, thereby alleviating anxiety.

NURSING DIAGNOSIS

Altered oral mucous membrane related to adverse reactions to antipsychotic medications

Nursing priority

Help the client maintain a moist, intact oral mucous membrane while taking antipsychotic medications.

Psychotic disorders

Patient outcome criteria

As treatment progresses, the client, family, or both should be able to:
- demonstrate no mouth sores
- reduce the sensation of dry mouth by utilizing medication management strategies.

Interventions

1. Determine the client's hydration status by assessing oral mucosa, fluid intake and output, and urine specific gravity.

2. Encourage an adequate fluid intake of eight to ten 8-oz (240-ml) glasses of water or healthy, decaffeinated, nonalcoholic beverages daily, within the client's physical capabilities, and any fluid restrictions that exist due to a medical condition.

3. Monitor the client's fluid intake, and observe for signs and symptoms of water intoxication, including headaches, dizziness, vomiting, and coma.

4. Encourage good oral hygiene and lip lubrication.

5. Provide hard candy or sugarless gum.

Rationales

1. If the client's hydration status is inadequate, the nurse should implement appropriate interventions to improve it, such as offering beverages at regular intervals.

2. Adequate fluid intake can help prevent dry mucous membranes (within any fluid restrictions due to medical reasons).

3. The client may periodically overhydrate himself while taking antipsychotic medications.

4. Practicing good oral hygiene and lubricating the lips help prevent skin breakdown and maintain normal function and structure of mucous membranes.

5. Sucking on hard candy or chewing gum increases salivation and lubrication in the oral cavity, thereby decreasing dry mouth.

DISCHARGE CRITERIA

Nursing documentation indicates that the client:
- has demonstrated improved reality orientation
- has demonstrated an improved attention span and ability to concentrate
- can control impulses
- can use more adaptive coping skills
- has demonstrated improved social skills
- has reported a decrease in or absence of hallucinations.

Nursing documentation also indicates that the family:
- knows the signs and symptoms of relapse
- is aware of the client's aftercare needs and knows how to make the necessary arrangements
- understands the client's medication dosage and potential adverse reactions as well as how to manage those reactions
- knows who to contact should an emergency arise.

SELECTED REFERENCES

American Psychiatric Association. "Practice Guidelines for the Treatment of Patients with Schizophrenia," *American Journal of Psychiatry* 154(supplement 4):1-63, 1997.

Baker, K.P. "The Development of the Self Care Ability to Detect Early Signs of Relapse among Individuals Who Have Schizophrenia," *Archives of Psychiatric Nursing* 9:261, 1995.

Boyd, M.A., and Nihart, M.A. *Psychiatric Nursing: Contemporary Practice*. Philadelphia: Lippincott-Raven Pubs., 1998.

Breier, A. *Antipsychotic Drugs*. Washington, D.C.: American Psychiatric Association, 1995.

Diagnostic and Statistical Manual of Mental Disorders, 4th ed. Washington, D.C.: American Psychiatric Association, 1994.

Junginger, J. "Common Hallucinations and Predictions of Dangerousness," *Psychiatric Services* 46(9):91, 1995.

Klausner, M., and Brecker, M. "Risperidone Guidelines," *Psychiatric Services* 46(9):950, 1995.

Lotterman, A. *Specific Techniques for the Psychotherapy of Schizophrenic Patients*. Madison, Conn.: International Universities Press, 1995.

McGlashan, T.H. "Psychosocial Treatments of Schizophrenia: The Potential Relationships," in *Schizophrenia: From Mind to Molecule*. Edited by Andreasen, N.C. Washington, D.C.: American Psychiatric Association, 1994.

Nihart, M.A. "Neurobiology of Schizophrenia," *Journal of the American Psychiatric Nurses Association* 2(5):174, 1996.

Torrey, E.F. *Surveying Schizophrenia: A Manual for Families, Consumers and Providers,* 2nd ed. New York: Harper Perennial, 1995.

Yudofsky, S.C., and Hales, R.E. *Textbook of Neuropsychiatry*. Washington, D.C.: American Psychiatric Association, 1997.

Zarate, C.A., et al. "Algorithms for the Treatment of Schizophrenia," *Psychopharmacology Bulletin* 31:461-67, 1995.

Delusional disorder

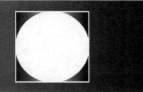

DSM-IV classification
297.1 Delusional disorder

INTRODUCTION

Description

Delusional disorder is a psychotic disorder characterized by stable, logical, and systematized, nonbizarre delusions that occur in the absence of other psychiatric disorders. The delusions occur without the prominent hallucinations (blunted affect, catatonia, thought disorganization, or functional deterioration) present in schizophrenia. Delusions are false, firmly fixed beliefs that are outside the individual's social, cultural, and religious background. In delusional disorder, the nonbizarre delusions are characterized by adherence to situations that could possibly occur in real life (that is, being followed, poisoned, or infected or being deceived by a friend or spouse). The primary symptom is the delusion, and this may or may not interfere with the individual's ability to function socially or occupationally.

Delusional disorder is relatively uncommon in clinical settings (inpatient). This disorder accounts for 1% to 2% of psychiatric hospitalizations. The estimated prevalence is about 0.03%; however exact information is not readily available. Delusional disorder may begin in adolescence, although it usually occurs in middle to late adulthood. Most studies have reported that women were more likely to experience delusional disorder than men. However, women do better at follow up, whereas men come into conflict with the law and are often found in forensic environments for diagnosis and treatment. Many individuals with this disorder are able to function in the workforce unless they become stressed, especially in the area of their delusion. There are several types of delusions that have been identified. (See _Subtypes of delusional disorder._)

Subtypes of delusional disorder

Erotomanic delusions

Erotomanic delusions concern romantic or spiritual love. The client believes there is a shared, idealized (rather than sexual) relationship with someone of higher status than himself (a superior at work, a celebrity, an anonymous stranger). The client will try to contact the person through calls, letters, gifts, spying, and even stalking. The client may attempt to rescue the beloved person from imagined danger. Clients with erotomanic delusions commonly harass public figures and often come to the attention of law enforcement officials.

Grandiose delusions

Grandiose delusions concern a belief that the client has great unrecognized talent, special insight, or prophetic power or has made an important discovery. To achieve recognition, the client may contact government agencies. If the client is experiencing a religious-oriented delusion, participation in a cult may become important. Additionally, a client may believe that he shares a special relationship with a well-known personality, such as a rock star or a world leader. The client may assume the identity of the famous person, believing that the famous person is really an impostor.

Jealous delusions

Jealous delusions focus on fidelity and betrayal. The client believes, without cause, that a lover has been unfaithful, then launches a search for evidence to justify the delusion. The "evidence" is usually misinterpreted normal daily occurrences. The client may confront the person, try to control their movements, follow them, or even track down the suspected paramour. The client may become physically aggressive and attack.

Persecutory delusions

Persecutory delusions cause the client to believe that he's being followed, harassed, plotted against, poisoned, mocked, or deliberately prevented from achieving long-term goals. The client may develop a simple or elaborate persecutory scheme. The client who develops a delusional system may interpret slight offenses as part of the scheme. The client perceiving injustice may file numerous lawsuits or seek redress from government agencies (querulous paranoia). The client who becomes resentful and angry may lash out violently against the perceived injurer. These delusions are difficult to treat and control.

Somatic delusions

Somatic delusions involve bodily functions or sensations. These individuals believe they have a physical ailment. This subtype of delusion occurs in the absence of other medical and psychiatric conditions. Somatic delusions focus on foul odors perceived to come from the skin, mouth, rectum, or vagina; an infestation of insects on or in the skin; that a certain body part is distorted or ugly; or that part of the body is not functioning.

Unspecified delusions

There is no one predominant delusional theme. The individual presents with two or more delusional themes.

Mixed type

This subtype applies when no one delusion theme is predominant.

Etiology and precipitating factors

The cause of delusional disorder is still unknown. Biological theories of causation focus on neuropathologic, genetic, and biochemical research. Magnetic resonance imaging (MRI) studies of individuals with delusional disorder reveal a subtle degree of temporal lobe asymmetry. It is not clear whether this represents a neurodegenerative process or is part of the normal aging process. Presently, there is no evidence of localized brain pathology. Genetic and biochemical hypotheses have not been fully explored. It has been suggested that a complex dopaminergic system may lead to delusions. This could support the hypothesis that a particular delusion depends on the "circuit" that is not functioning. Finally, research based on psychological or social theories have not produced significant insights into the disorder.

Potential complications

If left untreated, delusional disorder can cause aggressive, sometimes violent behavior as well as weight loss and fluid and electrolyte imbalances from self-imposed dietary restrictions.

Assessment guidelines

Nursing history (functional health pattern findings)

Health perception–health management pattern
• Denial of illness, problems, or stressors

Nutritional-metabolic pattern
• Concern about or evidence of weight loss secondary to fear that food is tampered with, poisoned, or rotten
• Dehydration evidenced by dry mucous membranes, poor skin turgor, or concentrated urine

Activity-exercise pattern
• Activity changes secondary to social withdrawal
• Extreme anxiety and agitation

Sleep-rest pattern
• Concern over or evidence of sleep disturbance secondary to fear, especially fear of harm

Cognitive-perceptual pattern
• Belief that others are trying or want to inflict hurt
• Actual incidents from which delusional beliefs are derived
• Hypervigilance or scanning of the environment accompanied by misperceived observations
• Lack of insight or understanding
• Inability to acknowledge inaccurate perceptions
• Use of projection as a primary defense for managing anger, resentment, and hostility unacceptable to the ego

Self-perception–self-concept pattern
• Low self-esteem
• Feelings of being victimized or persecuted

Role-relationship pattern
• Difficulty relating to others
• Inability to trust others
• Poor social skills
• Avoidance of social interactions or situations

Coping–stress tolerance pattern
• Difficulty coping with anxiety
• Increased paranoid thinking and behavior with high stress
• Agitation or violence during stressful situations

Value-belief pattern
• Belief that punishment is deserved

Physical findings

Cardiovascular
• Excess perspiration
• Increased heart rate
• Increased or decreased blood pressure
• Orthostatic changes with psychotropic medications

Gastrointestinal
• Constipation
• Dry mouth

Genitourinary
• Amenorrhea
• Difficulty achieving or maintaining erection
• Retarded ejaculation
• Diminished sex drive

Musculoskeletal
• Body posture alterations
• Balance disturbance
• Gait disturbances
• Muscle tension
• Restlessness

Neurologic
• Catatonia
• Dilated pupils
• Hyperreflexia
• Parkinsonian movements (such as tremors and pill-rolling finger movements)
• Sensory abnormalities (such as hyperesthesia, hypoesthesia, or paresthesia)
• Sleep disturbances (such as difficulty sleeping or staying asleep)

Psychological
• Ambivalence
• Anger
• Anxiety
• Apathy
• Argumentativeness
• Delusions
• Emotional lability
• Lack of facial expression
• Hallucinations
• Paranoia

NURSING DIAGNOSIS

Social isolation related to an inability to trust others

Nursing priority

Help the client develop and use social skills and an effective support system.

Patient outcome criteria

As the treatment progresses, the client, family, or both should be able to:
• demonstrate improved socialization skills
• report feeling less suspicious
• practice using alternative coping strategies
• identify early signs and symptoms of increasing anxiety.

Interventions

1. Encourage the client to talk about feelings, but do not expect immediate trust.

2. Encourage the client to reveal delusions without engaging in a power struggle over their content.

3. Agree to do only realistic, possible things, and then follow through with the plan. Inform the client in advance if you are changing the plan.

4. Use a supportive, empathic approach to focus on the client's feelings about troubling events, situations, and conflicts.

5. Minimize the number of health care providers on the client's care team, establishing a primary nurse or case manager.

6. Collaborate with the client when developing the plan of care and setting goals.

7. When setting limits on client behavior, communicate care and acceptance of the client as a worthwhile person.

8. Encourage and provide opportunities for participation and socialization in groups and group activities.

9. Respond positively when the client participates in social activities and interacts successfully with others.

Rationales

1. In the initial stages of treatment, the client lacks the capacity to trust; therefore, the nurse should work to ensure a predictable, honest, and safe environment.

2. Struggling over content may cause the client to perceive the nurse as a threat. Avoiding such struggles can foster trust between the nurse and client.

3. By demonstrating consistency and reliability with the client, the nurse can help establish a trusting and therapeutic relationship. For example, you might agree to allow the client to take a walk with a staff member every Wednesday morning.

4. A supportive approach fosters trust. Focusing on feelings may eventually help the client to identify and reveal their causes

5. Assigning a regular care team provides consistency and continuity for the client, which in turn decreases anxiety and promotes trust.

6. Including the client in planning can help diminish suspicion while increasing the client's self-esteem and sense of control.

7. The client should feel cared for as a person even though behavior is unacceptable.

8. A suspicious and paranoid client needs encouragement to engage in social activities. Reality testing in selective, supportive group activities can increase socialization success.

9. Rewarding adaptive behavior can enhance self-esteem and increase the likelihood that the behavior will continue.

Psychotic disorders

10. Be aware of the client's personal space, and use touch judiciously.

10. The client may feel trapped if the nurse moves in too closely. This feeling can lead to insecurity, increased anxiety, and violence. The client also might interpret attempts at touch as aggression and respond violently.

11. Recognize signs and symptoms of increased anxiety and take appropriate measures to prevent its escalation.

11. Early intervention, such as providing emotional support and decreasing environmental stimuli, can prevent anxiety from escalating to violent levels.

12. Teach the client alternative methods of coping with increased anxiety.

12. Alternative coping methods, such as verbalization of feelings, diversionary activities, rest periods, and relaxation techniques, represent new and useful skills. Learning them can enhance the client's self-esteem and self-control.

13. Help the client to identify behaviors that alienate others.

13. The client needs to understand that people usually interpret guarded and suspicious behavior as threatening and that this perception causes them to behave in a wary and cautious manner. Such a pattern only serves to reinforce the client's inaccurate perceptions.

14. Teach the family ways to cope with the client's paranoid thinking.

14. Family members may be frightened, confused, or angered by the content of the client's delusions. Teaching them effective coping methods such as not challenging the client about the content of the delusions can increase their sense of control.

15. Provide the client and family with information about aftercare options, appointments, and emergency services, and opportunities for increasing social contacts.

15. Effective discharge teaching makes the client and family aware of options, decreases discharge anxiety, and facilitates a smoother transition.

Nursing diagnosis

Altered nutrition: less than body requirements related to a fear of eating

Nursing priority

Help the client maintain adequate food and fluid intake.

Patient outcome criteria

As treatment progresses, the client, family, or both will be able to:
• eat food that they have supervised the preparation of
• begin to recognize food as safe
• maintain a weight within normal limits
• maintain hydration.

Interventions

1. Monitor the client's food and fluid intake and weight.

2. Give the client some control over food and dining location selection. When possible, serve the food in closed or original containers.

Rationales

1. Careful monitoring can alert the nurse that the client may be refusing to eat for fear of food tampering.

2. Allowing the client to select the food and dining location can provide a sense of control and decrease fears of food tampering. Offering the food in closed or original containers may allay fears and increase food intake, thereby maintaining adequate nutrition.

3. Provide the client with preferred fluids frequently throughout the day.

4. Ensure that the client is taking medications as prescribed.

3. Adequate fluid intake ensures adequate hydration.

4. The client may be reluctant to take medications. Administering them in liquid form and checking the client's mouth to see that all the medication has been swallowed can help ensure compliance.

DISCHARGE CRITERIA
Nursing documentation indicates that the client:
• has demonstrated improved reality testing
• has demonstrated less suspicious behavior
• can use alternate coping strategies
• can identify signs and symptoms of increased anxiety
• is aware of follow-up plans and support resources.
Nursing documentation also indicates that the family:
• reports the client is exhibiting less withdrawn and isolated behavior
• has been referred to the appropriate community support resources
• has scheduled follow-up appointments
• knows how to obtain emergency help.

SELECTED REFERENCES

Baker, P.B., et al. "Delusional Infestation: The Interference of Delusions and Hallucinations," *Psychiatric Clinics of North America* 18(2):345-61, 1995.

Chiu, H.F. "Delusional Jealousy in Chinese Elderly Psychiatric Patients," *Journal of Geriatrics, Psychiatry, and Neurology* 8(1):49-51, 1995.

Diagnostic and Statistical Manual of Mental Disorders, 4th ed. Washington, D.C.: American Psychiatric Association, 1994.

Harmon, R.B., et al. "Obsessional Harassment and Erotomania in a Criminal Court Population," *Journal of Forensic Science* 40(2):188-196, 1995.

Psychotic disorders

Miscellaneous psychotic disorders

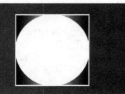

DSM-IV classifications

295.40	Schizophreniform disorder
295.70	Schizoaffective disorder
291.3	Alcohol-induced psychotic disorder with hallucinations
291.5	Alcohol-induced psychotic disorder with delusions
298.80	Brief psychotic disorder
297.3	Shared psychotic disorder (Folie a deux)
293.xx	Psychotic disorder due to a general medical condition
298.9	Psychotic disorder not otherwise specified

INTRODUCTION

Description

Schizophreniform disorder has similarities with schizophrenia. However, unlike schizophrenia, schizophreniform disorder has a duration of less than 6 months, about one-third of clients so diagnosed will recover. The other two-thirds will progress to a diagnosis of schizoaffective disorder.

Schizoaffective disorder is a complex psychotic disorder. It is diagnosed when there is an uninterrupted period of illness that includes a major depressive, manic, or mixed episode in conjunction with two of the following symptoms of schizophrenia: delusions, hallucinations, disorganized speech, catatonia, or disorganized behavior or negative symptoms (affective flattening, alogia, or avolition). Positive symptoms of schizophrenia must be present without the mood symptoms. The episodic presentation of schizoaffective disorder is central to the illness. There are intervals of exacerbation and quiescence in which psychosocial functioning is adequate. The disorder usually occurs from early adulthood to late in life. It is less common than schizophrenia, but due to the difficulty of diagnosis, reports of prevalence range from 0.5% to 13.6% of the population.

Brief psychotic disorder is characterized by sudden onset of a short episode that lasts at least 1 day but no more than 1 month. The disorder includes at least one of the positive symptoms of criteria A for schizophrenia, which include delusions, hallucinations, disorganized speech, grossly disorganized or catatonic behavior, and negative symptoms, such as affective flattening, alogia or avolution. Although episodes are brief, the individual may be impaired enough to require medical supervision. This disorder is uncommon and generally appears in early adulthood. The individual's ethnocultural background needs to be considered in relation to the social or religious context of symptoms.

Shared psychotic disorder (Folie a deux) occurs when an individual develops delusions as a result of a close relationship with another person (the inducer or primary case) who already has a psychotic disorder with prominent delusions. The individual, who is usually healthier and less impaired than the inducer, begins to share the inducer's delusional belief, and is later dominated by the inducer. Shared psychotic disorder is rarely diagnosed in an inpatient setting; it is more likely to arise in a home care or long-term care environment where the two individuals may live together for along time and the delusion may be easier to assess. It may be somewhat more common in women than in men.

Psychotic disorder due to a general medical condition has essential features, including prominent hallucinations or delusions, that directly result from the physiologic effects of a general medical condition, as shown by the client's history, physical examination, and laboratory findings. Although substance-induced psychotic disorder also manifests prominent hallucinations and delusions, they must be judged to be caused by the direct physiologic effects of a substance (illicit or prescribed medications, over-the-counter medications, or toxic exposures).

Etiology and precipitating factors

Numerous studies have examined the relationship of schizoaffective disorders to schizophrenia and bipolar disorder; however, the etiology of schizoaffective disorder itself remains unresolved. There is some evidence for a strong genetic factor, and the episodic nature of schizoaffective disorder suggests both structural and neurochemical components. Environmental, psychological, psychodynamic, and interpersonal factors appear to have a precipitating and influencing role when they occur with a biomedical alteration that creates vulnerability.

Schizophreniform disorder, brief psychotic disorder, and shared psychotic disorder have not received any research attention that attempts to discover an etiologic foundation, and their causes remain unknown at this time.

Potential complications

If left untreated, the client's condition may progress to aggressive, violent behavior, posing an immediate danger to the client and others.

The nurse should be aware that some disorders cause signs and symptoms similar to those of psychosis. An undiagnosed medical condition can lead to serious, even life-threatening problems. (*See Disorders associated with psychosis.*)

Disorders associated with psychosis

The disorders listed below can produce signs and symptoms similar to those of psychosis:

Abstinence phenomena
- Alcohol withdrawal
- Barbiturate withdrawal
- Delirium tremens

Endocrine disorders
- Addison's disease
- Cushing's syndrome
- Hyperparathyroidism
- Hypoparathyroidism
- Hypothyroidism

Heavy metal poisoning
- Lead
- Manganese
- Mercury
- Thallium

Infections
- Bacterial meningitis
- Cerebrovascular syphilis
- Central nervous system infection
- Human immunodeficiency virus
- Parasitic and postencephalitic syndrome

Intoxications
- Alcohol (hallucinosis, pathological intoxication)
- Anticholinergic compounds
- Barbiturates
- Bromide, carbon disulfide, other industrial agents
- Carbon monoxide
- Hallucinogens
- Opiates
- Organic phosphates (insecticides)
- Phencyclidine (PCP)
- Stimulants (amphetamines, cocaine, ketamine)

Medication toxicity
- Corticosteroids
- Digitalis glycosides
- disulfiram [Antabuse]
- indomethacin
- isoniazid [Ianiazid]
- levodopa [Dopar]
- methyldopa [Aldomet]
- phenylbutazone
- procainamide
- propranolol
- Sedatives-hypnotics

Metabolic
- Adult phenylketonuria
- Cardiac failure
- Fluid-electrolyte imbalance
- Folate-responsive homocystinuria
- Hepatic failure
- Hyperglycemia
- Hypoglyemcia
- Ketoacidosis
- Periodic catatonia
- Porphyria
- Renal failure
- Respiratory failure
- Wilson's disease

Neurologic
- Delirium
- Dementia
- Head trauma
- Narcolepsy
- Seizure (psychomotor, complex partial)

- Space occupying lesions (tumors, hydrocephalus)
- Vascular lesions

Vitamin deficiencies
- niacin
- Pernicious anemia
- pyridoxine
- Thiamine deficiencies (Wernicke-Korsakoff syndrome)

Systemic illnesses
- Carcinomatosis
- Collagen and autoimmune diseases
- Dehydration
- Exposure
- Heatstroke
- Mononucleosis
- Starvation
- Viral syndromes

ASSESSMENT GUIDELINES

Nursing history (functional health pattern findings)

Health perception–health management pattern
- Concern about abrupt symptom onset
- Denial of symptoms or illness
- Lack of concern about symptoms
- History of noncompliance with previous treatment or aftercare
- Presence or severity of symptoms
- Need for treatment
- Poor physical health secondary to psychotic symptoms and disorganized thoughts
- Weight loss
- Poor hygiene and grooming

Nutritional-metabolic pattern
- Weight loss secondary to apathy and lack of appetite or hyperactivity and distractibility
- Fear of food tampering

Elimination pattern
- Constipation secondary to poor nutritional status or medication use

Activity-exercise pattern
- Psychomotor agitation or retardation
- Concern over symptoms interfering with ability to carry out normal daily activities or with usual functional level
- Pacing to relieve anxiety
- Hypervigilance
- Decreased motivation and interest in activities
- Restlessness secondary to adverse reactions to medication or psychotic symptoms
- Disorganized or bizarre behavior and posturing

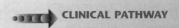 CLINICAL PATHWAY

Psychotic disorders

	Day 1	Day 2

Clinical assessment	• Suicide or homicide risk
	• Multidisciplinary assessment initiated
	• Physical examination initiated
	• Initial family meeting scheduled
	• Appetite deficit
	• Sleep deficit
	• Activities of daily living (ADLs) deficit
		• Suicide or homicide risk
		• Assessments completed:
		  – care level
		  – nursing
		  – multidisciplinary
		  – physical examination
		  – psychiatric

Tests	• SMA-6, complete blood count (CBC), liver function tests (LFT) • Urinalysis and urine toxicology (if applicable) • Thyroid stimulating hormone • Other:_____	• Laboratory results: Normal Abnormal • SMA-6, CBC, LFT? __ __ • TSH __ __ • Other: _____ __ __
Treatments	• Initiate contact with outpatient • Orient to level system • Evaluate group appropriateness	• Increase participation in programs and groups • 1:1 support

Patient and family education and patient rights	• Orient to unit
	• Patient rights, consent, and confidentiality
	• Release of information
	• Relaxation techniques
		• Patient discusses:
		  – diagnosis
		  – treatment options
		  – discharge planning

Discharge planning	• Initiate discharge plan	• Home or resource assessment • Discharge plan presented to team, patient, and significant other • Liaison with outpatient care providers
Psychosocial supports	• Psychosocial assessment • Assessment of stressors • Assessment of coping skills • Discuss outside resources patient can access during symptom exacerbation	• Assessment of illness progression

Medication	• Assessment of:
	  – current medications
	  – AIMS test
	  – symptoms
	  – history
	• Continue or start medication and teaching
		• Continue teaching related to medication and its adverse effects
		• Monitor response to medication including evaluation for presence of extrpyramidal symptoms

Nutrition, hydration, and elimination	• Assess bowel and bladder functions • Monitor intake t.i.d. • Regular diet • Nutritional assessment • Vital signs • Weight	• Assess bowel and bladder functions • Monitor intake t.i.d. • Regular diet • Nutritional assessment • Vital signs • Weight
Activity	• Level 2	• Assess for level advance • Full engagement in unit activities

Day 3	Day 4 (Discharge)	Discharge outcomes

• Suicide or homicide risk
• Assessments completed:
  – social work
  – occupation therapy (OT)
	• Suicide or homicide risk
	• Biopsychological summary completed
	• Adequate sleep, appetite, ADLs
		• Assessment for discharge readiness:
		  – affect appropriate
		  – mood stabilized
		  – no evidence of thought disorder
		  – denies homicide or suicide ideation
		  – adequate behavioral and impulse control

• As indicated	• As indicated	• Laboratory values within normal limits
• Continue to increase participation in programs and groups	• Outpatient transition begun	• Patient verbalizes importance of compliance with outpatient follow-up
• Teaching protocol completed	• Continue to reinforce teaching	• Patient identifies reportable signs and symptoms of relapse • Patient verbalizes understanding of teaching
• Continue to discuss and finalize discharge plans	• Continue to discuss and initialize discharge plans	• Patient and family verbalize discharge plan • Patient is discharged • Follow-up referrals
• Focus on posthospital plans and support system	• Engage posthospital support system	• Patient sets realistic goals and demonstrates willing attempt to reach them • Identifies resources outside of the hospital to utilize when experiencing symptom exacerbation
• Continue teaching related to medication and its adverse effects • Monitor response to any medication changes or adjustments	• Continue teaching related to medication and its adverse effects • Monitor response to any medication changes or adjustments	• Discharge preparation • Prescription(s) • Instructions • Verbalizes knowledge of schedule, desired effects, and adverse effects for each medication
• Assess bowel and bladder functions • Monitor intake t.i.d. • Regular diet • Nutritional assessment • Vital signs • Weight	• Assess bowel and bladder functions • Monitor intake t.i.d. • Regular diet • Nutritional assessment • Vital signs • Weight	• Verbalizes relevant dietary restrictions • Adequate intake
• Assess for level advance	• Assess for level advance	• Demonstrates willingness to interact with others around treatment issues

Adapted with permission from Danbury (Conn.) Hospital.

Psychotic disorders

Sleep-rest pattern
• Increased sleeping
• Decreased sleeping caused by early morning awakening or insomnia
• Insomnia secondary to hallucinations or delusions
• Sedation secondary to medication

Cognitive-perceptual pattern
• Concern about disturbed thinking
• Hallucinations
• Delusions
• Decreased attention span
• Difficulty concentrating
• Disturbed thought processes (such as blocking, loose associations, flight of ideas, tangentiality, and ideas of reference)
• Lack of insight or denial of illness

Self-perception–self-concept pattern
• Grandiose thoughts
• Feelings of powerlessness
• Inability to meet expectations
• Low or exaggerated self-esteem
• Feelings of persecution

Role-relationship pattern
• Disturbed interpersonal relationships secondary to symptom development
• Altered ability to perform role of spouse, parent, or worker
• Inability to trust others
• Feelings of loneliness

Sexual-reproductive pattern
• Hypersexuality
• Decreased libido
• Sexual dysfunction
• Discomfort about masturbation

Coping–stress tolerance pattern
• Feelings of being overwhelmed
• Symptom exacerbation during stressful times
• Escalation of symptoms from exposure to specific stressors

Value-belief pattern
• Feelings of worthlessness, hopelessness, or helplessness
• Paranoia or grandiose delusions
• Delusions of having a different identity
• Overreliance on or identification with religion or religious figures

Physical findings
Cardiovascular
• Excessive perspiration
• Increased heart rate
• Increased or decreased blood pressure
• Orthostatic changes secondary to psychotropic medications

Gastrointestinal
• Constipation secondary to psychotropic medications
• Dry mouth secondary to psychotropic medications

Genitourinary
• Amenorrhea
• Difficulty achieving or maintaining erection
• Retarded ejaculation
• Diminished sex drive

Musculoskeletal
• Altered body posture
• Balance disturbance
• Gait disturbances
• Muscle tension
• Restlessness

Neurologic
• Catatonia
• Dilated pupils
• Hyperreflexia
• Parkinsonian movements (such as tremors and pill-rolling finger movements)
• Sensory abnormalities (such as hyperesthesia, hypoesthesia, or paresthesia)
• Sleep disturbances (such as inability to sleep or difficulty staying asleep)

Psychological
• Ambivalence
• Anger
• Anxiety
• Apathy
• Argumentativeness
• Delusions
• Emotional lability
• Absence of facial expression
• Hallucinations
• Paranoia

NURSING DIAGNOSIS

Ineffective individual coping related to misinterpretation of environment and impaired communication style

Nursing priority

Help the client develop and use adaptive coping skills.

Patient outcome criteria

As the treatment progresses, the client, family, or both should be able to:

$ report feeling less suspicious and fearful of others

• describe the signs and symptoms of increasing anxiety

• demonstrate alternative coping methods (communication of feelings, asking for validation and feedback) to manage misinterpretations of the environment.

Interventions

1. Provide the client with information and realistic feedback about symptoms.

2. In a nonjudgmental manner, encourage the client to verbalize feelings.

3. Encourage the client to explore adaptive behaviors that help in socializing and accomplishing normal daily activities.

4. Administer medication as ordered and monitor the client's response.

5. Teach the client and family about the illness and treatment.

6. Ensure the safety of the client and others.

7. Collaborate with the client to establish a balanced daily schedule of activity and rest.

Rationales

1. By speaking frankly and accurately about the disorder, the nurse can develop trust and a therapeutic alliance with the client.

2. Talking about feelings can develop the client's awareness and understanding of emotional reactions.

3. Developing useful adaptive behaviors can enhance the client's self-esteem.

4. Medications can help diminish psychotic symptoms.

5. An informed client and family are more likely to comply with the treatment plan.

6. Because any psychotic client can become aggressive toward self and others, the nurse must implement interventions to ensure safety. Providing a safe, secure environment also increases client trust.

7. Because the client may exhibit disrupted sleep and activity patterns, establishing a balanced schedule can help restore optimal functioning.

NURSING DIAGNOSIS

Altered health maintenance related to an inability to meet basic health needs consistently

Nursing priority

Teach the client strategies for assuming health maintenance responsibilities.

Patient outcome criteria

As treatment progresses, the client, family, or both should be able to:

• initiate interactions with health care providers to assist them in determining health care needs

• maintain a relationship with the primary care provider

• follow up with outpatient therapy and maintain a medication regimen.

Psychotic disorders

Interventions

1. Assess the client's health maintenance knowledge and capacity for self-care.

2. Teach and rehearse with the client behavior modification strategies.

3. Collaborate with the client to determine appropriate community support referrals.

Rationales

1. Such assessment can help the nurse and client plan for the cognitive and perceptual restructuring necessary to change client behavior.

2. Concrete problem-solving and cognitive strategies, such as cueing, behavioral contracting, anticipatory guidance, positive reinforcement, and keeping a daily journal, can help the client control inappropriate health-related behaviors.

3. External support systems, such as a local mental health center or the National Alliance for the Mentally Ill, can help the client maintain changes that promote health.

DISCHARGE CRITERIA

Nursing documentation indicates that the client:
• has demonstrated improved reality orientation
• has demonstrated an improved ability to perform normal daily activities
• has demonstrated a decline in or absence of violence directed at self and others
• has demonstrated improved psychomotor behavior within acceptable limits
• is able to use alternative coping methods and socialization skills
• is aware of aftercare needs and plans.
Nursing documentation also indicates that the family:
• can identify symptoms of illness exacerbation
• has been referred to the appropriate community resources
• can cope with the client's illness
• has scheduled necessary follow-up appointments
• knows how to obtain emergency assistance if needed.

SELECTED REFERENCES

Diagnostic and Statistical Manual of Mental Disorders, 4th ed. Washington, D.C.: American Psychiatric Association, 1994.

Henry, A., and Coster, W. "Predictors of Functional Outcome among Adolescents and Young Adults with Psychotic Disorder," *American Journal of Occupational Therapy* 50(3):171-181, 1995.

Kendler, K.S., and Walsh, D. "Schizophreniform Disorder, Delusional Disorder and Psychotic Disorder Not Otherwise Specified: Clinical Features, Outcome and Familial Psychopathology," *Acta Psychiatrica Scandinavica* 91(6):370-78, 1995.

O'Connell, K. "Schizoaffective Disorder? A Case Study," *Journal of Psychosocial Nursing* 33(10):35-42, 1995.

Part 5

Personality
disorders

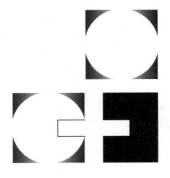

Cluster A personality disorders

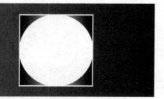

DSM-IV classifications
301.00   Paranoid personality disorder
301.20   Schizoid personality disorder
301.22   Schizotypal personality disorder

Psychiatric nursing diagnostic class
Relatedness disruptions

INTRODUCTION

Cluster A personality disorders, which generally begin in early adulthood, share certain characteristics, including eccentric behavior, suspicious ideation, and social isolation. In addition, these personality disorders have their own unique features. (For an overview of cluster A personality disorders and their respective patterns along with etiologic factors, see *Classifying personality disorders*.)

Clients with *paranoid personality disorder* have a pervasive and unwarranted perception that others are deliberately deceiving, exploiting, or harming them. Paranoid individuals usually are secretive, hypervigilant, and argumentative. They have difficulty confiding in others and search for any evidence of an impending attack. Generally, they do not seek psychiatric assistance on their own but may be encouraged to seek it by their family or health care providers, especially at times of increased stress.

Schizoid personality disorder is characterized by a pervasive indifference to social relationships and a stable but restricted emotional range. Individuals with this disorder are typically "loners" who have no close friends and are not close to their family. They usually engage in solitary activities and display little if any desire for sexual relations. They may be able to perform adequately in the workplace if the occupation promotes social isolation (for example, a night security guard) and makes few demands on their abilities.

The distinguishing characteristics of *schizotypal personality disorder* include peculiar ideas such as superstitious beliefs and eccentric appearance and behavior. These deviations, however, are not severe enough to meet schizophrenia criteria. Under extreme stress, schizotypal individuals may experience psychotic symptoms, including paranoid ideation, suspicion, ideas of reference (belief that certain events are directly related to an individual), odd beliefs, magical thinking, and digressive, vague, and inappropriately abstract speech.

Etiology and precipitating factors

No single theoretical explanation for the development and persistence of personality disorders exists. Research suggests that familial associations and inheritable personality characteristics play a role in cluster A personality disorders. Much more research is needed to determine how economic, sociocultural, neurobiological, and family dynamics factors contribute to abnormal personality development.

Potential complications

Certain features of paranoid personality disorder, such as suspicion and hypersensitivity, can predispose the client to delusional disorder or schizophrenia (paranoid type).

ASSESSMENT GUIDELINES

Nursing history (functional health pattern findings)
Health perception–health management pattern
• Minimal concern about general health
• No history of psychiatric disturbance
• No perceived need or desire for psychiatric intervention
• Inability or reluctance to follow up on health care recommendations

Nutritional-metabolic pattern
• Concern about using food to soothe self
• Peculiar eating rituals or patterns (such as eating particular foods in a set order)

Elimination pattern
• Constipation secondary to medication use

Activity-exercise pattern
• Hypervigilance
• Inability to relax
• Significant self-restriction of daily activity

Sleep-rest pattern
• Sleep disruption during times of stress
• Excessive sleeping to avoid conflict

Cognitive-perceptual pattern
• Transient ideas of reference
• Absentmindedness
• Magical thinking
• Unusual perceptual experiences (clairvoyance and telepathy)
• Illusions
• Indecisiveness
• Poor decision-making abilities

Classifying personality disorders

Cluster and descriptor		Characteristics
CLUSTER A: ODD, ECCENTRIC	**Paranoid** (Suspicious pattern)	• Pattern of distrust and suspiciousness • Hypersensitivity, frequent feelings of being mistreated and misjudged • Preoccupied with unjustified doubts about others loyalty, reluctant to confide in others
	Schizoid (Asocial pattern)	• Pattern of detachment from social relationships • Restricted range of expression of emotions • Does not desire or enjoy close relationships, including being part of a family • Lacks close friends or confidants, takes pleasure in few things • Pattern of acute discomfort in close relationships • Cognitive and/or perceptual distortions (magical thinking, ideas of reference, odd thinking, bodily illusions)
	Schizotypal (Eccentric pattern)	• Eccentricities in behavior • Pattern of excessive emotionality and attention seeking • Egocentric, craves being the center of attention • Interactions are often characterized by sexually seductive and provocative behavior
CLUSTER B: DRAMATIC, EMOTION-AL, ERRATIC, IMPUL-SIVE	**Histrionic** (Gregarious pattern)	• Rapidly shifting and shallow expression of emotions • Suggestible and easily influenced by others or circumstances
	Antisocial (Aggravating pattern)	• Pattern of disregard for and violation of the rights of others • Failure to conform to social norms, frequent altercations with justice and law enforcement systems • Deceitfulness, impulsivity, or failure to plan ahead • Inability to maintain close interpersonal relationships, especially a sexually intimate one • Lack of remorse, indifference to causing hurt or suffering in another
	Narcissistic (Egoistic pattern)	• Pattern of grandiosity, need for admiration, and lack of empathy • Preoccupation with fantasies involving power, success, wealth, beauty, or love • Sense of entitlement • Requires constant and excessive admiration and attention • Displays arrogant, haughty behaviors and attitudes
	Borderline (Unstable pattern)	• Pattern of instability in interpersonal behavior, self-image, and affect • Marked impulsive and unpredictable behavior • Identity disturbance, unstable sense of self • Recurrent suicidal behavior, self-mutilation
CLUSTER C: ANXIOUS, FEARFUL	**Obsessive-Compulsive** (Conforming pattern)	• Pattern of preoccupation with orderliness, perfectionism, and control • Excessively devoted to work and productivity • Preoccupation with rules, trivial details, and other expressions of conformity • Overconscientious, scrupulous, and inflexible about morality, ethics, or values • Displays rigidity and stubbornness
	Dependent (Submissive pattern)	• Pattern of submissive and clinging behavior • Excessive need to be taken care of, feels uncomfortable or helpless when alone • Difficulty in decision making and problem solving • Difficulty expressing disagreement, fearful of being left alone to care for self
	Avoidant (Withdrawn pattern)	• Pattern of social inhibition • Feelings of inadequacy and hypersensitivity to criticism or negative evaluation • Social withdrawal accompanied by longing for close relationships • Views self as socially inept, personally unappealing, and inferior to others

Self-perception–self-concept pattern
- Perception of self as a "loner"
- Desire to be left alone
- Self-centeredness
- Guardedness
- Secretiveness
- Belief that others are to blame for personal mistakes
- Eccentric behaviors

Role-relationship pattern
- Need for rigid routines to function in occupation
- Difficulties functioning at work
- Fear of intimacy
- Fear or suspicion of others
- Anxiety in social settings
- Avoidance of family gatherings
- Few if any significant personal relationships

Sexual-reproductive pattern
- Little or no desire to have sexual relations

Coping–stress tolerance pattern
- Anger when stressed
- Fear of losing control
- Indifference to criticism
- Psychotic symptoms when stressed

Value-belief pattern
- Belief that others are threatening or trying to inflict harm
- Belief in clairvoyance, telepathy, or a sixth sense
- Belief that others are capable of eavesdropping on the client's thoughts and feelings

Physical findings

Cardiovascular
- Increased heart rate
- Increased blood pressure

Respiratory
- Increased respiratory rate when stressed and if psychotic symptoms develop

Gastrointestinal
- Dry oral mucous membranes secondary to psychotropic medication use
- Increased gastric acidity
- Increased salivation

Genitourinary
- Frequent urination

Integumentary
- Bruises resulting from banging or hitting things

Musculoskeletal
- Clenched fists
- Muscle tension

Neurologic
- Hypervigilance

Psychological
- Aloofness
- Anger
- Anxiety in social settings
- Unusual perceptual experiences (such as sensing that someone who is not present is actually in the room)
- Feelings of constriction
- Eccentric behavior or appearance
- Digressive, vague, or overly abstract speech
- Jealousy
- Odd beliefs (such as belief in the ability to predict the future)
- Paranoid ideation
- Desire for social isolation
- Suspicion of others
- Little or no desire to forgive others

NURSING DIAGNOSIS

Impaired social interaction related to disorganized thinking

Nursing priority

Help the client identify feelings that inhibit social interaction.

Patient outcome criteria

As treatment progresses, the client, family, or both should be able to:
- verbalize factors that cause impaired social interactions
- identify feelings that inhibit social interactions
- attend and actively participate in group and social activities.

Interventions

1. Establish a working relationship by listening and responding to the client and showing respect for thoughts and feelings.

2. Collaborate with the client to develop a schedule of specific social interactions and activities.

3. Review with the client the family's social behaviors and the ways family members relate among themselves. Identify any behavioral rules or expectations that the client may have learned from the family.

4. Encourage the client to participate in social interactions and provide objective feedback on individual behavior and its effects on others.

5. Encourage the client to identify personal behaviors that cause discomfort in social situations, thereby inhibiting socialization.

6. Teach the client strategies for changing undesirable social behaviors, such as teaching the client how and when to ask others for help. Allow the client to rehearse these strategies by role playing specific social situations. This can be done alone with the client or, if appropriate, in a group setting.

7. Help the client to assume responsibility for personal behavior. Suggest keeping a daily journal and making entries describing social situations, related feelings, socializing strategies, and degrees of success achieved.

8. Refer the client to appropriate community programs, support groups, and self-help lectures and programs. Encourage participation in these programs.

9. Encourage the client and family to participate in ongoing psychotherapy.

Rationales

1. A trusting relationship between the nurse and client helps to establish a safe environment in which the client can practice social interaction skills and prepare for future socialization.

2. Such a schedule can reduce the client's anxiety about social interactions and activities; it also helps to ensure participation in such activities.

3. Examining family behavior can help the nurse identify and understand the client's dysfunctional social behaviors.

4. The client who begins to comprehend how others perceive types of behaviors may feel more comfortable interacting socially.

5. Identifying factors that impair the client's social interactions can help the nurse develop appropriate interventions and help the client understand and overcome a desire for social isolation.

6. Rehearsing socializing strategies in a safe environment provides the client with immediate feedback, including praise for successes and recommendations for changing or revising behaviors.

7. Keeping a journal can help the client identify behavioral patterns and their causes. The journal also enables the client to evaluate the success of implemented socializing strategies.

8. Participation in such programs can reinforce positive behaviors, expand the client's social support network, and decrease opportunities for social isolation.

9. Ongoing psychotherapy can promote and maintain positive change for the client and family.

NURSING DIAGNOSIS

Ineffective individual coping related to the client's inability to trust others, self-absorption, or unusual perceptions and communication patterns

Nursing priority

Help the client cope with the current situation and feel safe and comfortable about changing behaviors.

Patient outcome criteria

As treatment progresses, the client, family, or both should be able to:
• verbalize and demonstrate decreased suspicion
• demonstrate and report increased security
• demonstrate the ability to establish new relationships.

Interventions

1. Inform the client about the norms and expectations of therapy and hospitalization.

2. Introduce the hospitalized client to the psychiatric unit or mental health center personnel, providing each person's name, title, role, and duties.

3. During the client's hospital stay, establish daily meetings and meet all scheduled commitments on time.

4. Communicate clearly and concisely with the client.

5. During interactions with the client, keep in mind that any client resistance to recommended changes is symptomatic of the condition and not a personal challenge.

6. Collaborate with the client and multidisciplinary team to establish a reward system for achieving clearly defined expectations.

Rationales

1. Explaining procedures and expectations can help foster a trusting relationship between the nurse and client. Such a relationship can make the client feel more secure and help prevent unnecessary surprises.

2. Knowing staff members can decrease the client's anxiety about uncertainty.

3. Establishing and maintaining a daily schedule creates a secure, predictable environment for the client and fosters trust.

4. Direct, unambiguous communication helps prevent misunderstanding and misinterpretation, which in turn enhances social interaction.

5. Responding to client resistance in a nonchallenging and nonthreatening way can foster a trusting relationship.

6. Tangible reinforcement for meeting expectations can strengthen the client's positive behaviors.

DISCHARGE CRITERIA

Nursing documentation indicates that the client:
• has demonstrated the ability to engage in social exchanges
• has demonstrated an ability to receive and use constructive criticism
• can use newly acquired coping strategies in social situations
• is aware of available community and family support resources
• has demonstrated a willingness to participate in follow-up therapy.
Nursing documentation also indicates that the family:
• understands the client's diagnosis, treatment, and expected outcomes
• can use new coping strategies to handle the client's condition
• has agreed to participate in a follow-up therapy program
• has been referred to the appropriate community resources.

SELECTED REFERENCES

Bernstein, D., et al. "Childhood Antecedents of Adolescent Personality Disorders," *American Journal of Psychiatry* 153:7, 1996.

Boyd, M.A., and Nihart, M.A. *Psychiatric Nursing: Contemporary Practice.* Philadelphia: Lippincott-Raven Pubs., 1998.

Diagnostic and Statistical Manual of Mental Disorders, 4th ed. Washington, D.C.: American Psychiatric Association, 1994.

Millon, T. *Disorders of Personality: DSM IV and Beyond.* New York: John Wiley & Sons, 1996.

Cluster B personality disorders

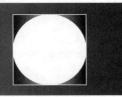

DSM-IV classifications
301.50 Histrionic personality disorder
301.71 Antisocial personality disorder
301.81 Narcissistic personality disorder
301.83 Borderline personality disorder

Psychiatric nursing diagnostic class
Altered self-concept

INTRODUCTION

Cluster B personality disorders are typically experienced as dramatic, emotional, or erratic behavioral patterns. Individuals with these personality disorders crave immediate gain and satisfaction; often they act impulsively, without first critically thinking, identifying, and weighing the consequences of their actions. They may direct verbal and physical outbursts of anger and rage at other persons, objects, or themselves. Because of such behaviors, clients with cluster B personality disorders are often in conflict with society, and they may not receive appropriate treatment until they have been incarcerated and diagnosed. (See *Classifying personality disorders*, page 119, for more information on these disorders.)

Histrionic personality disorder is characterized by dramatic, controlling, attention-seeking behaviors and an intense level of emotionality. Men with histrionic personality disorder are more likely to also experience substance abuse disorders whereas women are more likely to experience depressive episodes, suicide attempts, and several somatic symptoms. This disorder is estimated to occur in 2% to 3% of the general population and in 10% to 15% of people being treated for mental illnesses.

Antisocial personality disorder is characterized by a complete lack of empathy toward and total disregard of others' thoughts and feelings. Clients with this disorder become easily enraged ("murderous rage") and may boast without remorse of physically or emotionally hurting others. In addition, those with antisocial personality have little or no ability to postpone gratification, and they reject routines, compromises, and anything that may involve authority figures. They frequently change jobs or schools, habitats, and relationships. Risk taking and an accident history are prevalent among such individuals.

Persons with *narcissistic personality disorder* seem socially engaging, confident, and successful; however, when involved in a relationship, they may be exploitative and even overdependent, oscillating between idealizing and disdaining their loved one. When their "narcissistic confidence" is shaken, they briefly display rage, shame, or emptiness before utilizing blaming and alibis to place themselves in the best light. This disorder occurs in 1% of the general population and is estimated to occur in 2% to16% of the mental health clinical population.

The client with *borderline personality disorder* typically experiences several forms of dysregulation, including affective (mood), behavioral, cognitive, self, and interpersonal dysregulation. Affective dysregulation includes mood instability and difficulties with anger. Behavior dysregulation involves impulsiveness, suicidal behaviors, threats, and self-mutilation. Cognitive dysregulation is manifested by dissociative responses and paranoid ideation. Interpersonal dysregulation is demonstrated by chaotic relationships and fear of abandonment. Self-dysregulation realm is evidenced by identity disturbance, difficulties with a sense of self, and an overpowering sense of emptiness. A client with borderline personality disorder reacts strongly to separation and isolation in angry, mercurial, and self-damaging ways. Excessive stress can cause the client to regress to developmentally earlier levels of anxiety tolerance, social adaptation, and impulse control, which can produce significantly regressed behavior from an adult or adolescent.

Etiology and precipitating factors
No single theoretical explanation exists for the development and persistence of personality disorders. Research suggests that familial associations and inheritable personality characteristics play a role in cluster B personality disorders.

Sociocultural influences and family dynamics have an impact on these personality disorders, but it is unclear to what extent due to the lack of empirical evidence, on the development of personality. There is a substantial need for focused research into these aspects of personality disorder development.

Potential complications
Undiagnosed medical reasons for anxiety symptoms may lead to the exaggeration of previously problematic yet adaptive behaviors. Furthermore, explosiveness, dramatic behavior, social withdrawal, and self-absorp-

tion may indicate cranial changes associated with such conditions as tumors or aneurysms.

ASSESSMENT GUIDELINES

Nursing history (functional health pattern findings)

Health perception–health management pattern
- Real or perceived crises
- Substance abuse
- Fear of losing control, "going crazy," or being abandoned
- Anxiety
- Restlessness or irritability
- Tendency to attribute difficulties to anyone else but self
- Frustration with not being understood by health care providers
- Denial of the extent of drug or alcohol use

Nutritional-metabolic pattern
- Finickiness about or lack of interest in food
- Weight gain or loss
- Anorexia, bulimia, or bulimarexia

Elimination pattern
- Frequent use of laxatives or cathartics
- Diarrhea, flatulence, or irritable bowel
- Excessive focus on elimination patterns
- Frequent urination

Activity-exercise pattern
- Decreased energy
- Excessive exercise
- Exhaustively detailed descriptions of activities
- Withdrawn or seclusive feelings
- Difficulties relaxing and engaging in leisure activities

Sleep-rest pattern
- Insomnia, early morning awakening, nightmares, or unusually vivid dreams
- Substance use or abuse to aid sleep
- Fears related to going to bed (hypervigilance, difficulty sleeping alone, sleeping on couch or floor, or needing a nightlight)
- Expectation of being exempt from hospital unit schedule

Cognitive-perceptual pattern
- Disturbed body image
- Difficulty concentrating
- Difficulty with recent memory
- Suspicion or paranoia about interview with nurse or doctor
- Vague somatic complaints such as generalized muscle aches
- Impaired social judgment

Self-perception–self-concept pattern
- Poor self-esteem and feelings of worthlessness or emptiness
- Poor frustration tolerance
- Increased irritability
- Increased anxiety
- Feelings of powerlessness, helplessness, or hopelessness
- Exaggerated sense of abilities
- Distorted body image
- Ambivalence regarding self and decision-making and task-completion abilities
- Confusion about gender, gender role, or sexual orientation

Role-relationship pattern
- Feelings of not being understood or supported by loved ones
- Detachment from loved ones
- Tendency to deny or minimize relationship's importance
- History of multiple relationships
- History of physical or sexual abuse
- Being overinvolved with or estranged from family
- Being overwhelmed by work or school
- History of multiple jobs
- Feeling adequate or competent only at work or school
- Social withdrawal and increased sense of isolation
- Suspicious, guarded, seductive, irritable, controlling, or condescending behaviors
- Being victimized in abusive relationships
- Frequent crises in relationships

Sexual-reproductive pattern
- Difficulties with intimacy
- Engaging in indiscriminate sex, sometimes with multiple partners at one time or when the risk of "getting caught" is high
- Sporadic or no use of contraception
- Little or no satisfaction with sexual relationships

Coping–stress tolerance pattern
- Chronic or acute muscle tension in back, neck, or back of head
- Poor frustration tolerance
- Chronic irritability
- Impulsive engagement in high-risk activities (such as mountain climbing or hang gliding)
- Chemical substance use for stress relief
- Self-mutilation as means of stress relief
- Inability to identify stress or how to cope with it
- Frequent suicidal thoughts
- Alternating social withdrawal and overinvolvement

Value-belief system
- Religious fanaticism or magical thinking
- Perception of self as superior to or having no need for religion
- Hopelessness

- Spiritual distress
- Rage concerning spiritual issues
- Guilt caused by spiritual distress

Physical findings
Cardiovascular
- Cold, clammy skin
- Elevated blood pressure
- Hot and cold flashes
- Increased heart rate
- Palpitations
- Sweating
- Tingling sensation

Respiratory
- Increased respiratory rate
- Shortness of breath
- Smothering sensation
- Choking sensation

Gastrointestinal
- Dry mouth
- Abdominal distress
- Nausea
- Vomiting
- Diarrhea
- Difficulty swallowing

Genitourinary
- Frequent urination

Musculoskeletal
- Increased fatigue
- Muscle aches, pains, or soreness
- Muscle tension
- Restlessness
- Shakiness
- Trembling
- Twitching

Neurologic
- Dilated pupils
- Dizziness or faintness
- Light-headedness
- Paresthesia
- Restlessness

Psychological
- Feeling keyed up or on edge
- Inability to concentrate
- Irritability
- Blank mind
- Sleep disturbance (such as insomnia or early awakening)

NURSING DIAGNOSIS

Risk for violence, self-directed or directed at others, related to depression or low self-esteem

Nursing priority

Ensure that the client will not harm self or others.

Patient outcome criteria

As treatment progresses the client, family, or both will be able to:
- demonstrate adherence to an agreed upon plan not to harm self or others
- verbalize when beginning to experience feelings of lack of control
- seek assistance from appropriate, supportive persons who can assist the client to not act violently toward self, others, or property.

Interventions

1. Establish a contract by which the client agrees to inform the staff when the client feels out of control.

2. Search the client's belongings and remove sharp objects, belts, and medications that can be used harmfully.

Rationales

1. Such an agreement can increase the client's self-control and understanding that behavioral choices are available.

2. Removing potentially harmful objects provides a safe environment for the client and others and communicates to the client that the staff is concerned about personal safety.

3. Clearly define for the client treatment expectations and boundaries as well as the consequences of noncompliance.

4. Document and communicate the plan of care to all staff and enlist their cooperation.

5. Use an appropriate degree of observation, seclusion, or restraints and prescribed medications to prevent the client from harming self or others.

6. Observe the client for verbal and nonverbal cues indicating increased agitation.

7. Work with the client to establish a meeting schedule. Be sure to arrive promptly for any scheduled meeting.

8. Work with the client when in a calm, nonagitated state, preferably during a planned meeting, to identify events that trigger harmful behavior.

3. Communicating directly and clearly helps the client understand that external controls will ensure safety even when personal controls are collapsing, which can make the client feel more secure.

4. Communication among the members of the treatment team helps to ensure consistency and increases predictability during treatment.

5. Providing external controls and structure reduces the client's potential for impulsive harm.

6. If the nurse intervenes early to prevent violent and harmful behavior, the client may be permitted to remain in a less restrictive environment.

7. Collaboration between the nurse and client can increase predictability and reinforce normal behavior by decreasing the client's need for attention.

8. Identifying internal triggers that lead to harmful behaviors can enhance the client's sense of self-control and decrease feelings of powerlessness.

Nursing diagnosis

Fear related to impulsiveness, poor judgment, or feelings of hopelessness, helplessness, powerlessness, or low self-esteem

Nursing priority

Help diminish incapacitating anxiety and allow the client to feel safe.

Patient outcome criteria

As treatment progresses, the client, family, or both should be able to:
• demonstrate reduced manipulative behaviors to alleviate anxiety
• discuss events, situations, and feelings in a consistent manner to different staff members
• report and exhibit a decrease in impulsivity
• report being less fearful.

Interventions

1. When interacting with the client, use a direct, calm, and consistent approach.

2. Use a professional approach, and respect the client's sense of personal space.

3. Define expected client behaviors and explain why they are desired.

Rationales

1. The nurse must guard against becoming upset by the client's behavior to ensure the client's sense of safety and security.

2. Professional and respectful nursing behavior, both physical and verbal, helps to decrease the client's confusion about boundaries. It also helps to decrease client suspicion while increasing trust.

3. By clearly defining expected behaviors, the nurse increases predictability for the client.

4. Consistently maintain the limits set for client behaviors, and expect the client to test these limits frequently.

5. Avoid confrontations and power struggles by establishing clear expectations for client behavior in various settings.

6. Hold the client responsible for behavior.

7. Work with the client to schedule meetings. After assessing the risk for self-harm, cancel meetings when the client is acting out.

4. Maintaining behavioral limits increases predictability and communicates to the client that the nurse is in control.

5. The client may attempt to involve the nurse in many power struggles. The nurse must decide which ones are important and require follow-up interventions.

6. Insisting on such responsibility can help the nurse develop a collaborative as opposed to an adversarial relationship with the client. Doing so also gives the client a sense of self-control.

7. Regularly scheduled meetings increase predictability; not meeting with a client who is acting out reinforces normal behavior. It is important to establish that the client is not in a high self-harm situation before deciding not to meet with them. Identify and encourage them to use resources, such as other staff members, writing in a journal, exercise and recreational activities, until your established meeting time.

NURSING DIAGNOSIS

Impaired social interaction related to behaviors that produce hostility in others, low self-esteem, or poor social skills

Nursing priority

Help the client learn more appropriate behaviors.

PATIENT OUTCOME CRITERIA

As treatment progresses, the client, family, or both should be able to:
• participate in social and group activities on the unit and in the community
• report a decrease in levels of anger and hostility
• demonstrate an increase in sense of self-esteem
• engage in discussions with family members in a respective and calm manner, using active listening skills.

Interventions

1. Identify nonverbal behaviors that the client uses when acting out or manipulating others, such as throwing hands up in the air, winking, or smiling.

2. Set appropriate expectations for social interaction, being careful not to fall short of or tax the client's abilities.

3. Teach the client appropriate behaviors through role playing, suggestions, and written assignments such as listing desired objects or activities and the means to acquire them.

4. Expect a decrease in "splitting" behavior rather than total elimination.

Rationales

1. By recognizing these behaviors and not responding positively to them, the nurse can avoid unintentionally reinforcing the client's dysfunctional behaviors.

2. The client will quickly interpret low expectations as demeaning. Expectations exceeding the client's abilities will frustrate both the nurse and client.

3. The client needs to learn new appropriate behaviors to replace those that are being discarded.

4. Long-term therapy is usually necessary before splitting (a core element of personality disorders) can be brought under control.

5. Provide a structured setting in which the client and family can talk calmly with each other about the disorder and its ramifications.

5. A supportive environment, both before and after discharge, promotes client progress.

NURSING DIAGNOSIS

Ineffective individual coping related to feelings of loneliness, emptiness, boredom, poor impulse control, poor frustration tolerance, or fear of abandonment

Nursing priority

Help the client make connections among thoughts, feelings, and behaviors.

Patient outcome criteria

As treatment progresses, the client, family, or both should be able to:
• refer to the self as "I" or "me"
• arrive punctually for therapy sessions
• demonstrate acceptance of some responsibility for present difficulties
• identify some connections among thoughts, feelings, and behaviors.

Interventions

1. Collaborate with the client to schedule meetings. Avoid meeting when the client is acting out.

2. Use a professional approach, and respect the client's sense of personal space.

3. Discuss with the client the consequences of behavior, such as keeping others at a distance; during calm periods, suggest some effective alternatives. Keep in mind that you may have to identify some effects on others because the client may be incapable of empathizing with others and understanding their feelings.

4. Encourage the client to use the words "I" and "me" when referring to self.

5. Work with the client, preferably during planned meeting times, to identify events that trigger acting-out behaviors.

6. Help the client to identify manipulative behaviors, focusing on observable behaviors.

7. Limit interactions with the client to a few consistent staff members.

Rationales

1. Regularly scheduled meetings increase predictability; refusing to meet with a client who is acting out can reinforce normal behavior.

2. Professional and respectful nursing behavior, both physical and verbal, helps to decrease the client's confusion about boundaries. It also helps to decrease client suspicion while increasing trust.

3. Frank but supportive conversations provide the client with objective responses to behavior and may encourage some behavioral risks. Such conversations also may provide the client with evidence that not all interactions result in rejection.

4. Using the words "I" and "me" helps to reverse the dissociative process and forces the client to assume responsibility for personal feelings.

5. Identifying behavioral triggers can help the client see relationships between internal and external events and behaviors. This new understanding allows the client to have more choices in behaviors and increases their sense of self-control.

6. Helping the client to view behavior more objectively can decrease the perception of others as extensions of the self.

7. Limited interactions can increase the client's sense of predictability, which in turn promotes trust.

DISCHARGE CRITERIA

Nursing documentation indicates that the client:
• has regularly exhibited nonviolent behavior
• has demonstrated the ability to seek help from staff as an alternative to self-destructive behaviors
• has demonstrated a desire not to harm self or others and to learn other coping behaviors
• has demonstrated an ability to make some connections among thoughts, feelings, and behaviors
• consistently refers to self as "I" and "me"
• is aware of available appropriate community resources.

Nursing documentation also indicates that the family:
• has demonstrated the ability to identify sources of internal and external support
• verbalizes an understanding of the client's diagnosis, treatment, and expected outcomes
• verbalizes an understanding of usual and unusual responses to any prescribed medication
• understands when, why, and how to contact the appropriate health care professional in case of an emergency
• has been referred to appropriate community and family support groups
• demonstrates a willingness to participate in follow-up therapy.

SELECTED REFERENCES

Boyd, M.A., and Nihart, M.A. *Psychiatric Nursing: Contemporary Practice.* Philadelphia: Lippincott-Raven Pubs., 1998.

Burgess, A. *Advanced Practice: Psychiatric Nursing.* Stamford, Conn.: Appleton & Lange, 1998.

Constantino, J. "Intergenerational Aspects of the Development of Aggression: A Preliminary Report," *Journal of Developmental and Behavioral Pediatrics* 17(3):176-82, 1996.

Cook, D. "Psychopathic Personality in Different Cultures: What Do We Know? What Do We Need to Find Out?" *Journal of Personality Disorders* 10(1): 23-40, 1996.

Diagnostic and Statistical Manual of Mental Disorders, 4th ed. Washington, D.C.: American Psychiatric Association, 1994.

Favazza, A. *Bodies Under Siege: Self-mutilation and Body Modification in Culture and Psychiatry.* Baltimore: Johns Hopkins University Press, 1996.

Flynn, P., et al. "Comorbidity of Antisocial Personality and Mood Disorders among Psychoactive Substance Dependent Treatment Clients," *Journal of Personality Disorders* 10(1):56-57,1996.

Goldstein, R., et al. "Gender Differences in Manifestations of Antisocial Personality Disorder among Residential Drug Abuse Treatment Clients," *Drug and Alcohol Dependency* 41(1):34-45, 1996.

Hamburger, M., et al. "Psychopathology, Gender and Gender Roles: Implications for Antisocial and Histrionic Personality Disorders," *Journal of Personality Disorders* 19(1):41-55, 1996.

Hampton, M. "Dialectical Behavior Therapy in the Treatment of Persons with Personality Disorder," *Archives of Psychiatric Nursing* 11:96, 1997.

Isometsa, E., et al. "Suicide among Subjects with Personality Disorders," *American Journal of Psychiatry* 153:667, 1996.

Laporte, L., and Galtman, H. "Traumatic Childhood Experiences as Risk Factors for Borderline and Other Personality Disorders," *Journal of Personality Disorders* 10(3):247-59, 1996.

Link, P. *Clinical Assessment and Management of Severe Personality Disorders.* Washington, D.C.: American Psychiatric Association, 1996.

Stein, K. "Affect Instability in Adults with a Borderline Personality Disorder," *Archives of Psychiatric Nursing* 10(1):32-40, 1996.

Cluster C personality disorders

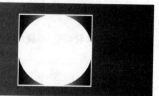

DSM-IV classifications
301.40 Obsessive-compulsive personality disorder
301.60 Dependent personality disorder
301.82 Avoidant personality disorder
301.90 Personality disorder not otherwise specified

Psychiatric nursing diagnostic class
Relatedness disruption

INTRODUCTION

Cluster C personality disorders typically begin in adolescence or earlier and continue through adulthood. These disorders share certain common characteristics, including fearfulness and high anxiety. Individuals with cluster C disorders are anxious and fearful and usually have some degree of social and occupational impairment due to restricted affect, lack of assertiveness, difficulty expressing feelings, and their unrealistic expectations of others. They also experience the lack of problem-solving and decision-making abilities. (See *Classifying personality disorders,* page 119, for additional information.)

Individuals with *obsessive-compulsive personality disorder* typically are rigid, inflexible, indecisive, ruminative, perfectionist, moralistic, and highly judgmental of themselves and others. They generally are unable to express emotions and use rituals and rules to maintain control and to manage feelings of helplessness and powerlessness.

Dependent personality disorder is characterized by dependent and submissive behavior. Individuals with this disorder experience significant difficulty making everyday decisions and require excessive advice, direction, and reassurance from others. They have difficulty initiating projects, experience devastation and helplessness when close relationships end, and are preoccupied with the fear of being abandoned. Their self-esteem is determined by and can be controlled by others.

Individuals with *avoidant personality disorder* generally develop a fear of negative evaluation and timidity in early adulthood. They usually expect rejection and are self-deprecating, easily hurt by criticism, and devastated by disapproval. Typically, they have few or no close friends other than first-degree relatives and are unwilling to become involved unless they can be certain of being liked by the other person. Once a relationship is established, they become very clinging and fearful of losing it.

A diagnosis of *personality disorder not otherwise specified* is used when features of the disorder do not meet the full criteria of any one personality disorder type but significantly interfere with social or occupational functioning.

Etiology and precipitating factors

There is little evidence to support a biological cause of obsessive-compulsive personality disorder. Family theory proposes that parental overcontrol and overprotection establishes distinct limitations on the child's behavior. The child learns from parental feedback that play and not being productive at most times is shameful and the child experiences guilt when not being totally responsible. This is commonly referred to as being an over-responsible child.

Similarly, there is little biological data for the development of avoidant personality disorder. Psychopharmacologic studies suggest that individuals with this disorder experience aversive or toxic stimuli more intensely due to an overabundance of neurons in the aversive center in the limbic system. Symptoms are significantly reduced when these individuals are treated with benzodiazepines, beta-blockers, or monoamine oxidase inhibitors, only to return when the medication is discontinued.

Individuals with avoidant personality disorder have repeatedly experienced rejection and humiliation. This may severely decrease the person's self-esteem and deflate their self-worth.

Dependent personality disorder is usually explained as a result of parental genuine caring, affection, and attachment that has become overprotective. The child learns to rely on others to meet their basic needs but does not learn sufficient skills to become autonomous and independent.

Potential complications

If untreated, cluster C personality disorders can lead to impaired occupational functioning. Additionally, social phobia may result from avoidant personality disorder. Major depression is a common complication of dependent personality disorder. Obsessive-compulsive personality disorder could lead to hypochondriasis and major depression.

ASSESSMENT GUIDELINES

Nursing history (functional health pattern findings)

Health perception–health management pattern
• Anxiety
• Numerous minor, chronic physical complaints or illnesses
• Fatigue from compulsive working
• Inability to assume responsibility for behavior
• History of physical or sexual abuse

Nutritional-metabolic pattern
• Dietary deficiencies and imbalances
• Concern about weight
• Skin problems (rashes or hives)

Elimination pattern
• Concern over GI disturbances
• Frequent or urgent urination
• Difficulty controlling urination
• Excessive perspiration

Activity-exercise pattern
• Restlessness
• Withdrawn behavior
• Desire for isolation
• Inability to engage in leisure activities
• Compulsive work habits excluding leisure activities and family life
• Apathy

Sleep-rest pattern
• Inability to sleep restfully
• Sleeping to avoid conflict
• Reliance on sleeping medications

Cognitive-perceptual pattern
• Inability to concentrate because of overwhelming problems
• Forgetfulness
• Preoccupation with work

Self-perception–self-concept pattern
• Dependency and indecisiveness
• Excessively ordered, rigid, or controlling behavior
• Concern over perfectionistic behavior
• Feeling overly conscientious and loyal
• Perception of self as incompetent and powerless
• Inflexible
• Perception of self as overly sensitive to criticism
• Perception of self as a procrastinator

Role-relationship pattern
• Fear of developing relationships
• Family-taught traits (such as an inability to talk about feelings)
• Avoidance of social situations and close relationships
• Devastation when close relationships end
• Dependence on and fear of being abandoned by family or friends

• Desire to obstruct the efforts of family members, friends, or coworkers by failing to perform tasks or work duties

Sexual-reproductive pattern
• Difficulty expressing affection
• Difficulty with intimacy
• Concern about involvement in high-risk sexual behavior (such as unprotected sex or promiscuity)
• History of sexual or physical abuse

Coping–stress tolerance pattern
• Exhausted by the mere effort of getting to a social event
• Exaggerated concern over potential difficulties
• Frequent perception of events as catastrophes
• Feelings of helplessness when alone
• Preoccupation with details, rules, lists, order, or schedules to cope with uncertainty and anxiety
• Inability to refuse the requests of others
• Extremely sensitive to criticism from others
• Concern about doing things for others to obtain approval and acceptance

Value-belief pattern
• Inability to discard worn-out or worthless objects, even those without sentimental value
• Feeling powerless to achieve life goals
• Lack of self-regard
• Avoidance of job promotions that require increased social demands
• Inability to believe in anything or anyone
• Intolerance of others' beliefs
• Exaggerated involvement in religion

Physical findings

Cardiovascular
• Elevated blood pressure
• Flushed face
• Increased heart rate
• Palpitations
• Sweating

Respiratory
• Increased respiratory rate
• Increased respiratory infections

Gastrointestinal
• Abdominal pain
• Diarrhea
• Increased salivation
• Nausea
• Ulcerative colitis

Genitourinary
• Frequent urination
• Infections
• Sexually transmitted diseases

Musculoskeletal
• Frequent falls and bruising
• Clenched fists

- Exhaustion
- Increased fatigue
- Muscle aches, pains, or soreness
- Muscle tension
- Jaw tension

Neurologic
- Dizziness or faintness
- Headaches
- Restlessness
- Sleep disturbance (such as insomnia, early morning awakenings, difficulty staying asleep)

Psychological
- Annoyance
- Anxiety

- Argumentativeness
- Decreased self-esteem
- Forgetfulness
- Irritability
- Loneliness
- Disbelief about diagnostic study findings
- Obsessive thinking
- Overachievement
- Restricted interests and knowledge
- Ruminative thinking
- Scornfulness

NURSING DIAGNOSIS

Altered family process related to rigidity in functions, roles, and rules

Nursing priority

Help the client and family identify and alter family rules that are growth inhibiting and unhealthy and learn new strategies to increase role flexibility.

Patient outcome criteria

As treatment progresses, the client, family, or both should be able to:
- verbalize and share fears and anxieties
- identify rigid family rules and explain how these rules affect each member
- identify specific areas requiring change.

Interventions

1. Work with the client and family to identify specific roles and behavioral rules that they have established for one another. Concentrate on behaviors that supposedly protect the family from emotional outbursts.

2. Explore with the client and family the effects of rigid and inflexible behaviors on family, friends, and coworkers. Use concrete examples and role playing to make these effects more vivid.

3. Work with the client and family to plan role and function changes and to develop healthful family rules.

Rationales

1. Identifying roles and behaviors that might be causing family dysfunction is necessary before the client and family members can affect changes.

2. Explanations and dramatizations can clarify how dependency and rigid adherence to constricted role behaviors produce rigidity and a lack of spontaneity within the family.

3. By working together to renegotiate their relationships with one another, family members can gain a sense of control over their situation. Working together also provides family members with opportunities to interact in an effective and balanced manner.

NURSING DIAGNOSIS

Altered thought processes related to indecision or doubt over decisions

Nursing priority

Help the client learn and use a problem-solving approach to decision making.

Patient outcome criteria

As treatment progresses, the client, family, or both should be able to:
• identify ritualistic behaviors
• demonstrate the use of problem-solving and decision-making skills to manage anxiety.

Interventions

1. Encourage the client to make decisions.

2. Examine how the client avoids or makes decisions, and discuss the negative consequences of indecision with the client.

3. Teach, model, and rehearse with the client problem-solving processes and decision-making behaviors.

4. Respond clearly and directly to the client's efforts to learn new coping strategies.

5. Help the client to identify anxiety related to the need for perfection or for knowing everything as well as the origin of this behavior (possibly a parent or other family role model).

6. Explain to the client how ritualistic behaviors are used to decrease anxiety about being imperfect and inadequate.

Rationales

1. Encouraging self-determination can help dispel the client's perception of being inadequate and a failure.

2. Understanding how the client avoids decisions and where the coping strategies were learned can help the nurse develop effective and appropriate interventions for managing client anxiety.

3. Learning how to conceptualize a problem, develop options, select the most reasonable option, evaluate and revise the plan if necessary can decrease the anxiety that fosters avoidance. Modeling behaviors and role playing can provide the client with immediate evidence that these strategies can work.

4. Responding to the client's efforts and to positive behavioral change can increase and reinforce client self-awareness and confidence.

5. Finding causes for seemingly inexplicable behaviors or needs increases client awareness and helps the client to make connections between feelings and certain behaviors or beliefs.

6. Knowing the rationale behind ritualistic behaviors, such as creating "to-do" lists or schedules and compulsive reading, can help the client begin to identify an underlying fear of being exposed as incompetent or inadequate.

NURSING DIAGNOSIS

Ineffective individual coping related to the inability to ask for help, the need always to be right and perfect, verbal manipulation, and the need to use rules and routines to maintain a secure environment

Nursing priority

Teach the client new adaptive coping strategies.

Patient outcome criteria

As treatment progresses, the client, family, or both should be able to:
• demonstrate the use of problem-solving and decision-making skills to manage anxiety previously managed by avoidance, dependency, passivity, or perfectionism
• demonstrate a decrease reliance on negative coping mechanisms (manipulation, blaming, rituals).

Interventions

1. Discuss any fears the client has about seeking help. Teach and rehearse ways of asking for help.

2. Discuss past instances in which the client asked for help. Evaluate the client's behavior and feelings as well as responses from others and the outcome of these incidents.

3. Avoid any power struggles with the client.

4. Encourage the client to accept responsibility for behavior and to explore how behavior affects others. Also encourage the client to monitor or check behaviors with trusted family members or loved ones.

5. Discuss what exactly the client thinks will happen if one is wrong about something. Work with the client to identify both realistic and unrealistic outcomes. Encourage the client to discuss what the family has taught its members about being right or wrong.

6. Help the client to develop a sense of humor about the use of perfectionism to cope with tension and anxiety. Point out that being able to regard oneself with humor is a valuable trait.

7. Accept the client's self-image and respect personal rights.

8. Maintain established routines and keep scheduled appointments with the client.

9. Give positive reinforcement of the client's diminishing use of rules and routines and eventual use of healthier coping strategies.

Rationales

1. The client should realize that fear of rejection may make seeking help impossible. Learning adaptive strategies for seeking help can progressively decrease any related anxiety.

2. Self-appraisal of behaviors and feelings as well as appraisal of others' responses help the client to look at fears more realistically.

3. Power struggles are unresolvable and reinforce the client's maladaptive behavior pattern.

4. The client may develop a more realistic view of how individual behavior affects others, and this may support self-initiated behavioral changes.

5. Such discussion allows the client to explore and challenge dysfunctional messages learned in the family. The client also may begin to understand that perfectionism can have destructive outcomes.

6. Humor and laughter can be therapeutic, providing pleasurable physical sensations that reduce tension and anxiety. Humor also can decrease a person's emotional distance from others, while enhancing a general sense of well-being.

7. Through acceptance and respect, the nurse can enhance the client's self-worth and promote feelings of adequacy.

8. Consistency and predictability create a secure environment for the client and consequently decrease anxiety.

9. When abandoning old rules and routines, the client may fear rejection and experience anxiety and guilt. To allay such fears, the nurse maintains a supportive, secure relationship with the client.

Nursing diagnosis

Powerlessness related to perfectionistic behavior that protects against inferiority feelings or to intellectualization or denial of feelings as a means to gain self-control

Nursing priority

Decrease the client's use of perfectionistic behaviors, intellectualization, or denial to manage anxiety and gain self-control.

Patient outcome criteria

As treatment progresses, the client, family, or both should be able to:
• identify and express feelings as they occur
• demonstrate realistic self-appraisal
• report increased ability and comfort in use others for feedback and validation of feelings.

Interventions

1. Encourage the client to identify perfectionistic behaviors and to consider how these behaviors suppress anxiety and feelings of helplessness and powerlessness. Slowly and deliberately encourage the client to consider the feelings associated with these behaviors.

2. Assign and review home or group exercises that require the client to experience a mistake or imperfect behavior and to describe in a journal anticipated consequences and what actually occurred.

3. Collaborate with the client to establish realistic, attainable goals and a definitive, achievable plan for managing stress.

4. Refer the client to appropriate support groups and activities, including a comprehensive stress management program, an intensive program for the children of alcoholics or members of dysfunctional families, and other support groups, such as Adult Children of Alcoholics (ACOA) and Codependents Anonymous (CODA).

Rationales

1. The client needs to experience a safe environment and relationship with the nurse before beginning the anxiety-producing process of linking behaviors and feelings.

2. Such exercises can help the client realize that the consequences of imperfect behavior are not usually as dire as expected and are commonly mild or neutral. Recording observations in a journal enables the client to review and revise distorted thinking.

3. Attainable goals and a structured anxiety management plan can help the client to perceive capabilities and limitations more realistically and to learn concrete skills for managing stress.

4. Knowing about appropriate support groups and activities can decrease the client's sense of loneliness, uniqueness, and isolation.

NURSING DIAGNOSIS

Social isolation related to an inability to establish and maintain relationships

Nursing priority

Help the client develop skills for establishing and maintaining at least one new relationship.

Patient outcome criteria

As treatment progresses, the client, family, or both should be able to:
• demonstrate beginning attempts to establish and maintain a new relationship
• report decreased level of anxiety when attending social or group activity.

Interventions

1. Assess the client's present socialization pattern, and encourage the client to relate to you.

2. After establishing a mutually agreed upon time to meet, begin at the client's interaction level and do not prematurely move to a higher level.

3. Cautiously invite the client to interact with you and another carefully selected person. Initially invite participation in a neutral, nonthreatening, and noncompetitive activity.

Rationales

1. Assessing the client's socialization pattern can help the nurse determine both the duration of the disturbance as well as the probable time needed for treatment. As an objective, trustworthy, nonthreatening person, the nurse can promote a successful personal interaction.

2. Building a trusting relationship with the client requires the nurse's consistency and reliability. Forcing or pursuing complex interactions prematurely will heighten the client's fear of failure and produce social withdrawal and avoidance.

3. The nurse's support and activity planning provide the client opportunities for gradually expanding interaction to a social group. Nonthreatening activities, such as watching television or going for a walk, allow the client to practice socialization skills.

DISCHARGE CRITERIA

Nursing documentation indicates that the client:
• has demonstrated an increased ability to distinguish between thoughts, feelings, and actions
• has demonstrated a decreased reliance on ritualistic behaviors and activities
• understands the diagnosis, treatment, and expected outcomes
• is aware of available community and family resources
• can use alternative coping skills.
Nursing documentation also indicates that the family:
• understands how family rules affect the client
• can identify appropriate internal and external support resources
• demonstrates an ability to use alternative coping skills
• has demonstrated a willingness to participate in an ongoing therapy program
• has been referred to the appropriate community and family resources

• has scheduled necessary follow-up appointments
• understands when, why, and how to contact appropriate health care professionals in case of an emergency.

SELECTED REFERENCES

Boyd, M.A., and Nihart, M.A.. *Psychiatric Nursing: Contemporary Practice.* Philadelphia: Lippincott-Raven Pubs., 1998

Diagnostic and Statistical Manual of Mental Disorders, 4th ed. Washington, D.C.: American Psychiatric Association, 1994.

Link, P. *Clinical Assessment and Management of Severe Personality Disorders.* Washington, D.C.: American Psychiatric Association, 1996.

Millon, T. *Disorders of Personality: DSM IV and Beyond.* New York: John Wiley & Sons, 1996.

Varcarolis, E.M. *Foundations of Psychiatric Mental Health Nursing,* 3rd ed. Philadelphia: W.B. Saunders Co., 1998.

Dissociative disorders

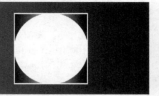

DSM-IV classifications
300.12 Dissociative amnesia
300.13 Dissociative fugue
300.14 Dissociative identity disorder
300.15 Dissociative disorder not otherwise specified
300.60 Depersonalization disorder

Psychiatric nursing diagnostic class
Identity disturbance

INTRODUCTION

Dissociative disorders range in severity from dissociative amnesia to dissociative identity disorder.

Dissociative amnesia is characterized by an inability to recall important personal information, usually of a traumatic or stressful nature. Several types of memory disturbances have been described in dissociative amnesia, including localized amnesia, selective amnesia, generalized amnesia, continuous amnesia and systemized amnesia. (See *Dissociative amnesia: Types of memory disturbances* for more information.)

The client with *dissociative fugue* wanders or travels and assumes modified identities, usually in response to a painful circumstance or acute stress. The fugue state may end abruptly, and the individual may experience partial or complete memory loss of the time period. The prevalence rate is 0.2% in the general population, and it may increase during times of extremely stressful events, such as natural disasters, bombings, and wars.

The client with *dissociative identity disorder* exhibits two or more distinct personalities (up to 200 personalities have been reported). Each personality manifests a separate memory, value and belief system, behavioral pattern, attitudes, and self-image. Usually there is a primary "host" identity that carries the individual's given name and is passive, dependent, guilty and depressed. The host may display partial awareness of the other personalities. Clients with this disorder experience frequent memory gaps for both remote and recent personal history. Transitions between identities are often triggered by psychosocial stress.

Dissociative disorder not otherwise specified is one in which the exhibited dissociative symptoms do not meet the criteria for the other dissociative disorders. Examples include trance states, characterized by an altered consciousness with diminished responsiveness to stimuli.

Depersonalization disorder is characterized by feelings of detachment or estrangement from one's mental processes or body. Other symptoms include sensory anesthesia and a sense of not being in control of one's actions. Depersonalization is a common experience, and this diagnosis is made only when the symptoms are severe enough to cause marked distress or impaired functioning.

Etiology and precipitating factors
Current research suggests that the limbic system may be involved in the development of dissociative disorders. Traumatic memories are processed in the limbic system and stored in the hippocampus. Traumatic events experienced in early childhood appear to impact neurotransmitters, particularly serotonin. This area needs much more extensive research.

Several studies suggest that dissociative identity disorder is more common among the first-degree biological relatives of persons with the disorder that in the general population. Learning theory proposes that dissociative disorders can be learned methods for avoiding

Dissociative amnesia: Types of memory disturbances

Localized amnesia
Individual fails to recall events that occurred during a circumscribed period of time, usually first few hours after a profoundly disturbing event

Selective amnesia
Individual can recall some part but not all of the events during a circumscribed period of time

Generalized amnesia
The individuals failure to recall encompasses their entire life. Individuals with this rare disorder usually present to emergency departments, general hospital consultation liaison services or to the police

Continuous amnesia
Inability to recall events subsequent to a specific time up to and including the present

Systematized amnesia
Individual experiences a loss of memory for certain categories of information, such as all memories about a specific person or their family

stress and high levels of anxiety. When stress becomes intolerable, the individual may consciously use dissociation to "tune out" the painful or offending event.

Potential complications
If left untreated, dissociative disorders can cause aggressive behavior toward the self or others. Such behavior might include assaults, depression, hypochondriasis, posttraumatic stress disorder, psychoactive substance abuse disorder, rape, self-mutilation, and suicide attempts. Dissociative amnesia must be differentiated from amnestic disorder due to a general medical condition or amnestic disorder due to a brain injury; otherwise, these disorders will only worsen without correct diagnosis and focused treatment.

ASSESSMENT GUIDELINES
Nursing history (functional health pattern findings)
Health perception–health management pattern
• History of headaches
• Palpitations
• Loss of consciousness
• Anxiety or panic symptoms
• Substance abuse

Nutritional-metabolic pattern
• Weight loss secondary to appetite loss

Activity-exercise pattern
• Lethargy
• Loss of interest in usual activities

Cognitive-perceptual pattern
• Impaired recall
• Amnesia
• Hearing own thoughts spoken aloud
• Hearing others talking in head
• Sudden awareness of being in strange surroundings with no memory of getting there
• Feeling of being outside the body

Self-perception–self-concept pattern
• Perception of the self as "we"
• Awareness of "other parts" of self
• Feeling like a different person at times
• Low self-esteem

Role-relationship pattern
• Incidents of being approached by strangers who claim or seem to claim to be acquaintances or friends
• Difficulty maintaining relationships
• Difficulty functioning at work

Coping–stress tolerance pattern
• Memory lapses when stressed or anxious
• Sudden trips away from familiar surroundings

Value-belief pattern
• Hearing from others about allegedly engaging in behaviors that would conflict with personal values or beliefs
• Inability to accomplish life goals

Physical findings
Cardiovascular
• Cold, clammy skin
• Elevated blood pressure
• Hot and cold flashes
• Increased heart rate
• Palpitations
• Sweating
• Tingling sensation

Respiratory
• Increased respiratory rate
• Shortness of breath
• Smothering sensation
• Choking sensation

Gastrointestinal
• Dry mouth
• Abdominal distress
• Nausea
• Vomiting
• Diarrhea
• Difficulty swallowing

Genitourinary
• Frequent urination

Musculoskeletal
• Increased fatigue
• Muscle aches, pains, or soreness
• Muscle tension
• Restlessness
• Shakiness
• Trembling
• Twitching

Neurologic
• Dilated pupils
• Dizziness or faintness
• Light-headedness
• Paresthesia
• Restlessness

Psychological
• Feeling keyed up or on edge
• Inability to concentrate
• Irritability
• Blank mind
• Sleep disturbance (such as insomnia or early morning awakening)

NURSING DIAGNOSIS

Personal identity disturbance related to underdeveloped ego, threat to self-concept, or childhood abuse or trauma

Nursing priority

Help the client understand the relationship between anxiety and dissociation and to learn to use adaptive coping skills.

Patient outcome criteria

As treatment progresses, the client, family, or both should be able to:
• demonstrate a decrease or absence of amnesia
• verbalize an awareness of previously dissociated material
• demonstrate that no alternate identities are dominant.

Interventions

1. Develop an honest, nonjudgmental relationship with the client.

2. Assess the client for memory loss.

3. Assess the client for homicidal or suicidal thoughts or impulses.

4. Assess the client for auditory hallucinations.

5. Share and analyze findings with all members of the treatment team.

6. Discuss the diagnosis and treatment plan with the client.

7. Explain to the client with dissociative identity disorder that the treatment goal is the integration of the alternate identities, and establish a contract with the client to work toward that goal.

8. Establish contact with the client's alternate identities and work with them toward integration.

9. Develop a contract with the client that identifies the treatment team members and the client's alternate identities that are to participate in treatment, the treatment expectations, and limits on aggressive behavior toward self or others.

Rationales

1. A client with a dissociative disorder typically exhibits extreme difficulty establishing trusting relationships, especially with authority figures. This difficulty is probably the result of having been betrayed in the past by a parent or loved one.

2. The client probably will be amnestic about periods when a modified or distinct personality is dominant.

3. Aggressive behavior, especially toward the self, and self-mutilation commonly occur during dissociative states.

4. Unlike schizophrenics, who usually hear voices as if they were in the external world, clients with dissociative disorder typically perceive voices arguing inside their own heads. Full-blown auditory hallucinations would suggest another problem such as schizophrenia.

5. Strong, consistent teamwork can help ensure successful treatment.

6. An open and honest discussion of the diagnosis and treatment helps to establish trust between the nurse and client. Such trust can induce the client to cooperate in the treatment.

7. The integration process is usually lengthy, and active client participation increases the chances for success.

8. It is important to include the alternate identities in any treatment contract. Communicating with and eliciting the cooperation of the client's alternate identities is essential to integration.

9. A contract can promote safety when angry, hostile, or aggressive alternate identities dominate the client.

10. Obtain a client history that includes when and why each alternate identity was created, where each fits chronologically in the client's life, what function each serves, and when and how each is triggered.

11. Try to establish communication between or among the client's alternate identities, taking care not to overwhelm the client with information or memories.

12. Avoid focusing on the communication barriers between alternate identities. Instead, explore the reasons why such barriers exist.

13. Help the client to incorporate the dissociated material into conscious memories by encouraging the sharing of painful, repressed memories. Usually, abreaction (verbal disclosure of repressed thoughts or emotions) of painful memories effectively leads to this incorporation.

10. Developing a history that includes alternate identities helps to fill in any gaps in the client's conscious history and may subsequently reveal the traumatic events that caused the dissociative state.

11. The client's alternate identities are shields from painful memories. To maintain client trust and cooperation, the nurse must take care to reveal these dissociated memories in a nonthreatening, supportive manner and environment.

12. Focusing on why barriers between alternate identities exist can make crossing them less threatening for the client.

13. After the memory is identified, the client needs to verbalize the memory and repressed emotions. This time-consuming process must occur with each alternate identity and for each dissociated event.

NURSING DIAGNOSIS

Ineffective individual coping related to a severe level of repressed anxiety

Nursing priority

Help the client learn and use new coping skills.

Patient outcome criteria

As treatment progresses, the client, family, or both should be able to:
• verbalize feelings of improved self-esteem
• demonstrate adaptive coping skills
• verbalize an understanding of dissociation as a way of coping
• report an absence of voices.

Interventions

1. Remain with the client and reassure him that he is safe and secure.

2. Identify stressors that caused the client's severe anxiety and explore feelings related to the stressors.

3. Collaborate with the client to identify alternative methods of coping with identified stressors. Identify which responses are adaptive and which are dissociative.

Rationales

1. The presence of a trusted individual such as the nurse can help to create a secure environment and alleviate the client's fear of a dissociative event.

2. The nurse must obtain information about stressors to develop a relevant plan of care. Explaining that others experience similar feelings in similar situations can reinforce the client's self-esteem.

3. When extremely anxious, the client may be unable to evaluate the appropriateness of behavior and may require assistance with solving problems and making decisions. By providing such information, the nurse helps the client to change inappropriate behavior and adopt new coping strategies.

Personality disorders

4. Help the client to learn and use new coping strategies (such as talking with someone or practicing relaxation techniques) for managing stressful events.

5. Acknowledge and reinforce the client's attempts at change.

6. Provide information, education, and support to the client's family or loved ones during treatment.

7. Inform and educate the client about the need for long-term follow-up therapy.

4. The client must replace dissociation with new, more constructive coping strategies to prevent regression.

5. Positive reinforcement can enhance the client's self-esteem and encourage him to continue desired behaviors.

6. Family members and loved ones should know about the disorder and how to cope with it because they probably will be the ones confronted by the client's alternate identities. Furthermore, the more family and loved ones know about the disorder, the more likely they will support treatment.

7. Because the client is going to be facing previously avoided issues, such as relationships, sexuality, and work, he will need ongoing support to cope effectively.

DISCHARGE CRITERIA

Nursing documentation indicates that the client:
• has demonstrated a decrease in or absence of control by alternate identities
• understands that dissociation is a way of coping
• has demonstrated an absence of aggressive or self-destructive thinking and behavior
• can identify and describe the signs and symptoms of relapse
• has demonstrated improved self-esteem
• understands the need for long-term follow-up treatment
• is aware of available community and family resources.
Nursing documentation also indicates that the family:
• has verbalized an understanding of the client's diagnosis, treatment, and expected outcomes
• can use alternative coping skills in dealing with the client's alternate identities
• understands the long-term nature of the integration process
• knows when, why, and how to contact the appropriate health care professional in case of an emergency
• has been referred to the appropriate community and family resources
• has demonstrated a willingness to participate in a follow-up therapy program.

SELECTED REFERENCES

Bryant, D., and Kessler, J. *Beyond Integration: One Multiple's Journey.* New York: W.W. Norton & Co., 1996.
Burgess, A.W. *Advanced Practice Psychiatric Nursing.* Stamford, Conn.: Appleton & Lange, 1998.
Diagnostic and Statistical Manual of Mental Disorders, 4th ed. Washington, D.C.: American Psychiatric Association, 1994.
Michelson, L.K., and Ray, W.J. *Handbook of Dissociation.* New York: Plenum Publishing Corp., 1996.
O'Reilly, M. "From Fragmentation to Wholeness: An Integrative Approach with Clients Who Dissociate," *Perspectives of Psychiatric Care* 32:5, 1996.
Ross, C.A. *Dissociative Identity Disorder: Diagnosis, Clinical Features and Treatment of Multiple Personality.* New York: John Wiley & Sons, 1997.
Spira, J.L. *Treating Dissociative Identity Disorder.* San Francisco: Jossey-Bass, 1996.
Stuart, G.W,. and Laraia, M.T. *Principles and Practices of Psychiatric Nursing,* 6th ed. St. Louis: Mosby–Year Book, Inc., 1998.
Turkus, J.A., and Cohen, B.M. *Multiple Personality Disorder: Continuum of Care.* New York: Jason Aronson, 1997.
Varcarolis, E.M. *Foundations of Psychiatric Mental Health Nursing,* 3rd ed. Philadelphia: W.B. Saunders Co., 1998.

Part 6

Adjustment disorders

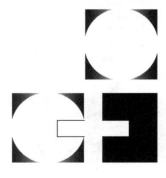

Adjustment disorders

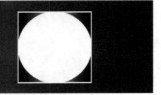

DSM-IV classifications
309.00 Adjustment disorder with depressed mood
309.24 Adjustment disorder with anxiety
309.28 Adjustment disorder with mixed anxiety and
      depressive mood
309.30 Adjustment disorder with disturbance of con-
      duct
309.40 Adjustment disorder with mixed disturbance of
      emotions and conduct
309.90 Adjustment disorder not otherwise specified

Psychiatric nursing diagnostic class
Altered self-concept

INTRODUCTION
Adjustment disorders are generally characterized by mal-adaptive reactions to identifiable psychosocial stressors, such as job loss, relationship termination, academic problems, and family or work problems. The intensity of the individual's reaction, which typically occurs within 3 months of stressor onset and persists no longer than 6 months, is not always proportionate to the intensity of the stressor.

Adjustment disorder with depressed mood includes feelings of hopelessness and tearfulness. *Adjustment disorder with anxiety* is predominantly characterized by nervousness, worrying, and jitteriness.

Adjustment disorder with mixed anxiety and depressive mood represents a combination of anxiety and depression or other emotional responses. *Adjustment disorder with disturbance of conduct* is characterized by conduct that violates the rights of others or age-appropriate societal norms and rules. Behaviors include truancy, vandalism, fighting, defaulting on legal obligations, and reckless driving. *Adjustment disorder with mixed disturbance of emotions and conduct* has both emotional symptoms, such as anxiety and depression, and conduct disturbances, such as truancy and fighting.

Adjustment disorder not otherwise specified involves maladaptive reactions to psychosocial stressors. For example, an individual's intense reaction to a medical diagnosis could produce pathologic denial or noncompliance.

Etiology and precipitating factors
Many factors can inhibit an individual's ability to adjust to life changes, thereby causing an adjustment disorder. One person may have difficulty trusting friends or fami-ly; another may perceive change as a threat to the self or family. Other factors include inadequate communica-tion, inability to use health care resources, lack of fami-ly support, satisfaction with current situation, lack of motivation, and unrealistic or incongruent goals. Un-met dependency needs, retarded ego development, fixa-tion in an earlier developmental stage, and low self-es-teem also can contribute to adjustment disorder devel-opment.

Other factors related to the family may play a part in the development of these disorders. As children, indi-viduals with adjustment difficulties may have received inadequate or nonexistent role modeling in dysfunc-tional or shame-based families. Such experiences inhibit the development of self-esteem, adequate coping skills, and self-regulation skills.

Potential complications
An undiagnosed physical problem can sometimes close-ly resemble an adjustment disorder, thereby delaying appropriate treatment and leading to more serious physical deterioration. Adjustment disorders that occur with medical illness may exacerbate the medical illness, or the illness may promote more serious symptoms that may develop into an anxiety or depressive disorder.

ASSESSMENT GUIDELINES
Nursing history (functional health pattern findings)
Health perception–health management pattern
• Concern over acute or chronic illness or disability
• Numerous somatic complaints (such as headaches, backaches, or stomachaches) with or without diagnostic validation
• Numerous illnesses, colds, flu, or general fatigue
• Aches and pains
Nutritional-metabolic pattern
• Concern over eating behaviors
• Appetite changes
• Weight loss or gain
• Healing difficulties secondary to a chronic health problem
• Skin problems secondary to a chronic health problem
Elimination pattern
• Bowel and urinary elimination problems
Activity-exercise pattern
• Concern about being easily fatigued

- Difficulty performing normal daily activities
- Withdrawn or apathetic behavior
- Diminished interest or ability to participate in leisure activities

Sleep-rest pattern
- Fatigue after sleep
- Difficulty falling asleep or staying asleep
- Early morning awakening

Cognitive-perceptual pattern
- Learning difficulties that inhibit work or academic performance
- Concentration difficulties that inhibit work or academic performance
- Impaired memory
- Vision or hearing dysfunction
- Acute or chronic pain

Self-perception–self-concept pattern
- Perception of self as dependent and indecisive
- Perception of self as inadequate and anxious
- Perception of self as angry and hostile
- Concerns about body image, self-esteem, and self-worth
- Fear, anxiety, resentment, or general disappointment

Role-relationship pattern
- Concern over relationships with family and loved ones
- Manipulative or limit-testing behavior or behavior that plays family members or friends against one another
- Concern over the lack of support for necessary lifestyle changes from family and friends
- Refusal to interact with others or a preference for isolation
- Intense need to be independent and self-reliant

Sexual-reproductive pattern
- Difficulty with intimacy
- Dissatisfaction with sexual relations
- Concern about involvement in high-risk sexual behavior (such as promiscuity)
- Concern about involvement with high-risk partners (such as I.V. drug users and homosexual or bisexual partners)

Coping–stress tolerance pattern
- Inappropriate expressions of anger
- Difficulties in academic or work performance
- Depressed, tense, jittery, or tearful appearance
- Inability to identify persons or measures that would help the condition
- Presence of one or several psychosocial stressors in the past year
- Substance use or abuse

Value-belief pattern
- Feeling unable to achieve life goals
- Disbelief about present situation

Physical findings

Cardiovascular
- Cold, clammy skin
- Elevated blood pressure
- Hot and cold flashes
- Increased heart rate
- Palpitations
- Sweating
- Tingling sensation

Respiratory
- Increased respiratory rate
- Shortness of breath
- Smothering sensation
- Choking sensation

Gastrointestinal
- Dry mouth
- Abdominal distress
- Nausea
- Vomiting
- Diarrhea
- Difficulty swallowing

Genitourinary
- Frequent urination

Musculoskeletal
- Backache
- Fatigue
- Muscle aches and pains

Neurologic
- Headaches
- Nervousness

Psychological
- Ambivalence
- Anger
- Depression
- Hopelessness
- Tearfulness
- Worrying

Adjustment disorders

NURSING DIAGNOSIS

Impaired adjustment related to inadequate support systems, disability requiring lifestyle changes, unresolved grieving, or impaired cognition

Nursing priority

Help the client develop new strategies for coping with limitations or losses.

Patient outcome criteria

As treatment progresses, the client, family, or both should be able to:
- identify stressful situations that lead to impaired adjustment and articulate specific actions for dealing with them
- initiate necessary lifestyle changes appropriate to the disorder
- report or demonstrate progress in coping with grief.

Interventions

1. Assess the client's physical and psychosocial status to determine the degree of impaired function.

2. Encourage the client to explore feelings and to talk about perceived inabilities to adapt to the present situation.

3. Have the client identify significant past stressors and coping methods used. Acknowledge the client's efforts to cope and adjust.

4. Teach and rehearse with the client this problem-solving approach: Identify and isolate the problem, seek out alternatives and resources, determine the pros and cons of each alternative, make an appropriate decision, and reevaluate it. Encourage the client to select another solution if the first option does not succeed.

5. Collaborate with the client to identify available and appropriate support systems.

6. With the client and family, develop and implement a plan for meeting immediate and future needs. Also, encourage them to anticipate future changes and to develop a preventive plan.

7. Help the client to become aware of appropriate additional resources, such as occupational therapy, vocational rehabilitation training, and physical therapy.

Rationales

1. An accurate assessment can help the nurse develop a more appropriate plan of care and can make the client more aware of how the condition affects lifestyle.

2. Helping the client to express feelings and perceptions can foster trust between the client and nurse. Doing so also helps the nurse more clearly understand the client's condition.

3. Recalling previous successes with coping and adjusting can improve the client's confidence and ability to manage present situations.

4. The client may need specific education about solving problems logically and systematically. Supporting the client in problem-solving efforts, including unsuccessful attempts, can build self-confidence and give the client a more realistic perspective on behavior.

5. The client may feel more relaxed and, therefore, may benefit more when working from within a supportive family or community network.

6. Working together to solve problems and make appropriate adjustments can give the client and family an increased sense of control over the immediate situation and the future.

7. Knowing about support resources and how to obtain referrals provides the client with new skills and strategies for managing lifestyle and health status changes and for making realistic plans.

NURSING DIAGNOSIS

Dysfunctional grieving related to a real and perceived but uncertain loss, multiple losses and bereavement processes, or inhibited grieving

Nursing priority

Help the client verbalize feelings associated with the usual stages of grief.

Patient outcome criteria

As treatment progresses, the client, family, or both should be able to:
• participate in activities of daily living
• demonstrate active self-care
• verbalize hope for the future.

Interventions

1. Determine the client's stage of grief and identify specific behaviors associated with it.

2. Speak clearly and honestly when communicating with the client, and keep any commitments made.

3. Encourage the client to discuss feelings about the loss or losses. Allow the client to direct the discussion, and accept unconditionally any emotional responses, unless expressed aggression or violence requires intervention.

4. Arrange for and monitor physical activities that allow the client to vent anger, such as walking, jogging, exercising, biking, playing volleyball or basketball, and using a punching bag.

5. Encourage the client to examine and discuss realistically the lost person or object.

6. Collaborate with the client to identify appropriate strategies for coping with loss. Provide reinforcement and feedback when the client tries new strategies.

7. Collaborate with the client and family to develop a plan that incorporates cultural and religious beliefs that might help the client cope with loss. Involve a religious leader if this is appropriate.

8. Explain to the client that loss can have physiologic effects, and stress the importance of maintaining physical well-being through good nutrition, rest, exercise within limits, proper hydration, regular elimination patterns, and regular physical examinations.

Rationales

1. An accurate baseline assessment enables the nurse to form an effective plan of care.

2. These strategies form the basis of a trusting and therapeutic relationship.

3. Verbalizing feelings, especially anger, in a nonthreatening and supportive environment can help the client understand that responses to the loss are legitimate. Doing so also can help the client resolve unfinished issues.

4. Physical exercise can provide a safe, effective outlet for relieving stored-up muscle tension and anger.

5. Relinquishing idealized perceptions while acknowledging and accepting both negative and positive aspects of the lost person or object can help the client resolve grief.

6. Reinforcing efforts and successes can enhance self-esteem, confidence, and self-reliance and encourage the client to incorporate positive behaviors.

7. A culturally sensitive plan of care may facilitate grief resolution, especially if the client gains strength from spiritual support.

8. Instituting health practices to correct any adverse physiologic effects of stress and grief can help prevent physical illness.

Adjustment disorders

NURSING DIAGNOSIS

Defensive coping related to inadequate support systems, work overload, unmet expectations, or personal vulnerability

Nursing priority

Help the client reduce the sense of distress.

Patient outcome criteria

As treatment progresses, the client, family, or both should be able to:
• assume responsibility for actions, achievements, and failures
• establish and maintain relationships
• describe appropriate alternative coping strategies.

Interventions

1. Assess the client's anxiety and functional levels and ability to comprehend the present situation. Determine what is stressful or threatening to the client.

2. Identify the client's usual coping mechanisms (such as blaming, projection, or rationalization) and in which circumstances they are used. Observe the client's interactions with others and discuss these observations, using role playing when necessary to clarify meaning.

3. Provide safe outlets and opportunities for the client to socialize with others. Encourage involvement in activities and classes in which new skills, especially assertiveness skills, can be learned and practiced.

4. Collaborate with the client to set realistic, attainable, and concrete goals. Acknowledge accomplishments toward defined goals.

Rationales

1. This assessment can help the nurse to evaluate the client's capacity to learn new coping strategies and to make appropriate suggestions for change.

2. Clear and honest communication about the nurse's observations can give a more realistic perspective on the client's behavior and help him appraise behaviors and situations more realistically.

3. Participating in classes and social activities can help the client acquire knowledge and new skills, adjust distorted thinking, and improve self-esteem.

4. Encouraging realistic goals and conveying a belief in the client's ability to achieve these goals enhances confidence and self-esteem.

NURSING DIAGNOSIS

Impaired social interaction related to decreased perception of appropriate social behavior

Nursing priority

Help the client learn an effective social interaction style.

Patient outcome criteria

As treatment progresses, the client, family, or both should be able to:
• establish and maintain relationships
• identify factors and feelings that lead to impaired social interactions
• report or demonstrate a decreased manipulation of others for personal gratification.

Interventions

1. Encourage the client to verbalize feelings rather than acting them out or internalizing them.

2. Set limits on client behaviors that adversely affect social interaction with peers, family members, or visitors, such as making embarrassing comments or ridiculing others.

3. Encourage the client to engage in support, psychoeducation, or activity groups.

Rationales

1. Verbalizing feelings represents straightforward behavior, which can allow for appropriate social interactions.

2. Inappropriate behavior can alienate the client from peers and family and may result in frustration, hostile outbursts, or social withdrawal.

3. Attending and participating in group activities, such as games or crafts, can decrease the client's sense of isolation and reinforce behavioral change.

DISCHARGE CRITERIA

Nursing documentation indicates that the client:
• can use newly learned skills to manage adjustment problems
• has verbalized an understanding of the loss and grief
• understands the diagnosis, treatment, and expected outcome
• is willing to participate in an ongoing follow-up psychotherapy program
• can use alternative coping skills
• is aware of available community and family resources.
Nursing documentation also indicates that the family:
• understands the client's diagnosis, treatment, and expected outcome
• has developed a realistic plan for adjusting to the client's present and future condition
• demonstrates a willingness to participate in an ongoing psychotherapy program
• verbalizes an understanding of the potential psychophysiologic responses to bereavement
• can use alternative coping skills
• has been referred to the appropriate community and support resources
• has scheduled the necessary follow-up appointments
• knows when, why, and how to contact appropriate emergency health care.

SELECTED REFERENCES

Aguilera, D.C. *Crisis Intervention: Theory And Methodology*, 8th ed. St. Louis: Mosby–Year Book, Inc., 1998.

Barry, P. D. *Psychosocial Nursing: Care of Physically Ill Patients and Their Families,* 3rd ed. Philadelphia: Lippincott-Raven Pubs., 1996.

Diagnostic and Statistical Manual of Mental Disorders, 4th ed. Washington, D.C.: American Psychiatric Association, 1994.

Feldman, M.D., and Christensen, J.E. *Behavioral Medicine in Primary Care: A Practical Guide.* Stamford, Conn.: Appleton & Lange, 1997.

Rundell, J.R., and Wise, M.G. *Textbook of Consultation Liaison Psychiatry.* Washington, D.C.: American Psychiatric Association, 1996.

Watkins, A. *Mind-Body Medicine: A Clinician's Guide to Psychoneuroimmunology.* New York: Churchill Livingstone Inc., 1997.

Adjustment disorders

Part 7

Age-specific disorders

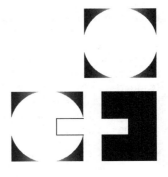

Attention deficit hyperactivity disorder

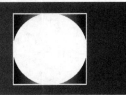

DSM-IV classifications
314.00 Attention deficit hyperactivity disorder — predominantly inattentive type
314.01 Attention deficit hyperactivity disorder — predominantly impulsive type
314.01 Attention deficit hyperactivity disorder — combined type
314.90 Attention deficit hyperactivity disorder not otherwise specified

Psychiatric nursing diagnostic class
Altered attention

INTRODUCTION

Attention deficit hyperactivity disorder (ADHD) is characterized by a persistent pattern of inattention and hyperactivity-impulsivity that is more frequent and severe than is typically seen in individuals at a comparable level of development. Inattentiveness may manifest as difficulty maintaining focus on school or occupational tasks, difficulty following through on instructions, and easy distractibility. Hyperactivity may be exhibited by fidgeting or squirming in the seat and inability to remain seated for a period of time. Impulsivity may be exhibited by impatience, difficulty in delaying responses, blurting out answers before a question has been asked, and frequently interrupting the speaker. Several subtypes of ADHD are now recognized.

Etiology and precipitating factors

It seems that ADHD is a heterogeneous disorder with multiple etiologies. No single cause has been found for ADHD. Contributing environmental factors may include perinatal insult, head injury, lead poisoning, and diet (for example, allergies to foods or additives); however, there is little research to substantiate these hypotheses.

There is some evidence that the frontal lobe has an essential role in attention, organization, planning, regulation of motor activity, and behavioral control. These so-called executive functions seem to be deficient in individuals with ADHD. Neuroimaging studies suggest that the function of the frontal lobe and the striatum (caudate and putamen) are involved in the pathophysiology of ADHD. Frontal lobe dysfunction may signal a primary problem in the prefrontal regions of the cortex in some circumstances.

Finally, genetic studies demonstrate that biological relatives of children with ADHD are more likely to be affected by ADHD than biological relatives of age-related controls.

Potential complications

If undetected or left untreated, ADHD can lead to possible physical injury from failure to control impulses. Additionally, poor grades in school can lead to academic failure.

ASSESSMENT GUIDELINES

Nursing history (functional health pattern findings)

Health perception–health management pattern
• Disproportionate concern about general health
• Lack of concern about a significant health problem
• Inordinate use of legal stimulants, such as caffeine, nicotine, and diet medication, to feel more focused
• No effect or a calming effect derived from stimulants
• Inconsistent approach toward health maintenance activities
• Inability to follow through on prescribed treatments

Elimination pattern
• GI irritability secondary to caffeine or nicotine intake

Activity-exercise pattern
• Constant activity or restlessness
• Poor coordination dating from childhood
• Irritability or anxiety when faced with unstructured time

Sleep-rest pattern
• Daytime sleeping
• Trouble making the transition from sleep to a conscious state
• Excessive movement during sleep (usually reported by the client's partner in adult, or reported by parent in child)

Cognitive-perceptual pattern
• Problems concentrating and sustaining attention dating from childhood
• Excessive shifting from one activity to the next
• Easy distractibility
• History of poor school performance secondary to dyslexia
• Diminished response to pleasurable or painful emotional experiences

Self-perception–self-concept pattern
• Perception of self as moody, difficult, irritable, short-tempered, impulsive, immature, lazy, or demanding
• Perception of self as an "underachiever"
• Inability to follow through on identified goals and tasks
• Fear of losing self-control
• Poor self-esteem
• External locus of control

Role-relationship pattern
• History of being the family troublemaker
• History of stormy interpersonal relationships
• History of erratic school and work performance
• Difficulty entertaining another person's point of view
• History of trouble with the law

Coping–stress tolerance pattern
• Being tense or "wired" most of the time
• Low stress tolerance and a restricted range of problem-solving skills or coping mechanisms
• Alcohol or illicit substance use to ease stress

Value-belief pattern
• Chronic dissatisfaction with life
• Feelings of powerlessness

Physical findings
Gastrointestinal
• Abdominal distress secondary to caffeine or nicotine intake

Musculoskeletal
• Muscular tension
• Restlessness
• Increased motor activity
• Minor physical anomalies (such as curved fifth digit or elongated middle toe)

Neurologic
• Posturing of upper extremities when walking with a heel-to-toe gait
• Diadochokinesis (ability to make antagonistic movements, such as pronation and supination of hands, in quick succession)
• Poor hand-eye coordination

Psychological
• Irritability
• Impulsiveness
• Hyperactivity
• Inattentiveness
• Low frustration tolerance

NURSING DIAGNOSIS

Knowledge deficit related to misinterpretation of information about the client's disorder and treatment plan

Nursing priority

Inform the client and family about the usual treatment plan for a client with ADHD and alleviate any misconceptions.

Patient outcome criteria

As treatment progresses, the client, family, or both should be able to:
• identify behavioral and cognitive symptoms related to ADHD
• identify and use coping methods that diminish impact of ADHD behavioral symptoms.

Interventions

1. Establish and maintain a trusting relationship with the client and family by actively listening and showing empathy and respect.

2. Assess the client's knowledge of ADHD and of appropriate diagnostic measures and interventions.

3. Create an educational plan that includes one-on-one sessions with the client as well as group sessions with family and loved ones.

Rationales

1. These strategies can decrease the client's and family's anxiety level and help to create an optimum learning environment.

2. Assessing the client's knowledge of ADHD enables the nurse to construct an individualized educational plan.

3. The ADHD client typically learns more effectively in an individualized, low-stimulus setting. Group sessions, however, can promote consensual understanding, enhance the client's sense of control, and minimize the use of scapegoating.

4. Include in the client's educational plan information about the biological theories of ADHD, impact of substances and stress on ADHD effects, the use of psychostimulants and antidepressants, and individual and family coping mechanisms that address psychophysiologic symptoms.

4. A comprehensive teaching plan best addresses the complex nature of ADHD. Furthermore, knowledge about the disorder can increase the client's sense of control.

Nursing diagnosis

Ineffective individual coping related to ADHD as evidenced by distracted or impulsive behavior, inability to delay gratification, inability to complete tasks, conflict-ridden relationships, and outbursts of rage

Nursing priority

Help the client identify effects of ADHD and learn effective coping mechanisms that diminish the impact of these effects.

Patient outcome criteria

As treatment progresses, the client, family, or both should be able to:
• identify and use health care interventions (medication and follow-up therapy) aimed at reducing educational and occupational impact of ADHD effects
• identify maladaptive coping mechanisms and behaviors that exacerbate ADHD symptoms.

Interventions

1. Acknowledge and manage any personal feelings about the client's behaviors while avoiding judgmental responses.

2. Provide the client with structured time and a low-stimulus atmosphere for tasks and interactions.

3. Encourage the client to identify previous adaptive and maladaptive coping strategies.

4. Help the client set realistic, short-term goals.

5. Respond positively to the client's goal setting as well as to any goal achievement.

6. Administer prescribed medications, such as psychostimulants and antidepressants, and monitor their effects on target symptoms, including inattention, impulsivity, and hyperactivity.

Rationales

1. In response to the client's behavior, the nurse may experience frustration and anger, feelings that may mirror those of the client or family. If not managed, these feelings can lead to power struggles with the client. Avoiding power struggles as well as judgmental responses enables the nurse to develop a direct, nonjudgmental, and supportive relationship with the client and promotes positive behavioral change.

2. A well-structured environment and decreased stimulation enhance the client's concentration ability.

3. Identifying both successful and unsuccessful coping strategies can help increase self-awareness and make the client feel more responsible for changing behavior.

4. Realistic, short-term goals can enhance the client's chances for success. Successful outcomes can in turn reinforce positive behaviors.

5. Positive reinforcement can promote behavioral change by enhancing the client's self-esteem and sense of control.

6. Close observation enables the nurse to provide the doctor as well as the client and family with information about medication efficacy.

7. Develop with the client a system for self-administering medications, and have the client rehearse this system before discharge.	**7.** The ADHD client's usual inability to attend to details can cause significant problems with medication administration. Consequently, the nurse may have to work creatively with the client and family to ensure medication compliance.

NURSING DIAGNOSIS

Self-esteem disturbance related to the client's condition as evidenced by excessive criticism of self and others, performance of scapegoat or clown role in family and social situations, and self-defeating behavior

Nursing priority

Help the client identify and address causes of diminished self-esteem.

Patient outcome criteria

As treatment progresses, the client, family, or both should be able to:
• use coping strategies that enhance self-esteem
• acknowledge successes in school or occupational performance.

Interventions	**Rationales**
1. Acknowledge the client's struggle with impact of ADHD effects.	**1.** Acknowledgment and validation can promote the self-regard necessary for behavioral changes.
2. Help the client identify behaviors that diminish self-esteem and prevent growth.	**2.** Recognizing these behaviors, such as taking the role of scapegoat or clown at school, work, or within the family and community, can enhance the client's sense of control and promote self-awareness.
3. Encourage the client to identify personal strengths, including personality traits and behaviors.	**3.** Identifying personal strengths can help the client adjust certain distorted self-perceptions. Correcting self-perceptions can enhance the client's feelings of self-worth and power.
4. Offer encouragement, support, and coaching as the client addresses difficult behaviors.	**4.** By being supportive during therapy, the nurse can help the client realize that behaviors, not people, are unacceptable and that such behaviors can be changed.
5. Encourage and help the client to set focused and attainable daily goals that provide opportunities for interaction and task completion.	**5.** Successful experiences will refute the client's self-perceptions of worthlessness and powerlessness.

NURSING DIAGNOSIS

Altered family processes related to the client's inattention or disruptive behaviors as evidenced by a history of unresolved conflict, by family members' attempts to blame each other for problems, and by family members' inability to acknowledge each others' contributions or limitations

Nursing priority

Promote the family's participation in therapy that helps to establish positive behaviors.

Age-specific disorders

Patient outcome criteria

As treatment progresses, the client, family, or both should be able to:
• engage in family relationships that facilitate personal growth, mutual support, goal achievement, and enjoyment
• utilize specific learned communication techniques and behaviors that enhance family and social relationships.

Interventions

1. Provide or arrange for family therapy sessions in which members identify their own contributions, both adaptive and maladaptive, and identify current family interactions that may contribute to the ADHD effects becoming worse.

2. Encourage family members to credit one another and to hold one another accountable for change.

3. Help family members to explore and pursue behavioral options that can help make family life a vehicle for personal growth, mutual support, and enjoyment and decrease blaming and shaming.

Rationales

1. Identifying adaptive as well as maladaptive contributions can help family members accept both credit and responsibility for their role in family relating. Such therapy can diminish scapegoating and help to establish trust.

2. Giving credit and demanding that family members be responsible for their behavior helps to create a trusting environment and improve family relations.

3. Given the long-standing patterns of blame, conflict, and disengagement commonly associated with ADHD, family members may require the nurse's guidance in imagining new ways of relating.

DISCHARGE CRITERIA

Nursing documentation indicates that the client:
• can recognize ADHD symptoms
• has demonstrated an ability to use adaptive coping skills to diminish the impact of ADHD effects
• understands the diagnosis, treatment, and expected outcome
• is aware of available family and community resources
• has demonstrated a willingness to pursue follow-up therapy.
Nursing documentation also indicates that the family:
• understands the client's disorder, treatment, and expected outcome
• can use appropriate coping mechanisms and newly acquired communication strategies and behaviors to diminish the impact of ADHD effects
• has been referred to the appropriate community resources for families of ADHD clients
• has scheduled the necessary follow-up appointments
• understands when, why, and how to contact the appropriate health care professional in case of an emergency.

SELECTED REFERENCES

Barkley, R.A. *ADHD and the Nature of Self Control.* New York: Guilford Press, 1997.

Boyd, M.A., and Nihart, M.A. *Psychiatric Nursing: Contemporary Practice.* Philadelphia: Lippincott-Raven Pubs., 1998.

Diagnostic and Statistical Manual of Mental Disorders, 4th ed. Washington, D.C.: American Psychiatric Association, 1994.

Nathan, P.E., and Gorman, J.M. *A Guide to Treatments that Work.* New York: Oxford University Press, 1998.

Scahill, L., and DeGraft-Johnson, A. "Food Allergies, Asthma, and Attention Deficit Hyperactivity Disorder," *Journal of Child and Adolescent Psychiatric Nursing* 10:6-40, 1997.

Scahill, L., and French, P. "Nonstimulant Treatment of Attention Deficit-Hyperactivity Disorder," *Journal of Child and Adolescent Psychiatric Nursing* 9:39-43, 1996.

Stern, T.A., et al. *The MGH Guide to Psychiatry in Primary Care.* New York: McGraw-Hill Book Co., 1998.

Conduct disorder and oppositional defiant disorder

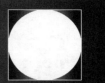

DSM-IV classifications
312.8 Conduct disorder
312.9 Disruptive behavior disorder not otherwise specified
313.81 Oppositional defiant disorder

Psychiatric nursing diagnostic class
Anger

INTRODUCTION

Disruptive behavior disorders are characterized by socially disruptive and problematic behaviors that are generally more troublesome to others than to the client exhibiting them. *Conduct disorder* typically manifests before or during adolescence and is characterized by behaviors that violate others' rights and that are more firmly entrenched and destructive than normal adolescent disruptions. Two subtypes of conduct disorder are recognized: childhood-onset type and adolescent-onset type. During the last decade, there has been a marked increase in the prevalence of conduct disorder.

Conduct disorder usually occurs with family members and friends as well as at school and lasts at least 6 months. Commonly, an adolescent with conduct disorder is identified and diagnosed with the problem when referred by school officials to school-based mental health clinicians, city or county health care providers, or the juvenile justice system.

Oppositional defiant disorder is marked by a persistent pattern of argumentativeness, angry outbursts, disobedience, reduced frustration tolerance, and blaming others. Individuals with this disorder experience difficulty making friends and generally find themselves in conflict with adults. Oppositional defiant disorder usually becomes evident before age 8 and no later than early adolescence. It almost always presents in the home setting but may not be evident in school or community.

Disruptive disorder, not otherwise specified, includes disorders characterized by conduct or oppositional defiant behaviors that do not meet the definition for conduct disorder or oppositional defiant disorder. However, the disorder produces clinically significant impairment.

Etiology and precipitating factors

Conduct disorder and oppositional defiant disorder appear to have both genetic and environmental causes. The risk of developing conduct disorder is increased in children with a biological or adoptive parent with antisocial personality disorder. Recent research has reported that among violent males with conduct disorder there is reduced binding of serotonin by platelets.

The family dynamics of children diagnosed with conduct disorder have demonstrated discipline that is harsh but inconsistent. Parental conflict is often severe, and supervision of children may be minimal or absent.

Potential complications

Without accurate assessment and intervention, children and adolescents with conduct disorder typically become involved in crime and end up in jail where they may not receive appropriate and necessary treatment. They also may develop a psychoactive substance abuse disorder, mood disorder, anxiety disorder, or somatoform disorder. Persistence of conduct disorder beyond adolescence, especially when the onset was early in life, may lead to adult antisocial personality disorder.

ASSESSMENT GUIDELINES

Nursing history (functional health pattern findings)

Health perception–health management pattern
- Anger toward and blame of others for own behavior
- Inability to control feelings and impulses
- General malaise
- Angry, hostile, or depressed manner

Nutritional-metabolic pattern
- Weight gain or loss
- Eating large quantities of food
- Drug or alcohol use

Activity-exercise pattern
- Infrequent physical and social activity participation
- Initiating fights with other children
- Hostility, physical aggression, disobedience, and defiance of authority when engaging in group activities
- Poor school performance

Sleep-rest pattern
- Inconsistent sleep patterns
- Biorhythm reversal (asleep in day, awake at night)

Cognitive-perceptual pattern
- Treating others as family treats self
- Little or no remorse for own behavior
- Denial of own behavior
- Difficulty focusing and concentrating

Self-perception–self-concept pattern
- Perception of self as victim of external forces
- Nervousness
- Self-hatred

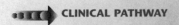 CLINICAL PATHWAY

Poor impulse control

	Day 1	Day 2

Monitoring and assessment	• Administration history and physical
	• Contraband search
	• Assess:
	  –mood, affect, irritability
	  –attention span, distractibility, impulsivity,
	  –aggression (verbal and physical)
	  –Mini-Mental State Exam, Child Depression Inventory, Connors scale for hyperactivity and conduct
	  –substance abuse
	  –interactions with peers, staff, and family
	• Monitor:
	  –sleep pattern
	  –activities of daily living (ADLs)
	  –energy level (EL)
	  –quiet room use.
		• Contraband search
		• Assess:
		  –mood, affect, irritability
		  –attention span, distractibility, impulsivity,
		  –aggression (verbal and physical)
		  –Mini-Mental State Exam, Child Depression Inventory, Connors scale for hyperactivity and conduct
		  –substance abuse
		  –interactions with peers, staff, and family
		• Monitor:
		  –sleep pattern
		  –ADLs
		  –EL
		  –quiet room use.

Medications	• Assess history of medication use and drug allergies.	• Assess need for medications.
Activity	• Unit-restricted for 48 hr • Restrictions and precautions • Level 1 Narcotics Anonymous (NA) for 48 hr	
Tests	• Urinalysis, toxicology, screen HCG • Purified protein derivative (PPD)	• Admission blood work: complete blood count, RPR, electrocardiogram

Diet	• Assess for:
	  –food allergies
	  –nutritional status & restrictions
		• Reassess as indicated

Consultations and referrals	• Social work assessment initiated	• Social work assessment continues • Schedule family session
Child life (CL)	• Discuss CL group activities with patient and family • Initiate CL evaluation • School—establish educational goals • Begin CL life group	• Patient begins education program and continues CL program • Initiate contact with home school
Occupational therapy (OT)	• Initiate OT interview evaluation with patient if possible • Discuss OT groups with patient and family • Patient will attend OT groups • Observe patient • Assess for psychological testing	• Complete initial evaluation and treatment plan • Identify if OT services are currently being received • Patient will attend OT groups • Begin assessing motor, visual, self-care functioning

Teaching	• Provide overview to family regarding:
	  –behavior management system used on unit
	  –explaining rules, time outs
	  –beginning discussion of discharge needs.
		• First family visit
		• Family teaching
		• Initiate parent handbook.
		• Patient demonstrates understanding of behavior system.

Discharge planning	• Begin discharge needs assessment. • Meet with family and patient if possible. • Arrange first meeting. • Family goals and expectations • Patient goals	• Social work initials discharge planning assessment

Day 3	Day 4	Day 5
• Assess need for medications	• Assess need for medications	• Assess need for medications
• Restrictions and precautions	• Restrictions and precautions	• Restrictions and precautions
• Read PPD	• As indicated	• As indicated
• Reassess as indicated	• Reassess as indicated	• Reassess as indicated
• Social work assessment continues.	• Social work assessment continues. • Family session	• Assessment completed • Goals identified • Services and counseling continue.
• Patient continues participating in education and CL program assessment.	• Patient continues participating in education and CL program assessment. • Finish CL assessment	• Patient continues participating in education and CL program assessment. • Begin school-return planning on discharge.
• Attend OT groups as indicated. • Continue assessment • Patient will attend OT groups.	• Attend OT groups as indicated. • Continue assessment • Patient will attend OT groups.	• Attend OT groups as indicated. • Continue assessment and evaluation as indicated. • Patient will attend OT groups.
• Family visits or contact	• Family visitor meetings	• Family visitor meetings
• Discharge planning continues with family and community agencies • Continue discharge planning needs	• Discharge planning continues with family and community agencies • Discuss patient goals for home	• Discharge planning continues with family and community agencies • Discuss family discharge goals and expectations

Adapted with permission from The Johns Hopkins Hospital, Baltimore, Md.

Age-specific disorders

- Difficulty articulating personal strengths
- External focus control

Role-relationship pattern
- Little to no relationships with family and peers
- Behaviors that violate others' rights (including stealing, lying, setting fires, destroying property)
- Runaway or truant behaviors
- Disruptive and socially unacceptable behaviors with peers, including initiating fights and cheating
- Dysfunctional family patterns
- Isolation from peers
- Lack of social skills

Sexual-reproductive pattern
- History of sexual abuse
- Sexual abuse of others
- Promiscuity

Coping–stress tolerance pattern
- Lack of impulse control
- Jittery feelings
- Aggressive behavior toward others with little or no provocation

Value-belief pattern
- Feelings that events are beyond personal control

Physical findings
Musculoskeletal
- Above- or below-average physical growth

Reproductive
- Early sexual experimentation
- Sexual aggressiveness

Psychological
- Anxiety symptoms during interactions
- Difficulty concentrating
- Feeling and appearance of being "wired"
- Cruelty to animals
- Low self-esteem
- Low frustration tolerance
- Lying
- Anxiety and depression
- Lack of remorse for misdeeds
- Drug abuse

Nursing diagnosis

Risk for violence, self-directed or directed at others, related to dysfunctional family relationships manifested by overt hostility, poor impulse control, overt aggressive acts, and self-destructive behavior

Nursing priority

Provide a safe environment that protects the client and others from harm.

Patient outcome criteria

As treatment progresses, the client, family, or both should be able to:
- engage in less disruptive interactions with peers and family
- report or display an absence of suicidal thinking
- report and display an absence of aggression toward others.

Interventions

1. Assess the client for past and present suicide attempts, suicidal ideation, homicidal thoughts, and degree of impulsivity. Implement suicide precautions if the client appears to be at high risk.

2. Work with the client to identify situations or events that have triggered past aggressive acts. Assess behaviors that indicate increased anxiety or anger.

Rationales

1. Suicide assessment gives the nurse an idea of the client's stress tolerance and coping capabilities. Precautions, such as removing objects that the client could use to harm self or others and frequent observation, decrease the chances of a successful suicide attempt.

2. Recognition and intervention before an aggressive outbreak can help to break the client's behavioral cycle and to maintain a safe environment.

3. Provide the client with other outlets for stress and anxiety.

4. Respond positively to the client's effective use of stress-relieving outlets.

5. If the client suddenly becomes physically aggressive or violent, use appropriate means to control the behavior. Use seclusion or restraints if the client cannot be controlled by other means.

6. Approach the client in a consistent manner to establish a trusting relationship.

7. Work with the client to set reasonable, realistic limits on the client's most problematic behaviors. Expect the client to test these limits.

3. Outlets, such as exercising, listening to music, or sitting quietly, can enable the client to decrease anxiety and stress by channeling aggressions appropriately.

4. A positive response reinforces the client's use of appropriate behavior.

5. Typically, the client's narrowed cognition and perception renders verbal and other interventions ineffective. The nurse must use external controls until the client regains internal control.

6. A level of trust between the client and nurse is necessary before the client can begin to articulate feelings and inner conflicts.

7. Setting limits communicates expectations for positive behavior while helping to create a secure environment.

Nursing diagnosis

Self-esteem disturbance related to dysfunctional family system, parental rejection, or family disruption caused by separation, death, or other events

Nursing priority

Help the client develop strategies that can improve self-esteem.

Patient outcome criteria

As treatment progresses, the client, family, or both should be able to:
• use coping strategies that enhance self-control and increase self-esteem
• identify and acknowledge personal strengths.

Interventions

1. Structure the client's routine to include activities that can be performed successfully. Encourage the client to help choose activities.

2. Spend a designated amount of time (perhaps 20 minutes per shift) with the client.

3. Work with the client to gradually explore feelings. Have the client describe events and situations that previously have led to disruptive behaviors. Ask the client to describe what he was thinking while acting out and how others might have viewed such behavior. Suggest that the client keep a daily journal.

Rationales

1. Success can enhance self-esteem and enable the client to relate to the staff and peers in less disruptive ways.

2. Routine visits help the nurse avoid interacting with the client only in response to negative behaviors. Clients then view people less negatively and enhance feelings of self-worth.

3. An adolescent with conduct disorder probably will have difficulty articulating feelings. Having the client describe events or situations can help to establish a more objective basis from which to examine and discuss feelings. Ultimately, identifying and expressing feelings decreases the client's need to act out.

Age-specific disorders

4. Help the client to identify personal strengths. Encourage the client to identify a new strength each day.	**4.** Identifying personal strengths and positive traits can enhance the client's self-esteem.

NURSING DIAGNOSIS

Impaired social interaction related to a lack of role models or a dysfunctional family system

Nursing priority

Help the client learn and participate in more productive relationships with family and peers.

Patient outcome criteria

As treatment progresses, the client, family, or both should be able to:
• use alternative strategies to cope with stressful situations in family and peer relationships
• identify feelings, events, or situations that trigger disruptive behavior
• utilize harm-reduction plan to decrease automatic response to triggers that promote disruptive behaviors.

Interventions

1. Assist client in identifying personal strengths.

2. Encourage the client to interact with the staff and peers by scheduling participation in supervised activities.

3. Assess the ways in which family members relate to one another and solve problems.

4. Help identify situations that make the client uncomfortable and cause stress.

5. Explore with the client how others perceive him.

6. Use role playing to help the client develop alternative behaviors for handling stressful situations.

7. Set behavior limits, provide feedback, and encourage the client to assume responsibility for social behavior.

Rationales

1. Identifying strengths can enhance self-esteem.

2. Providing safe, structured settings for activities, such as walks, team sports, and jogging, can improve the client's socialization skills. Participation in peer group activities promotes feelings of normalcy.

3. Examining family relationships and the family's ability to solve problems can help the nurse identify ways to improve social development.

4. Identifying stressful situations can help the client know when to take appropriate stress-reducing actions.

5. Recognizing how others perceive him is among the client's first steps toward changing behavior.

6. Role playing gives the client opportunities to learn and rehearse alternative ways of relating to others.

7. These interventions can enhance the client's personal identity and self-esteem, and improve social interactions.

DISCHARGE CRITERIA

Nursing documentation indicates that the client:
• can recognize causes of disruptive behavior
• can verbalize an understanding of the need to control disruptive behaviors
• can express anger and frustration productively
• can participate positively in peer activities
• is aware of family and community resources.
Nursing documentation also indicates that the family:
• understands the diagnosis, treatment, and outcome
• is willing to participate in therapy
• has been referred to community resources
• is willing to participate in follow-up therapy

• understands when, why, and how to contact the appropriate health care professional in case of a crisis.

SELECTED REFERENCES

Barkley, R.A. *Defiant Children: A Clinician's Manual for Parent Training.* New York: Guilford Press, 1997.
Diagnostic and Statistical Manual of Mental Disorders, 4th ed. Washington, D.C.: American Psychiatric Association, 1994.
Klykylo, W.M., et al. *Clinical Child Psychiatry.* Philadelphia: W.B. Saunders Co., 1998.

Dementia

DSM-IV classifications

Alzheimer-related dementia

290.0 Dementia of the Alzheimer type, with late onset, uncomplicated (after age 65)

290.10 Dementia of the Alzheimer type, with early onset, uncomplicated (before 65)

290.11 Dementia of the Alzheimer type, with early onset, with delirium

290.12 Dementia of the Alzheimer type, with early onset, with delusions

290.13 Dementia of the Alzheimer type, with early onset, with depressed mood

290.20 Dementia of the Alzheimer type, with late onset, with delusions

290.21 Dementia of the Alzheimer type, with late onset, with depressed mood

290.30 Dementia of the Alzheimer type, with late onset, with delirium

Vascular-related dementia

290.4x Vascular dementia

290.40 Vascular dementia, uncomplicated

290.41 Vascular dementia, with delirium

290.42 Vascular dementia, with delusions

290.43 Vascular dementia, with depressed mood

Dementia due to other medical conditions

294.9 Dementia due to human immunodeficiency virus

294.1 Dementia due to head trauma

294.1 Dementia due to Parkinson's disease

294.1 Dementia due to Huntington's disease

290.10 Dementia due to Pick's disease

290.10 Dementia due to Creutzfeldt-Jakob disease

Substance-induced persisting dementia

291.1 Alcohol-induced persisting dementia

292.82 Inhalant-induced persisting dementia

292.82 Sedative, hypnotic or anxiolytic-induced persisting dementia

292.82 Other (or unknown) substance-induced persisting dementia

Dementia due to multiple etiologies

Dementia with unidentified etiology

294.8 Dementia not otherwise specified

Psychiatric nursing diagnostic class

Impaired cognition

INTRODUCTION

The term *dementia* describes several cognitive deficits that are due to direct physiologic effects of a general medical condition, to the persisting effects of a substance, or to multiple biological etiologies. The essential feature of dementia is the development of multiple cognitive deficits that are severe enough to significantly impair the individual's social and occupational function.

Dementias can be classified as *cortical* and *subcortical* to delineate the location of the underlying pathology. Cortical dementias are characterized by amnesia, aphasia (alterations in language ability), apraxia (impaired ability to execute motor activities), and agnosia (failure to recognize or identify objects despite intact sensory function) resulting from disease that globally affects the cortex. Subcortical dementias are caused by deterioration or dysfunction of deep gray-matter or white-matter structures inside the brain and brain stem. The symptoms of subcortical dementias are more localized and disrupt arousal, attention, and motivation. Additionally, a variety of clinical behavioral manifestations can develop.

Alzheimer-related dementia (AD) is a cortical dementia that is degenerative and progressive. Although most common in older individuals (late onset subtype), AD has been diagnosed in individuals as young as age 35 years (early onset subtype)

Vascular-related dementia (also known as multi-infarct dementia [MID]) is seen in approximately 20% of individuals with dementia. This type of dementia occurs most commonly in persons ages 60 to 75 years and in slightly more men than women. Vascular dementia results after a series of small strokes (transient ischemic attacks) that damage or destroy brain tissue. The behavioral changes that result from vascular dementia are similar to those found in AD, but the onset of symptoms is more rapid.

Dementia caused by other medical conditions can occur in individuals of any age, race, or gender. The elderly are particularly vulnerable to the development of dementia due to a general medical condition, because approximately 75% of older persons are affected by one or more chronic medical illnesses.

Substance-induced persisting dementia results from the persisting effects of a substance, such as illicit or prescribed medications and exposure to toxins.

Etiology and precipitating factors

Researchers have not yet identified a definitive cause of AD. Indeed, AD may actually represent a group of interrelated disorders. Several theories are related to the etiology of AD. The biological theories involve neuroanatomic changes, biochemical disruptions, and genetic and environmental influences.

In the early phase of AD, the brain appears normal; as the disorder progresses, brain tissue atrophies, with a proliferation of neuritic plaques (β-amyloid protein material surrounded by axon and dendrite fragments) and neurofibrillary tangles (fibrous proteins wound around one another within the cytoplasm of abnormal neurons) located mainly in the frontal and temporal lobes.

Neurochemically, AD has been associated with decreased levels of choline acetyltranferase activity in the hippocampus and cortex. This particular enzyme is required for the synthesis of acetylcholine, a neurotransmitter associated with memory. Decreases in acetylcholine markers correlate with the degree of cognitive impairment in AD.

Several studies support a genetic transmission theory. Approximately 10% of individuals with AD report that other family members are also affected. Researchers had hoped to discover a single identifiable genetic basis for AD; however, even in early onset AD, genetic factors appear heterogeneous, having more than a single gene. Chromosomes 14, 19, and 21 have been implicated in the development of AD.

Environmental toxins, including lead, mercury, and manganese, have been suggested as being causative agents in dementia. More definitive research is necessary to determine what role aluminum and other heavy metals play in the development of AD. (See *Organic substances associated with dementia*.)

Multi-infarct dementia results when a series of small strokes damage or destroy brain tissue. There are several primary causes of stroke, including high cholesterol levels, heart disease, diabetes, and hypertension.

Individuals of any age or gender are at risk for developing dementia from a medical condition that causes cerebral pathology. However, the elderly are particularly vulnerable to the development of dementia from general medical conditions, such as HIV, head trauma, Parkinson's disease, Huntington's disease, Pick's disease, and Creutzfeldt-Jakob disease.

Substance-induced persisting dementia usually results from long-term persisting effects of a substance, such as drugs of abuse, alcohol, and prescribed medications, or exposure to toxins. Prescribed medications are the most common toxins in the elderly. Drugs of abuse are the most common toxins in young adults.

For more information, see *Causes of dementia*, page 167.

Potential complications

Without accurate diagnosis, reversible dementias can be missed, and the disorder can progress to a persistent state. In addition, falls, self-inflicted injuries, and violence can occur. Individuals with dementia may wander away from home and become lost or injured. They may insist on driving and become involved in a motor vehicle accident. They could experience financial difficulty if they continue to handle their own financial affairs as their ability to calculate becomes impaired. In advanced stages of dementia, the individual is prone to decubiti, falls, fractures, and dehydration.

ASSESSMENT GUIDELINES

Nursing history (functional health pattern findings)

Health perception–health management pattern
• Vague physical and emotional complaints
• Worry and frustration over inability to remember things
• Fear of losing mental faculties
• Fear of being institutionalized
• Worry about inability to follow medical regimen
• Concern about decline in overall functioning level
• Neglect of preventive medical care
• Inability to identify when difficulties first began

Nutritional-metabolic pattern
• Change in usual appetite
• Weight gain or loss
• Difficulty eating because of dental problems (such as ill-fitting dentures or lack of dental care)
• Lack of normal thirst
• Bruises and cuts from bumping into objects
• Slow healing
• Concern about physical appearance

Organic substances associated with dementia

Organic substance	Symptoms
Aluminum	Cognitive impairment, myoclonus, seizure, speech disturbance
Arsenic	Confusion, drowsiness, headache
Lead	Abdominal cramps, anemia, encephalopathy, peripheral neuropathy
Mercury	Ataxia, confusion, depression, extrapyramidal signs, tremors
Toluene (methyl benzene)	Ataxia, loss of vision and hearing, profound cognitive impairment

Elimination pattern
- Loss of bladder or bowel continence
- Constipation or diarrhea
- Urinary tract infection symptoms (such as frequent or painful urination)
- Body odor

Activity-exercise pattern
- Fatigue
- Difficulty performing normal daily activities
- Loss of interest in recreational and leisure activities
- Difficulty going up and down steps
- Difficulty maintaining balance
- Coordination difficulty
- Restlessness
- Repeating the same action or movement

Sleep-rest pattern
- Early morning awakening or insomnia
- Concern about disrupted sleep patterns
- Using sleep disturbances as a reason for decreased participation in daily activities
- Reversed sleep-awake cycle

Cognitive-perceptual pattern
- Hearing difficulty
- Visual disturbances (such as double-vision and visual field disturbances)
- Difficulty remembering to wear glasses
- Difficulty remembering places, names, and situations
- Difficulty concentrating
- Becoming lost frequently
- Repeating questions and statements
- Inability to understand written language
- Difficulty selecting words when speaking
- Inability to grasp abstract ideas
- Difficulty learning new things
- Difficulty following verbal commands
- Difficulty initiating and focusing on tasks
- Difficulty perceiving direction, distance, and spatial relationships
- Inability to recognize familiar symbols and objects

Self-perception–self-concept pattern
- Perception of self as useless and powerless
- Feeling like a family burden
- Sadness and anger over diminished cognition and physical functioning
- Annoyance, fear, or anxiety when needs are not met promptly

Role-relationship pattern
- Concern or annoyance with family's increased responsibilities and vigilance
- Feeling ignored, neglected, or forgotten by family
- Sadness or embarrassment over role-reversal with children
- Loneliness
- Longing for family or friends
- Concern over financial responsibilities

- Concern over not "fitting in"

Sexual-reproductive pattern
- Inappropriate flirting
- Inappropriate sexual behavior (such as disrobing or masturbating in public)
- Difficulty with intimacy

Coping–stress tolerance pattern
- Tension or anxiety in new situations
- Agitation in response to internal or external stimuli
- Feeling out of control
- Anxiety, restlessness, or frustration if unable to follow directions
- Inability to solve problems

Value-belief pattern
- Feeling that life goals are unattainable
- Loss of interest in religious affiliations
- Concern over changes in religious beliefs and practices

Physical findings
Cardiovascular
- Poor circulation
- Arrhythmias
- High or low blood pressure
- Increased or decreased heart rate

Gastrointestinal
- Constipation
- Diarrhea
- Difficulty chewing and swallowing
- Impactions
- Incontinence

Genitourinary
- Decreased urination
- Incontinence
- Urinary tract infections

Musculoskeletal
- Muscle aches and pains
- Decreased range of motion
- Easy fatigability
- Muscle rigidity and tension
- Muscle atrophy
- Pacing
- Shakiness
- Weakness

Neurologic
- Balance difficulty
- Dizziness
- Gait disturbance
- Restlessness
- Seizures
- Sleep disturbances (such as frequent waking or insomnia)

Psychological
- Agitation
- Confusion

- Decreased ability to think abstractly
- Decreased concentration
- Irritability
- Language deficits
- Memory loss

Respiratory
- Cough
- Increased respiratory rate
- Increased susceptibility to upper respiratory tract infections
- Shortness of breath
- Increased sputum production

Nursing diagnosis

Risk for injury related to cognitive deficits, debilitated state, impaired mobility, wandering behavior, balance and perceptual impairment, and depressed mood

Nursing priority

Provide a safe environment in which the client can maintain optimum independence and safety.

Patient outcome criterion

As treatment progresses, the client, family, or both should be able to:
- verbalize an understanding of the disorder and its effects.

Interventions

1. Assess the client's physical and cognitive impairment levels. (See *Assessing for dementia,* page 168.) Obtain information from both the client and family about the client's prior habits, activities, hobbies, and usual ways of coping with stress.

2. Facilitate the client's access to personal belongings by removing obstacles and hazardous objects from the client's path. Use reflective tape on steps.

3. Avoid rushing the client with activities of daily living (ADLs) and ambulation.

4. Provide adequate lighting in the client's room and keep a bathroom light on at night. At night, help the client to the toilet every 4 hours or as needed.

5. Provide the client with an identification bracelet and keep a photograph of the client in the chart. Introduce the client to the staff. Provide other environmental cues.

6. Provide the client with stimulating, supervised activities requiring physical activity as well as a safe, controlled environment in which the client can wander.

Rationales

1. Establishing a performance baseline can help the nurse develop appropriate strategies that allow the client to function at optimum levels.

2. A hazard-free environment can decrease the risk of falls and injury.

3. Because the client's ability to follow directions may be significantly reduced, rushing to complete tasks can increase anxiety and frustration. A slower pace and patience on the nurse's part will make the client more comfortable and facilitate ADLs.

4. Adequate nighttime lighting can help to reduce confusion. Helping the client to the toilet can prevent falls that might occur when the client is trying to get out of bed or is looking for the bathroom.

5. A client identification bracelet and photograph in the chart as well as familiarity with the staff can help ensure the client's safety. Providing environmental cues, such as clocks and calendars, large signs with the client's name next to his bedroom and on the door, and signs with arrows pointing to his room, can improve the client's orientation and reduce confusion.

6. The client may wander to release tension or decrease boredom, in response to psychotropic medications, or in search of security. Providing safe opportunities for wandering can help relieve the client's tension or frustration.

Causes of dementia

Cognitive disorders of the dementia type can result from numerous medical conditions, mineral deficiencies, poisoning, and injuries.

Brain injury
- Delayed postanoxic encephalopathy
- Delayed radiation encephalopathy
- Dementia pugilistica
- Postanoxic encephalopathy
- Subdural hematoma
- Traumatic dementia

Heredodegenerative disorders
- Adrenoleukodystrophy
- Alzheimer's disease
- Amyotrophic lateral sclerosis
- Cerebrotendinous xanthomatosis
- Diffuse Lewy body disease
- Hallervorden-Spatz disease
- Huntington's disease
- Meningitis
- Metachromatic leukodystrophy
- Multiple sclerosis
- Myotonic dystrophy
- Neoplasms
- Olivopontocerebellar degeneration
- Parkinson's disease
- Pick's disease
- Syphilis
- Wilson's disease

Endocrinologic disorders
- Hyperthyroidism
- Hypothyroidism

Immune-related disorders
- Limbic encephalitis
- Multiple sclerosis
- Sarcoidosis
- Systemic lupus erythmatosis

Infectious and inflammatory disorders
- Acquired immunodeficiency syndrome dementia
- Creutzfeldt-Jakob disease
- Cytomegalovirus encephalopathy
- Encephalitis lethargica
- Lyme disease
- Mycoses
- Neurosyphilis
- Progressive multifocal leukoencephalopathy
- Progressive rubella panencephalitis
- Subacute sclerosing panencephalitis
- Toxoplasmosis
- Tuberculosis
- Whipple's disease

Mass lesions and central nervous system disorders
- Brain abscess
- Brain tumor
- Hydrocephalus
- Normal pressure hydrocephalus

Metabolic disorders
- Acquired hepatocerebral degeneration
- Hypocalcemic encephalopathy
- Hypoglycemia

Metal poisoning
- Arsenic poisoning
- Dialysis-related dementia
- Lead encephalopathy
- Manganese dementia
- Mercury poisoning
- Thallium poisoning

Substance-related disorders
- Alcoholic dementia
- Inhalant drugs
- Marchiafava-Bignami disease

Vascular-related disorders
- Binswanger's disease
- Cerebral amyloid angiopathy
- Cranial arteritis
- Granulomatous angiitis
- Hypertensive encephalopathy
- Lacunar dementia
- Polyarteritis nodosa
- Vascular dementia (multi-infarct dementia)

Vitamin deficiency
- Folic acid
- Pellagra
- Vitamin B_{12}

Age-specific disorders

Assessing for dementia

When assessing a client for dementia, determine the answers to the following questions.

Memory function

• Does the client complain of memory loss or memory deficit?

• Does the client complain of forgetting the location of familiar objects or forgetting familiar names?

• How concerned is the client about memory loss?

• Who else has noticed their memory difficulties: family members, friends and employers?

• Has the client lost the ability to recall the content of a story, either read or heard?

• Does neuropsychiatric examination reveal evidence of memory deficits?

• Does the client remember telephone numbers, dates of important events, and names of close family members?

Attention and concentration function

• Does the client try to hide signs of impaired mentation?

• Does neuropsychiatric examination reveal evidence of concentration deficits?

• Can the client manage complex tasks?

Communication function

• Can the client hold a conversation or utter meaningful sounds?

• Can the client communicate in written form?

• Can the client communicate in only nonverbal gestures and motions?

Mood and affect

• Has the client exhibited lability of affect?

Orientation function

• Has the client become disoriented to time, person, and place?

• Can the client recognize individuals who are familiar to them (family: spouse, children)?

• Does the client know who they are, can they tell you their name?

Problem-solving function

• Can the client solve simple problems (know who to call if electricity goes off, if stove catches on fire what would they do, if they don't have any medication left in their bottle who do they call)?

Psychomotor function

• Can the client perform psychomotor tasks?

• Can the client walk unassisted, what type of assertive devices do they utilize?

Self-care function

• Is the client incontinent?

• Can the client bathe and manage hygiene measures independently?

• Can the client dress independently; how much help do they need to dress?

• Can the client prepare and eat meals independently?

• Can the client manage their home environment (such as cleaning, pets, and yard)?

Sleep and rest function

• Have the client's sleep and awake cycles changed?

• Does the client experience nighttime restlessness and agitation?

---

7. Provide the client with appropriate sensory or mobility aids, such as glasses, a hearing aid, or a walker.

8. Ensure that the client avoids complex tasks and activities involving the use of toxic materials or sharp implements that could accidentally cause injury. Encourage the client's participation in a music or exercise program.

9. Carefully monitor the client's mood and assess for suicidal feelings.

10. Avoid using restraints.

7. By improving the client's ability to see, hear, and walk, the nurse can help prevent dangerous situations and injury. Doing so also can increase the client's potential to be physically and socially active.

8. Providing simple, safe tasks helps to ensure success and avoids frustrating the client. Most clients find music and simple exercise programs enjoyable and physically stimulating.

9. Depression and suicidal feelings can occur with dementia.

10. Restraints impair mobility and promote skin breakdown. They also can increase client agitation and confusion, which may result in injury. Alternatives to restraints include bean bag cushions and foam cushion wedges.

NURSING DIAGNOSIS

Personal identity disturbance related to cognitive deficits

Nursing priority

Ensure the client's safety and the safety of others while continuing to meet the client's needs.

Patient outcome criteria

As treatment progresses, the client, family, or both should be able to:
• demonstrate feelings of security
• remain harm-free
• maintain some form of personal identification on them at all times.

Interventions

1. Make sure that the client is wearing an identification bracelet or name tag with his home address and with the unit location at all times.

2. Place a sign with the client's name in bold letters outside his room, preferably in a highly visible area such as on the wall opposite where the door swings open.

3. Check on the client frequently throughout the day. If possible, perform checks at 15-minute intervals.

4. When communicating with the client, gently reorient him to person, place, and time, and reassure him of his safety.

5. Have the client who is prone to wandering stay near the nurses' station and provide him with diversional activities.

6. Teach the client to check clocks, calendars, and watches frequently throughout the day.

7. Remind the client about mealtimes, bedtime, and group activities.

8. Ask family members to bring in recent photographs of the client; keep one in the client's chart and display any others in his room.

Rationales

1. Proper identification ensures that the client will be returned to the proper location if he should begin to wander.

2. Signs serve to remind the wandering or confused client where to return.

3. Frequent contact decreases the client's need to seek assistance and provides him with a sense of security and consistency. It also ensures the client's safety.

4. Reorienting (gently) and reassuring the client's safety serves as a reality test and helps decrease confusion.

5. Placing the client in a highly visible area enables more people to directly observe and interact with him, ensuring safety and decreasing isolation. Diversional activities help to structure the client's time and provide distraction from wandering.

6. This helps to keep the client oriented to time.

7. Some clients need to be reminded to attend to activities of daily living. Frequent reminders also help keep the client oriented and more responsive to structure.

8. A recent photograph can be used by staff or police to help identify a wandering client. Displaying the client's pictures keeps him self-oriented.

Age-specific disorders

NURSING DIAGNOSIS

Risk for violence, self-directed or directed at others, related to delusional beliefs, suspicion, inability to recognize persons and places, increased stress, or decreased coping skills

Nursing priority

Help prevent violence by minimizing sources of stress.

Patient outcome criteria

As treatment progresses, the client, family, or both should be able to:
• demonstrate a decrease or absence of threatening behavior towards others
• demonstrate improved behavioral control
• report feeling less agitated
• demonstrate an increased ability to tolerate frustration

Interventions

1. Assess the client's delusional beliefs in a supportive manner. Do not contradict or challenge the client with rational explanations.

2. Always approach the client from the front, using a slow, consistent, and calm manner. Remember to introduce yourself, and offer reassurance while you attempt to identify the client's needs. Respond nondefensively to any of the client's accusations, and avoid touching or crowding the agitated client.

3. Avoid taking the client into elevators, dining rooms, and other gathering areas.

4. Avoid talking to staff members about the client while in his presence. Do not tease or ridicule the client.

5. Should the client become verbally abusive, protect others from possible attack by having the client either calm down alone in his room or work alone or with a staff member until the behavior subsides.

6. Administer psychotropic medications as prescribed to decrease agitation. Monitor the client's vital signs and agitated behavior closely for positive and negative changes. Use overt agitation severity scale to evaluate the outcome of interventions.

7. Avoid restraining the agitated client.

Rationales

1. Assessing the client's state of mind enables the nurse to implement appropriate interventions. Trying to convince the client that delusional beliefs are unfounded will only increase agitation.

2. The client may interpret any gesture as an assault and may perceive large numbers of staff as an attack force. Both misconceptions can lead to violence. A calm, slow approach by the nurse can help prevent such an outbreak.

3. The client may feel as though personal space is being violated and become agitated.

4. The client may perceive whispers and information that he cannot decode because of brain dysfunction as a plot against him. Teasing decreases client self-esteem and may trigger emotional outbursts.

5. The demented client usually exhibits diminished impulse control. Verbal attacks may represent a response to internal sensations or to the situation rather than to any one person or thing in the environment. Calming the client usually relieves the situation.

6. Small doses of neuroleptic medications can help alleviate paranoid, belligerent behavior. Anxiolytic medications may reduce anxiety symptoms. Because drug metabolism is significantly altered in elderly persons, the client probably will require a smaller than usual dose.

7. Using restraints to control agitation can escalate the agitation, producing aggression and violent behavior and resulting in increased isolation, sensory deprivation, and decreased mobility.

Nursing diagnosis

Impaired physical mobility related to use of restraints due to problems with angry, aggressive outbursts

Nursing priority

Ensure the safety of the client and others while continuing to meet the client's need for food, fluids, toileting, and contact with others.

Patient outcome criteria

As treatment progresses, the client, family, or both should be able to:
• demonstrate no injury from or complications of physical immobility due to restraints
• demonstrate a reduction in the time spent in restraints and overall use of restraints.

Interventions

1. If the client must be restrained, make sure that adequate staff and the proper equipment are on hand to carry out the plan.

2. Make sure that the team leader communicates the plan of action and the specific roles of each staff member before attempting to restrain the client.

3. If the client is to be restrained in bed, make sure the client is placed face up on the bed with all four extremities attached securely to the bed frame. Secure one arm above the head and one arm at the client's side.

4. Assess circulation to all extremities immediately after applying restraints, then at least hourly until the restraints are removed. Make sure the client maintains good body alignment while restrained.

5. After the client has been restrained, check the fit of the cuffs. For a good fit, you should be able to insert only a fingertip between the cuff and the client's skin.

6. Provide the client with basic needs, including food, fluids, toileting, range-of-motion exercises, and skin care during the duration of restraint.

7. Offer the client emotional support and prescribed medications during the restraint period.

8. Establish clear behavioral expectations that the client must meet before the restraints can be removed.

9. Include several team members in the discussion to remove restraints and reintegrate the client into the milieu.

10. When the client meets all the established behavioral criteria and the decision to remove the restraints has been made, remove all the restraints at once.

Rationales

1. Adequate numbers of trained staff are required to preserve the therapeutic value of using restraints and to minimize the risk of injuring the client and others. If locking restraints are used, the nurse must ensure that the key is readily available in case of an emergency.

2. Poor communication or a poorly planned approach will increase the risk of injury to all involved.

3. Restraining the client in this position helps to lessen the client's fear and vulnerability and prevents the risk of suffocation. It also prevents the client from sitting up in bed. The client should be restrained only to the bed frame, never to the side rails, which could cause injury.

4. Restraints applied too tightly will impede the client's blood flow. Proper body alignment is necessary to prevent contractures and injury.

5. The client's cuffs may have been secured too tightly or loosely at first and may need to be adjusted.

6. A restrained client should never be denied the necessities of food, fluids, and toileting. Range-of-motion exercises and skin care are necessary to prevent injury and skin breakdown.

7. Support and contact with staff are important to help the client realize that restraints are therapeutic and not a punitive measure. Medication, particularly neuroleptic agents, can reduce the client's agitation and anxiety associated with being restrained. Music intervention may also promote a decrease in the client's agitation.

8. Setting expectations gives the client a sense of control and establishes clear, measurable criteria necessary for restraint removal.

9. This provides an opportunity for the staff to verbalize concerns and observations about the client's behavior. Staff members not included in decision-making processes may feel unsafe and unconsciously sabotage the client's freedom from restraint.

10. Removing only some of the restraints poses a serious danger to the client. For instance, the client who is partially restrained might attempt to get out of bed and fall. Also, removing only some of the restraints communicates lack of trust to the client.

Age-specific disorders

NURSING DIAGNOSIS

Altered thought processes related to memory loss, brain dysfunction, sleep deprivation, and conscious or unconscious conflicts

Nursing priority

Facilitate clear communication and provide a structured environment with reduced stimuli.

Patient outcome criteria

As treatment progresses, the client, family, or both should be able to:
• demonstrate optimum communication skills and an interest in the immediate environment
• verbalize an understanding of the disorder and its effects on the ability to think and communicate effectively.

Interventions

1. Using assessment tools and family reports, assess the client's cognitive impairment.

2. Help the client to maintain a consistent daily routine. Obtain information about the client's past routines from family members or the client's primary caregivers. Inquire about the client's daily schedule and the safety measures implemented in the home.

3. Introduce yourself to the client and explain your actions before providing care.

4. Face the client and make eye contact before speaking. Once you have the client's attention, speak slowly and clearly using simple, short sentences. Use various communication aids, such as verbal or written cues, gestures, and pictures.

5. Note the client's nonverbal attempts to communicate.

6. Provide adequate lighting and stimulation as well as seasonal orientation in the environment.

7. Learn the client's usual hiding places for personal belongings.

8. Respond to the client's view of reality with empathy and support. Do not contradict delusional beliefs.

Rationales

1. An initial assessment provides the nurse with a baseline against which to measure future behaviors.

2. A consistent routine can help to decrease the client's anxiety, reinforce old habits, and minimize memory deficits.

3. The client may have lost the ability to interpret stimuli accurately; for example, the client may misinterpret your touching while bathing as sexual advances. Careful explanations can help prevent this kind of confusion.

4. Because the client's comprehension and concentration abilities are probably greatly impaired, attention-getting and attention-maintaining techniques are necessary to ensure comprehension.

5. The client with language deficits may use nonverbal means, such as facial expressions and hand gestures, to communicate with others.

6. Adequate and appropriate environmental stimuli can help overcome the confusion and disorientation that may result from the client's social and physical isolation.

7. The client may be unable to distinguish personal belongings from those of others and may inadvertently take something belonging to someone else. Knowing the client's hiding places enables the nurse to locate such items.

8. The client's ability to evaluate reality may be severely impaired. Arguing will only decrease the client's trust in the nurse or increase agitation.

9. Closely monitor the client's response to medications.

9. Because drug metabolism and absorption are altered in elderly persons, the demented client can easily become delirious after drug administration.

Nursing diagnosis

Dressing or grooming self-care deficit related to cognitive impairment, weakness, memory impairment, and increased dependency needs

Nursing priority

Foster the highest level of client independence while promoting safety.

Patient outcome criterion

As treatment progresses, the client, family, or both should be able to:
• maintain adequate activity levels dependent on the stage of disease impact.

Interventions

1. Assess the client's ability to perform normal ADLs.

2. Give direct, one-step directions. Address the client by name and avoid the use of pronouns when referring to him. Repeat sentences, and discuss persons or objects that the client can readily observe.

3. When necessary, assist the client in performing ADLs, such as brushing his teeth or combing his hair. Provide frequent cues and encourage the client to complete the activities as independently as possible.

4. Provide the client with limited choices; for example, in the morning, let the client choose from two shirts.

5. Anticipate the client's refusal of nursing care.

Rationales

1. Establishing a performance baseline for ADLs enables the nurse to more accurately measure changes in behavior and dependence.

2. Communicating clearly and precisely increases the probability that the client will understand. Avoiding abstract topics can help maintain the client's attention.

3. Though the client may retain the ability to perform routine activities, such as brushing teeth and combing hair, he may require some help.

4. Being able to make choices can bolster self-esteem and increase the client's sense of control. Limiting the choices prevents the client from being overwhelmed, which can lead to agitation.

5. By refusing care, the client may be trying to achieve some sense of control. In addition, a suspicious client typically will refuse care.

Nursing diagnosis

Social isolation related to cognitive impairment, decreased social awareness, impaired language, multiple losses, lack of support systems, and depressed mood

Nursing priority

Help the client experience social connection with others.

Patient outcome criteria

As treatment progresses, the client, family, or both should be able to:
• report involvement in socialization groups and activities
• report increased interest and participation in their environmental surroundings.

Age-specific disorders

Interventions

1. Interview the client and family to assess the client's previous style of socializing and personality traits.

2. Provide the client with activities that stimulate multiple senses.

3. In a relaxed manner, encourage the client to participate in group activities such as singing; however, do not force participation.

4. Encourage the client and family to bring in personal articles, such as photographs, books, and clothing.

5. Regularly converse with the client using short, simple sentences and nonverbal aids such as smiling. Allow time for the client to respond.

6. Inform the client of current events, repeating information as needed. Avoid asking about facts, especially those related to recent events.

7. Assess the client's sense of hopefulness and offer reassurance.

8. Listen to the client's reminiscences and encourage or invite him to participate in a reminiscence group.

9. Encourage visits from the client's family and friends. Educate family members about the client's deficits.

Rationales

1. Knowing the client's past socialization patterns can help the nurse set realistic expectations for social activities.

2. Such activities stimulate not only the client's recall ability but also the senses of touch, sight, and smell; for example, you might hand the client an orange and ask him to identify it.

3. The client in the early stages of primary dementia of the Alzheimer's type may sense cognitive decline and feel ignored or left out of group activities.

4. Familiar objects may trigger the client's memory, facilitate conversation, and decrease feelings of isolation and alienation.

5. Conversation fosters a sense of connectedness. Patience on the nurse's part can prevent the client from feeling frustrated and increase interest in conversation.

6. Routine communication and repetition will not bore the client and can provide security. Because memory of recent events is typically affected first, the nurse should avoid asking the client to relay facts that he cannot remember.

7. A hopeful attitude contributes to the client's physical and mental well-being.

8. Sharing stories about the past can give the client a sense of connection with others, thereby decreasing feelings of isolation.

9. Regular visits from family and friends can decrease the client's feelings of isolation and enhance self-esteem. Knowing about the disorder can help family and friends to cope with the client's illness more effectively and sensitively.

Nursing diagnosis

Bowel incontinence and altered urinary elimination related to weak bladder or bowel muscle tone, confusion, disorientation, or lack of awareness of toileting needs

Nursing priority

Help the client maintain adequate elimination patterns and avoid bowel or urinary complications.

Patient outcome criterion

As treatment progresses, the client, family, or both should be able to:
• maintain adequate elimination patterns and skin integrity.

Interventions

1. Assess the client's usual elimination pattern and use of medications or enemas to maintain that pattern.

2. Check with the client about toileting needs every 2 hours during the day and every 4 hours or as needed at night.

3. Record the time, consistence, and amount of bowel movements.

4. Encourage the client to drink adequate amounts of fluid during the day, but limit fluid intake in the evening.

5. Encourage the client to eat a well-balanced diet that is rich in bulk and fiber and to exercise daily.

6. Administer prescribed stool softeners and monitor the client's response.

7. Be accepting and empathetic when the client is incontinent.

8. Help the client to maintain proper skin care.

9. Be aware of the client's use of nonverbal cues, such as searching or restlessness, that might indicate a toileting need.

Rationales

1. By reinforcing the client's usual elimination pattern, the nurse can help the client to remain aware of toileting needs and avoid confusion.

2. Establishing a regular pattern can help minimize incontinence.

3. The client may be unable to recall when he had a bowel movement or if he was constipated.

4. Adequate hydration prevents constipation and urinary tract infections.

5. Regular exercise, such as walking and stretching, and eating foods rich in bulk and fiber can help prevent constipation.

6. Because the client may have a history of laxative abuse, monitoring prescribed medications is essential. Psychotropic medications with anticholinergic effects can cause constipation.

7. By being empathetic, the nurse can minimize the client's embarrassment and preserve self-esteem.

8. Skin care can help preserve the client's skin integrity.

9. The client may be unable to recognize or articulate his toileting needs.

NURSING DIAGNOSIS

Sleep pattern disturbance related to disorientation, brain dysfunction, or reversed sleep-awake cycle

Nursing priority

Help the client achieve adequate sleep and rest.

Patient outcome criterion

As treatment progresses, the client, family, or both should be able to:
• maintain adequate rest and activity levels.

Interventions

1. Encourage the client to remain awake and active during the day, and provide short, scheduled rest periods.

2. Provide the client with a comfortable pillow, blankets, and loose-fitting bed clothes.

Rationales

1. By increasing his activity level, the client will be tired in the evening and better able to sleep. Short rest periods during the day help to refresh the client, thereby preventing daytime fatigue.

2. The client may be unable to verbalize that he is cold or in need of other comforts. Extra pillows may facilitate breathing, and comfortable bedding can help induce sleep.

Age-specific disorders

3. Assist the client to the toilet every 4 hours or more often if needed during the day. Limit the client's fluid intake in the evening.

4. Provide a night light, and keep the client's bathroom well lit.

3. Attending to the client's elimination needs during the day and limiting fluid intake in the evening can avert premature arousal.

4. Adequate night lighting helps keep the client oriented to the surroundings and provides security.

NURSING DIAGNOSIS

Altered nutrition, less than body requirements, related to chewing difficulties, smell and taste changes, memory loss, decreased coordination, and depressed mood

Nursing priority

Help the client maintain a nourishing diet.

Patient outcome criteria

As treatment progresses, the client, family, or both should be able to:
• maintain adequate nutritional intake and optimal body weight.

Interventions

1. Assess the client's food preferences, and collaborate with the dietitian in planning nutritious meals that include the client's favorite foods.

2. Prepare the client's food, but allow him to eat as independently as possible.

3. Tolerate the client's diminished table manners and unusual mixtures of food. If possible, avoid isolating the client when dining.

4. Assist the client with oral hygiene and denture care.

5. Weigh the client weekly.

Rationales

1. The client is more likely to eat foods that he enjoys and that are prepared to his liking.

2. Being self-sufficient to any degree can enhance client self-esteem.

3. As the client's dementia progresses, he will probably regress and forget learned social behavior.

4. Providing oral hygiene and denture care enables the client to chew more effectively and to improve dietary intake.

5. The nurse should monitor the client for weight fluctuations, which may indicate poor food or fluid intake.

NURSING DIAGNOSIS

Ineffective family coping related to the client's personality changes, behavior, and diminished functioning level

Nursing priority

Help the family adapt to the disorder's impact.

Patient outcome criteria

As treatment progresses the client, family, or both should be able to:
• verbalize an understanding of the disorder and its effects
• verbalize a knowledge of signs and symptoms of increasing agitation or anxiety
• demonstrate the ability to adapt to client and family role changes
• demonstrate appropriate coping and stress-management strategies and problem-solving abilities
• demonstrate or verbalize more adaptive coping skills.

Interventions

1. Determine the relationship and roles of family members before the onset of the client's illness.

2. Educate family members about dementia, including its effects on the client and the family.

3. Listen empathetically to family members' fears and concerns regarding the client's condition and help them to solve problems.

4. Encourage family visits and involvement with the client.

5. Encourage family members to seek support for themselves. Suggest appropriate support groups or respite care.

6. Encourage the family's use of stress-management strategies, such as relaxation and respite care.

7. If the client is returning home, explain to the family what is involved in home care and provide referrals for community resources such as home health nursing.

Rationales

1. Establishing a baseline concerning the family's relationships and roles enables the nurse to more accurately determine the disorder's impact on the family and to implement appropriate interventions.

2. Family members can become frustrated or impatient when the client ceases to recognize them or becomes belligerent. By teaching the family about the disorder, the nurse can help prevent such reactions.

3. As roles shift, family members may be overwhelmed by increased responsibilities, and their problem-solving abilities can be compromised.

4. Participating in care can make the family feel useful and can strengthen family relationship and attachment.

5. Sharing their fears and concerns with other families in similar circumstances can help the client's family feel less alone and devastated.

6. By managing stress and improving their sense of well-being, family members can make themselves more available to the client.

7. The family may overestimate its ability to care for the client. Resource referrals can enable the family to obtain assistance such as a home health nurse.

NURSING DIAGNOSIS

Impaired home maintenance management related to cognitive deficits and increased dependency

Nursing priority

Help the client's family adapt to interpersonal and environmental changes, thereby facilitating care and maximizing the client's independence.

Patient outcome criteria

As treatment progresses, the client, family, or both should be able to:
• identify how specific cognitive deficits are impacting on the client's ability to maintain themselves in their home
• identify specific home- and community-based resources to assist the client and family to maintain the client in the home environment
• determine when it is time to consider another environment for care of the client.

Interventions

1. Assess the client's capabilities and the degree of supervision needed.

2. Educate the family members about the client's disorder. Advise them of techniques for coping with problem behaviors, such as wandering, hoarding, delusions, and agitation.

Rationales

1. Such assessment can help the nurse determine the client's needs and ensure both the client's and family's safety.

2. Proper teaching can help the family feel more capable of handling difficult behaviors and decrease their anxiety.

3. Recommend environmental modifications that accommodate the client's needs.

4. Work with the doctor to simplify the client's medication regimen.

5. Support the family's efforts at caring for the client, and encourage their involvement in respite care and Alzheimer's support groups.

3. Environmental modifications, such as moving the client's bedroom to the first level of the house and placing "safety locks" on doors and closets, can help to maintain the client's safety and facilitate the family's caregiving responsibilities.

4. A simplified medication regimen is less burdensome to the family and helps to ensure client compliance.

5. A well-developed network of professional and community resources can help caregivers to care for the client and manage stress more effectively.

DISCHARGE CRITERIA

Nursing documentation indicates that the client:
• has responded positively to treatment and care. It also indicates that the family:
• has verbalized an understanding of the client's diagnosis, treatment, and expected outcome
• is aware of the client's problematic behaviors and how to manage them
• has demonstrated an ability to interact with the client and to meet the client's needs
• has been referred to appropriate family and community resources
• has demonstrated the ability to identify follow-up needs
• has verbalized an understanding of the risks involved in client care and of how to maintain environmental safety
• understands when, why, and how to contact the appropriate health care professional in case of an emergency.

SELECTED REFERENCES

AHCPR. *Recognition and Initial Assessment of Alzheimer's Disease and Related Dementias: Clinical Practice Guideline*, vol. 19. Washington, D.C.: U.S. Department of Health and Human Services, 1996.

Borson, S., and Baskind, M.A. "Clinical Features and Pharmacologic Treatment for Behavioral Symptoms of Alzheimer's Disease," *Neurology* 48 (Suppl 6):S17-24, 1997.

Diagnostic and Statistical Manual of Mental Disorders, 4th ed. Washington, D.C.: American Psychiatric Association, 1994.

Folstein, M.F., et al. "Mini-Mental State: A Practical Method for Grading the Cognitive State of Patients for the Clinician," *Journal of Psychiatric Research* 12:189-98, 1975.

Franks, A.S., and Rawls, W.N. "Alzheimer's Disease: Clinical Features and Pharmacologic Management," *The American Journal of Managed Care* 4(4):595-604, 1998.

Peskind, E. "Neurobiology of Alzheimer's Disease," *Journal of Clinical Psychiatry* 57(Suppl 14):5-8, 1996.

Practice Guideline for the Treatment of Patients with Alzheimer's Disease and other Dementias of Late Life. Washington, D.C.: American Psychiatric Association, 1997.

Small, G.W., et al. "Diagnosis and Treatment of Alzheimer's Diseases and Related Disorders," *JAMA* 278:1363-71, 1997.

Stehman, J.M., et al. *Handbook of Dementia Care*. Baltimore: Johns Hopkins University Press, 1996.

Stewart, W.F., et al. "Risk of Alzheimer's Disease and Duration of NSAID," *Neurology* 48:626-32, 1997.

Taviot, P., et al. "Treating Alzheimer's Disease: Pharmacologic Options Now and in the Near Future," *Postgraduate Medicine* 101(6):73-76, 81, 84, 1997.

Trobe, J.D., et al. "Crashes and Violations among Drivers with Alzheimer's Disease," *Archives of Neurology* 53:411-16, 1996.

Yudofsky, S.C., and Hales, R.E. *Textbook of Neuropsychiatry*. Washington, D.C.: American Psychiatric Association, 1997.

Part 8

Addiction disorders

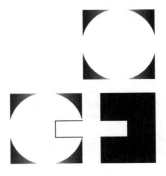

Alcohol-related disorders

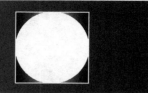

DSM-IV classifications
Alcohol use disorders
303.90 Alcohol dependence
305.00 Alcohol abuse
Alcohol-induced disorders
303.00 Alcohol intoxication
291.8 Alcohol withdrawal
291.0 Alcohol intoxication, with delirium
291.0 Alcohol withdrawal, with delirium
291.1 Alcohol-induced persisting amnestic disorder
291.x Alcohol-induced psychotic disorder
291.5 Alcohol-induced psychotic disorder, with delusions
291.3 Alcohol-induced psychotic disorder, with hallucinations
291.8 Alcohol-induced mood disorder
291.8 Alcohol-induced anxiety disorder
291.9 Alcohol-induced sleep disorder
291.9 Alcohol-related disorder not otherwise specified

Psychiatric nursing diagnostic class
Substance abuse

INTRODUCTION

Alcohol dependence is a common disorder that is progressive, debilitating, and often fatal. Individuals suffering from alcohol dependence experience recurring and persistent overpowering urges to drink. They continue to drink in spite of the psychophysiologic consequences that eventually produce irreversible organ damage. Additionally, these individuals and their families suffer serious personal, occupational, and financial problems. Once the pattern of compulsive use is established, individuals with alcohol dependence spend substantial time thinking about, obtaining, and consuming alcoholic beverages. (See *Alcohol screening test.*)

Alcohol abuse is a maladaptive pattern of alcohol use manifested by recurrent psychophysiologic, occupational, financial, and often legal consequences. Individuals with alcohol abuse often participate in physically hazardous situations while impaired, such as driving, operating potentially dangerous equipment, diving from high places, or swimming.

Alcohol intoxication is characterized by maladaptive behavioral or psychological changes that develop during or after the ingestion of alcohol. These changes are accompanied by slurred speech, incoordination, unsteady gait, nystagmus, impairment in attention or memory, stupor, or coma. (See *Effects of alcohol intake on blood alcohol levels and behavioral manifestations in nontolerant drinker.*)

Alcohol withdrawal is marked by a characteristic withdrawal syndrome that develops after cessation or reduction of daily, heavy, or prolonged alcohol ingestion. The syndrome includes some or all of the following symptoms: autonomic hyperactivity; increased tremor of the

Alcohol screening test

Several assessment tools, such as the **C**utting down alcohol consumption, **A**nnoyance by criticism of drinking, **G**uilty feelings associated with alcohol use, and **E**ye-openers, or early morning drinking (CAGE,1974), Michigan Alcoholism Screening Test (MAST,1971), and its shorter version, SMAST (1975), can help screen and identify the high-risk drinker who is abusing alcohol or is in danger of becoming dependent on alcohol. It is important in these hectic days to choose an assessment tool that has been tested in a variety of clinical settings and is "user friendly" and portable. We have chosen to instruct you on the CAGE for all of those reasons. To use this test, ask your client the following questions. For each positive response, score one point and then total the points. Generally, a score of two or more points indicates an individual who needs further evaluation of their drinking and definitive assessment for possible alcohol withdrawal syndrome.

Questions
1. Have you ever felt you should *cut down* on your drinking?
Yes   No

2. Have people *annoyed* you by criticizing your drinking?
Yes   No

3. Have you ever felt bad or *guilty* about your drinking?
Yes   No

4. Have you ever had a drink first thing in the morning to steady your nerves, get rid of a hangover *(eye-opener)*, or get your day started?   Yes   No

Scoring: Two or more positive answers to these questions strongly suggest alcohol dependence, physical dependence in relation to their inability to cut down on drinking, and the need for an awakening drink. Additional exploration should include the quantity of the alcohol and the frequency and in what circumstance do they drink. It is important to know if they think that they have experienced some form of alcohol withdrawal any time during a period of reduced drinking or abstinence.

Adapted with permission from Mayfield, D., et al. "The CAGE Questionnaire: Validation of a New Alcoholism Screening Instrument," *American Journal of Psychiatry* 131:1121, 1974.

Effects of alcohol intake on blood alcohol levels and behavioral manifestations in nontolerant drinker

Alcohol intake	Blood alcohol levels	Behavioral manifestations
1 to 2 drinks	0.05 mg %	• Mood and behavioral changes, impaired judgment
5 to 6 drinks	0.10 mg%	• Legal level of intoxication (in most states), slowed psychomotor action response time; clumsy voluntary motor action
10 to 12 drinks	0.20 mg%	• Depressed motor function area of cerebral cortex, ataxia and staggering, emotional lability
15 to 18 drinks	0.30 mg%	• Confusion, marked difficulty in thinking and problem solving, possible stupor
20 to 24 drinks	0.40 mg %	• Coma, possible respiratory depression
25 to 30 drinks	0.50 mg%	• Possible arrhythmias, death from respiratory depression due to brainstem depression

extremities; insomnia; nausea; vomiting; visual, tactile, or auditory hallucinations or illusions; psychomotor agitation; anxiety; and possibly seizure activity. The symptoms cause clinical distress or impairment in occupational, social, and behavioral functioning. Alcohol withdrawal is a syndrome with discrete and identifiable stages. An individual in stage 3 (severe withdrawal, often referred to as delirium tremens [DTs]) requires emergency medical management and an aggressive, collaborative treatment plan to reduce physiologic distress. (See *ANA standards of addictions nursing practice,* page 182.)

Alcohol-related disorder not otherwise specified is for disorders associated with the use of alcohol that do not meet the criteria for any other alcohol-related or alcohol-induced disorder.

Etiology and precipitating factors

Alcohol addiction and dependence have numerous biologic and psychological components. Neurochemical, neurophysiologic, and psychopharmacologic mechanisms common to alcohol and other drug addiction have been established. Although genetic evidence indicates that there is a familial predisposition to alcohol dependence, a common genetic marker for addiction or dependence has not yet been identified.

Neurobiologic studies suggest that alcohol and other drugs reinforce dependence by stimulating a "brain reward" mechanism located in the medial forebrain. This region is apparently served by axons associated with the mesotelencephalic dopamine system. Intoxication with alcohol or other drugs increases extracellular dopamine levels; the resulting dopamine related "high" becomes the reinforcement mechanism. The brain adjusts to the increased dopamine levels and causes a craving for increased amounts of the stimulant substance to reproduce the original pleasurable effect. In broad outline, this process is the engine that drives the addiction.

Alcohol dependence and abuse is also influenced by the individual's temperament and self-image as well as by environmental factors, such as family dynamics and peer pressures. Psychological theories suggest that some individuals are born with personality traits that render them increasingly susceptible to substance abuse, the so-called "addictive personality." Research is focusing on the behavioral characteristics of children and adolescents that predispose to substance abuse. Conduct disorders in children may be important behavioral risk factors for later substance abuse disorders. Hyperactivity has also been linked to alcohol and drug abuse. Recent evidence suggests that hyperactive boys are more likely to experience substance dependence or abuse in early adulthood.

Potential complications

Chronic alcohol use can cause various physiologic impairments, including peripheral neuropathy, Wernicke's encephalopathy, Korsakoff's syndrome, alcoholic car-

Addiction disorders

ANA standards of addictions nursing practice

In 1988, the American Nurses Association (ANA), with consultation from nurses working in the addiction field, developed a set of standards to be used when caring for clients who are addicted to alcohol and other drugs. These standards provide a guide for the practice of addictions nursing.

Standard I. Theory

The nurse uses appropriate knowledge from nursing theory and related disciplines in the practice of addictions nursing.

Standard II. Data collection

Data collection is continual and systematic and is communicated to the treatment team throughout each phase of the nursing process.

Standard III. Diagnosis

The nurse uses nursing diagnoses congruent with accepted nursing and interprofessional classification systems of addictions and associated physiologic and psychological disorders to express conclusions supported by data obtained through the nursing process.

Standard IV. Planning

The nurse establishes a plan of care for the client that is based upon nursing diagnoses, addresses specific goals, defines expected outcomes, and delineates nursing actions unique to each client's needs.

Standard V. Intervention

The nurse implements actions independently and/or in collaboration with peers, members of other disciplines, and clients in prevention, intervention, and rehabilitation phases of the care of clients with health problems related to problems of abuse and addiction.

Standard V-A. Intervention: Therapeutic alliance

The nurse uses the "therapeutic self" to establish a relationship with clients and to structure nursing interventions to help clients develop awareness, coping skills, and behavior changes that promote health.

Standard V-B. Intervention: Education

The nurse educates clients and communities to help them prevent and/or correct actual or potential health problems related to patterns of abuse and addiction.

Standard V-C. Intervention: Self-help groups

The nurse uses knowledge and philosophy of self-help groups to assist clients in learning new ways to address stress, maintain self-control or sobriety, and integrate healthy coping behaviors into their lifestyle.

Standard V-D. Intervention: Pharmacological therapies

The nurse applies knowledge of pharmacologic principles in the nursing process.

Standard V-E. Intervention: Therapeutic environment

The nurse provides structures and maintains a therapeutic environment in collaboration with the individual, family, and other professionals.

Standard V-F. Intervention: Counseling

The nurse uses therapeutic communication in interactions with the client to address issues related to patterns of abuse and addiction.

Standard VI. Evaluation

The nurse evaluates the responses of the client and revised nursing diagnoses, interventions, and the treatment plan accordingly.

Standard VII. Ethical care

The nurse's decisions and activities on behalf of clients are in keeping with professional codes of ethics and in accord with legal statutes.

Standard VIII. Quality assurance

The nurse participates in peer review and other staff evaluation and quality assurance processes to ensure that clients with abuse and addiction receive quality care.

Standard IX. Continuing education

The nurse assumes responsibility for his or her continuing education and professional development and contributes to the professional growth of others who work with or are learning about persons with abuse and addiction problems.

Standard X. Interdisciplinary collaboration

The nurse collaborates with the interdisciplinary treatment team and consults with other health care providers in assessing, planning, implementing, and evaluating programs and other activities related to addictions nursing.

Standard XI. Use of community health systems

The nurse participates with other members of the community in assessing, planning, implementing, and evaluating community health services that attend to primary, secondary, and tertiary prevention of addictions.

Standard XII. Research

The nurse contributes to the nursing care of clients with addictions and the addictions area of practice through innovations in theory and practice and participation in research, and communicates these contributions.

From *Standards of Addictions Nursing Practice with Selected Diagnoses and Criteria.* Washington, D.C.: American Nurses Association, 1988. Used with permission.

diomyopathy, esophagitis, esophageal varices, gastritis, pancreatitis, diabetes secondary to pancreatitis, alcoholic hepatitis, cirrhosis of the liver, cancer secondary to cirrhosis, and blood dyscrasias. Infants born to alcoholic women are at high risk for fetal alcohol syndrome. (For a more complete list of complications, see *Physiologic effects related to alcohol abuse,* page 184.)

ASSESSMENT GUIDELINES
Nursing history (functional health pattern findings)
Health perception–health management pattern
- Complaints of general pain and discomfort
- Headaches
- Distorted pain perception
- Depression

Nutritional-metabolic pattern
- Inadequate food intake
- Diminished taste
- Lack of interest in food
- Abdominal pain
- Poor muscle tone or skin turgor
- Weight loss or gain
- Pale mucous membranes

Elimination pattern
- Constipation or diarrhea
- Nausea and vomiting
- GI bleeding

Activity-exercise pattern
- Restlessness
- Difficulty performing normal daily activities
- Activity intolerance

Sleep-rest pattern
- Difficulty falling asleep
- Not feeling rested
- Sleep pattern reversal
- Early awakening
- Frequent nighttime awakenings
- Restlessness during sleep

Cognitive-perceptual pattern
- Disorientation about people, places, or time
- Confusion
- Slow information processing
- Slow and slurred speech
- Anxiety
- Poor short-term memory
- Bizarre thinking
- Exaggerated emotional responses

Self-perception–self-concept pattern
- Feelings of inadequacy, guilt, or shame
- Feelings of grandiosity
- Decreased self-esteem
- Derogatory statements about self
- Self-destructive behaviors

Role-relationship pattern
- Difficulty with intimacy
- Withdrawal from social contact
- Ineffective family communication
- Dysfunctional family roles
- Inability to express feelings
- Concerns about how family, friends, and coworkers will respond to the disorder

Sexual-reproductive pattern
- Actual or perceived limited sexual ability
- Decreased libido
- Lack of sexual satisfaction
- Disturbances in sexual relationships

Coping–stress tolerance pattern
- Withdrawal from relationships
- Tension, fearfulness, or nervousness
- Impaired ability to concentrate
- Feelings of helplessness or hopelessness
- Feeling that life is beyond personal control
- Financial stresses
- Need for attention, help, and reassurance

Value-belief pattern
- Feelings of hopelessness about addiction and treatment
- Desire to become more or less involved in spirituality or religion
- Lack of future plans
- Inability to believe in anything or anyone

Physical findings
Cardiovascular
- Arrhythmias
- Hypertension or hypotension
- Increased or irregular heart rate
- Shortness of breath

Respiratory
- Asymmetrical chest movements
- Diminished or loud breath sounds
- Elevated temperature
- Hypoxia
- Respiratory depression
- Tachypnea, especially during alcohol withdrawal

Gastrointestinal
- Ascites
- Diarrhea
- Hematemesis
- Hepatic pain
- Jaundice
- Esophageal mucosa inflammation
- Nausea and vomiting
- Esophageal varices

Genitourinary
- Sexual dysfunction
- Frequent urination

Physiologic effects related to alcohol abuse

Awareness of the complications of alcohol abuse is important in identifying, diagnosing, and treating the comorbid health problems in the individual with alcohol-related disorders.

Cardiovascular complications
- Alcoholic cardiomyopathy
- Increased systolic and pulse pressure
- Tissue damage, weakened heart muscle, and heart failure

Gastrointestinal complications
- Abdominal distention, pain, belching, and hematemesis
- Acute and chronic pancreatitis
- Alcoholic hepatitis leading to cirrhosis
- Cancer of the esophagus, liver, or pancreas
- Esophageal varices, hemorrhoids, and ascites
- Gastritis, colitis, and enteritis
- Gastric or duodenal ulcers
- Gastrointestinal malabsorption
- Hepatorenal syndrome
- Swollen, enlarged fatty liver

Genitourinary complications
- Hypogonadism, hypoandrogenization, hyperestrogenization in men
- Increased urinary excretion of potassium and magnesium (results in hypomagnesemia, hypokalemia)
- Infertility, decreased menstruation
- Prostate gland enlargement, leading to prostatitis and interference with urination
- Prostate cancer
- Sexual dysfunction (decreased libido, sexual performance decreased, and impotency)

Metabolic complications
- Hypoglycemia, hyperlipidemia, hyperuricemia
- Ketoacidosis
- Osteoporosis

Hematologic complications
- Abnormal red blood cells, white blood cells, and platelets
- Anemia and increased risk of infection
- Bleeding tendencies, increased bruising, and decreased clotting time
- Mineral and vitamin deficiencies (folate, iron, phosphate, thiamine)

Neurologic complications
- Wernicke-Korsakoff syndrome, Marchiafava-Bignami disease, cerebellar degeneration
- Peripheral neuropathy, polyneuropathy
- Seizures
- Sleep disturbances
- Stroke (increased risk of hemorrhagic stroke)

Respiratory complications
- Cancer of the oropharynx
- Impaired diffusion, chronic obstructive pulmonary disease, infection, and tuberculosis
- Respiratory depression causing decreased respiratory rate and cough reflex and increased susceptibility to infection and trauma

Trauma-related complications
- Burns, smoke inhalation injuries
- Injuries from motor vehicle crashes and falls

Musculoskeletal
- Ataxia
- Evidence of healed or new fractures
- Muscle aches, pains, or tension
- Trembling, shaking, or twitching

Neurologic
- Confabulation
- Confusion
- Impaired judgment
- Labile affect
- Memory deficits
- Sleep disturbances (such as insomnia or difficulty falling or remaining asleep)
- Seizures (most commonly tonic-clonic)

Integumentary
- Bruises
- Hematomas
- Jaundice
- Surface blood vessel vasodilation
- Petechiae

Psychological
- Anger
- Depression
- Manipulative behavior
- Restlessness
- Hostility or irritability
- Violence
- Mood swings

●▮▮▮◀ CLINICAL PATHWAY

Alcohol or drug dependence with rehabilitation

Plan	Day 1–3	Day 4 to 7	Day 8 to 15
Tests	• Chemistry 7 • Chemistry 12 • Complete blood count with differential • Rapid plasma reagin • Hepatitis profile • Urine drug screen • Urinalysis • Electrocardiogram • Urine test for pregnancy • Alcohol level	• As indicated	• As indicated
Treatments	• Chemical dependency groups • Occupational therapy groups • Group therapy	• Same as previous day	• Same as previous day
Medications	• Detoxification protocol	• As indicated	• As indicated
Consultations	• Consider: GYN if appropriate		
Interventions	• Vital signs per detoxification protocol • Monitor signs and symptoms of withdrawal. • Weight • Biological-psychological assessment q shift • Assess need for seizure precautions; implement protocol if indicated. • Set mutual goals for accomplishing activities of daily living. • Monitor hydration and elimination patterns • Suicide assessment • 1:1 contact per shift • Refer to chaplain for spiritual support.	• Same as previous day	• Same as previous day
Chemical dependency counselor	• Chemical dependency assessment	• Same as previous day	• Same as previous day
Diet	• Regular	• Regular	• Regular
Activity and safety	• Close side rails if delirium tremens	• Out to Narcotics Anonymous (NA) or Alcoholics Anonymous (AA) meetings with staff • To Psychiatric floor	• Same as previous day
Teaching	• Review program rules. • Begin relapse book. • Begin daily journal.	• Reinforce teaching.	• Reinforce teaching.
Discharge planning	• Contact referral source for update on patient status. • Make aftercare assessment.	• Explore discharge plans with patient. • Contact referral source. • Make aftercare plan.	• Same as previous day

Addiction disorders

Authored by Molly Metzler RN, BSN for Nanticoke Health Services. Licensed by The Center for Case Management, South Natick, Mass. Used with permission.

NURSING DIAGNOSIS

Sensory-perceptual alteration (visual, auditory, or tactile) related to alcohol consumption

Nursing priority

Help the client achieve detoxification and regain and maintain a normal level of consciousness.

Patient outcome criteria

As treatment progresses, the client, family, or both should be able to:
• remain safe and harm-free during the acute phase of alcohol withdrawal
• report diminished signs and symptoms of acute alcohol withdrawal.

Interventions

1. Assess the client's degree of alcohol intoxication and determine the withdrawal stage.

2. Observe the client's behavioral responses, especially noting any signs of disorientation, confusion, irritability, or sleeplessness.

3. Observe and document any auditory, visual, or tactile hallucinations exhibited by the client.

4. Provide a quiet, safe environment for the client.

5. Gently orient the client to people, place, and time. Do not argue or insist that the individual's answers are wrong. Inquire about how safe he feels in the place that he reports being; for example, if he reports ("I'm at home," the nurse may respond "Do you feel safe there?" and may remind him by telling him "Would you be surprised to learn that you are in the hospital and we are going to keep you safe?"

6. Teach the client about alcohol withdrawal symptoms.

Rationales

1. Determining the degree of intoxication and the withdrawal stage provides the nurse with baseline data for instituting appropriate nursing interventions for established medical protocols.

2. Sleep deprivation may aggravate disorientation and confusion. Worsening behavioral symptoms may indicate impending alcohol withdrawal syndrome (DTs) or possibly withdrawal from other drugs.

3. Hallucinations may occur during alcohol detoxification. Visual hallucinations commonly involve seeing insects or animals; tactile hallucinations involve feeling bugs crawling over the body; and auditory hallucinations involve hearing voices.

4. Decreasing environmental stimuli during the hyperactive stage of detoxification can help reduce the client's delirium. The nurse may need to institute safety precautions to protect the client from self-harm caused by a distorted sense of reality.

5. Orientation can help reduce the client's confusion and misinterpretation of external stimuli. Arguing or insisting that the client remembers his location will only increase his agitation. Frequent probing and asking orientation questions of an individual with alcohol-related delirium may precipitate further escalation of agitation and promote aggressive behavior (if they are not delirious).

6. Understanding the relationship between alcohol use and withdrawal symptoms may increase the client's readiness to continue with further treatment and enter alcohol rehabilitation after detoxification treatment is completed.

NURSING DIAGNOSIS

Sleep pattern disturbance related to alcohol abuse and decreased rapid eye movement (REM) sleep cycle

Nursing priority

Help the client recognize the relationship between alcohol use and sleep disturbance and to improve the client's sleep patterns.

Patient outcome criteria

As treatment progresses, the client, family, or both should be able to:
• describe the impact of alcohol ingestion on the sleep cycle
• use sleep hygiene interventions to facilitate sleep
• report an improved sleep pattern.

Interventions

1. Monitor the client's sleeping patterns and determine the type of sleep disturbance.

2. Establish a daily activity and rest schedule for the client.

3. Recommend appropriate dietary changes such as the elimination of caffeine.

4. Provide the client with a quiet, darkened room for sleeping.

5. Teach the client to use muscle relaxation techniques at bedtime.

Rationales

1. Knowing the precise sleep disturbance enables the nurse to plan appropriate sleep-inducing interventions.

2. Activity during the day, with rest but not naps, and a regular structured bedtime routine can help the client return to normal sleep patterns.

3. Rebound insomnia can occur during alcohol withdrawal, but extended abstinence usually resolves the problem. Coffee and other caffeine beverages can interfere with REM sleep.

4. A quiet environment reduces stimuli and induces relaxation; a darkened room can help induce sleep.

5. Reducing muscle tension can help alleviate anxiety and promote sleep.

NURSING DIAGNOSIS

Altered family processes related to role disruptions caused by the client's alcohol-related disorder

Nursing priority

Help the family recognize their own needs for information and support and to learn to use available resources.

Patient outcome criteria

As treatment progresses, the client, family, or both should be able to:
• report improved communication among family members
• acknowledge and discuss the impact of alcohol-related disorder on each family member
• actively participate in follow-up, family-focused care (Al-Anon, Al-Ateen, sibling group therapy, marriage therapy, or family therapy).

Addiction disorders

Interventions

1. Assess the interaction styles, communication patterns, and role behaviors within the family.

2. Assess the learning needs of family members.

3. Teach the family about the parts they may be playing in the client's alcohol-related disorder.

4. Encourage the family members to communicate openly and honestly with each other.

5. Inform the family about appropriate resources and programs.

Rationales

1. Understanding how the family functions can help the nurse to develop appropriate family interventions.

2. Family members usually need to be educated about alcohol-related disorders. In addition to teaching the family about the physiologic and psychological effects of alcohol abuse, the nurse should discuss alcohol-related disorder as a family disorder.

3. Family members may be unaware of the ways in which they contribute to the client's disorder. By informing them of their roles, the nurse can help family members adopt new, positive behaviors.

4. Communication is essential as changes occur in the family system. Learning to communicate openly is a slow process requiring long-term family therapy.

5. Groups such as Al-Anon, Al-Ateen, and Adult Children of Alcoholics provide support for maintaining family integrity and functioning.

NURSING DIAGNOSIS

Altered self-image related to unmet expectations, coping difficulties, guilt, and shame about alcohol abuse

Nursing priority

Help the client develop and maintain an enhanced self-concept.

Patient outcome criteria

As treatment progresses, the client, family, or both should be able to:
• demonstrate increased self-esteem and confidence
• recognize dependency needs and engage in health promoting and growth producing activities to meet them.

Interventions

1. Establish a trusting relationship with the client.

2. Assess the client's suicide risk.

3. Continually encourage the client to express their feelings.

4. Encourage the client to accept responsibility for managing their alcohol-related disorder.

Rationales

1. Establishing a trusting relationship with the client fosters a secure environment in which the client can discuss feelings of denial, shame, guilt, and helplessness. Such open discussions enable the nurse to help the client to develop a positive self-image.

2. Depression commonly accompanies alcohol intoxication and withdrawal. By assessing the client's suicide risk, the nurse institutes necessary measures to help prevent any self-harm to the client.

3. Ongoing expression of feelings can help the client to recognize what triggers certain feelings and ultimately to develop more constructive ways of handling them.

4. Assuming responsibility in managing their chronic disorder is an important step in developing self-regulation, self-responsibility, and a positive self-concept.

5. Help the client to explore and accept both positive and negative traits and behaviors.

6. Reinforce the client's positive efforts to cope with feelings.

7. Inform the client of support groups and programs.

5. A positive self-concept is based on a realistic appraisal and acceptance of one's strengths and weaknesses.

6. The nurse's reinforcement of positive behavior changes can help the client to recognize and value them.

7. Peer encouragement in group settings can enhance self-concept and support the client's efforts to remain sober. Support groups include Alcoholics Anonymous, Women for Sobriety, Men for Sobriety, Moderation Management Rational Recovery, Secular Organization for Sobriety/Save Our Selves (SOS), Self Management and Recovery Training (SMART).

Nursing diagnosis

Anxiety related to alcohol withdrawal, real or perceived threats to physical safety, or poor self-concept

Nursing priority

Help the client recognize anxiety and use adaptive coping mechanisms to cope with stress.

Patient outcome criteria

As treatment progresses, the client, family, or both should be able to:
• recognize anxiety and use adaptive coping mechanisms to decrease anxiety without resorting to alcohol (or other drugs)
• recognize the need for support, seek assistance, and use appropriate resources.

Interventions

1. Assess the client's anxiety level and coping skills.

2. Convey a sense of acceptance toward the client and a willingness to assist them toward a plan for recovery.

3. Encourage the client to talk about his anxious feelings.

4. Help the client to learn adaptive coping strategies that reduce anxiety, such as using relaxation techniques and verbalizing concerns.

5. Administer prescribed medications.

Rationales

1. During alcohol withdrawal, the client usually experiences moderate to severe anxiety. The nurse must be prepared to handle the client's anxious behavior.

2. The client probably will detect, be sensitive to, and respond defensively to condescending or biased attitudes or behaviors. Avoiding or controlling these attitudes and behaviors allows the nurse to diminish the client's anxiety and promote a trusting relationship.

3. Many clients with alcohol-related disorders fear being dependent or out of control. Being able to talk about this anxiety can help relieve it.

4. Learning new ways to cope with anxiety can encourage the client to accept personal responsibility for making and maintaining positive changes.

5. Benzodiazepines (such as lorazepam [Ativan], oxazepam [Serax], and chlordiazepoxide [Librium]) are typically used during acute alcohol withdrawal to diminish the autonomic hyperarousal state, reduce hyperactivity, and promote the client's sense of being in control.

Addiction disorders

6. Teach the client stress management techniques, including cognitive and relaxation techniques.	**6.** Stress management training involves not only muscle relaxation but also cognitive restructuring, problem solving, and real-life rehearsals. Successful stress management can help the client regain control and increase self-esteem.

NURSING DIAGNOSIS

Potential for injury related to alcohol withdrawal, seizures, depression, or suicidal ideation

Nursing priority

Prevent the client from self-injury and injury to others.

Patient outcome criteria

As treatment progresses, the client, family, or both should be able to:
• remain harm-free and injury-free, from suicidal behavior or seizures
• report a decrease in seizure activity
• report a decrease in suicidal ideation and behavior.

Interventions

1. Assess the client's alcohol withdrawal stage.

2. Monitor and document any seizures the client may experience.

3. Provide a safe environment for the client

4. Assess the client's suicide risk.

Rationales

1. Early assessment enables the nurse to implement appropriate interventions that may halt symptom progression and prevent injury.

2. Seizures in a client with no history of seizures usually stop spontaneously and require only symptomatic treatment. Generalized (tonic-clonic) seizures are most common.

3. Sensory-perceptual alterations, such as hallucinations, lack of coordination, confusion, and disorientation, can result in potentially dangerous behavior due to an incorrect appraisal of the situation. A client who is anxious and frightened may also become agitated and combative, striking out at property, other individuals, and especially their health care provider.

4. During intoxication and/or alcohol withdrawal, the client may become depressed and develop thoughts of suicide. Often clients who are depressed and intoxicated will attempt suicide.

NURSING DIAGNOSIS

Altered nutrition: less than body requirements, related to the client's poor dietary intake while consuming alcohol, the effects of chronic alcohol intake on the client's digestive organs, and the interference of alcohol in absorption and metabolism of nutrients

Nursing priority

Help the client change dietary patterns and improve nutrition.

Patient outcome criteria

As treatment progresses, the client, family, or both should be able to:
• verbalize an awareness that alcohol ingestion can reduce dietary intake and alter nutrition
• report an increased ability to eat healthy foods with decreased gastrointestinal symptoms
• demonstrate behavioral and lifestyle changes that will help maintain appropriate nutrition.

Interventions

1. Evaluate the presence and quality of the client's bowel sounds and note any signs of abdominal distention.

2. Assess the client for nausea, vomiting, and diarrhea.

3. Provide fluid along with frequent, small, and easily digested meals and snacks.

4. Provide the client with a protein-rich diet, ensuring that at least half of the daily calories come from carbohydrates.

5. Add vitamins and thiamine to the client's diet as needed.

Rationales

1. Irritated gastric mucosa may result in nausea and hyperactive bowel sounds. Early detection of gastric irritation can prevent unnecessary nausea and vomiting.

2. These symptoms typically occur early during alcohol withdrawal and may interfere with achieving adequate nutrition.

3. Such meals and snacks can limit gastric distress and enhance the client's dietary intake. As the client's appetite and food tolerance increase, the nurse can adjust the diet to increase calories and nutrients needed for cellular repair.

4. A diet high in protein and carbohydrates can help stabilize the client's blood glucose level, thereby reducing the risk of hypoglycemia while providing nutrition for energy needs and cellular regeneration.

5. Individuals with chronic alcohol-related disorders commonly experience vitamin (especially folic acid, thiamine, and magnesium) deficiencies. Focused use of vitamin therapy is recommended during recovery

DISCHARGE CRITERIA

Nursing documentation indicates that the client:
• has demonstrated an understanding of alcohol-related disorder, its signs and symptoms, and its effects on the family
• can use newly learned coping strategies and skills
• is aware of available community and family support services
• has arranged to participate in an ongoing recovery and therapy program.
Nursing documentation also indicates that the family:
• has verbalized an understanding of the diagnosis, treatment, and expected outcomes
• has demonstrated an ability to use newly acquired adaptive coping mechanisms to enhance the client's recovery
• has been referred to the appropriate community resources for continuing recovery and support
• plans to participate in an ongoing therapy program
• understands when, why, and how to contact the appropriate health care professional in case of an emergency.

SELECTED REFERENCES

Allen, K.M. *Nursing Care of the Addicted Client.* New York: Lippincott-Raven Pubs., 1996.
Diagnostic and Statistical Manual of Mental Disorders, 4th ed. Washington, D.C.: American Psychiatric Association, 1994.
Ewing, J.A. "Detecting Alcoholism: The CAGE Questionnaire," *JAMA* 252(14):1905-07, 1984.
Friedman, L., et al., eds. *Source Book of Substance Abuse and Addiction.* Baltimore: Williams & Wilkins Co., 1996.
Lowinson, J. H., et al. *Substance Abuse: A Comprehensive Text,* 3rd ed. Baltimore: Williams & Wilkins Co., 1997.
Mayfield, D., et al. "The CAGE Questionnaire: Validation of a New Alcoholism Screening Instrument," *American Journal of Psychiatry* 131:1121, 1974.
Mayo-Smith, M.F. "Pharmacological Management of Alcohol Withdrawal: A Meta-Analysis and Evidence-Based Practice Guideline," *JAMA* 278(2):144-51, 1997.
Miller, N.S., et al. *Manual of Therapeutics for Addictions.* New York: Wiley-Liss, 1997.
Nathan, P.E., and Gorman, J.M. *A Guide to Treatments that Work.* New York: Oxford University Press, 1998.
Standards of Addictions Nursing Practice with Selected Diagnoses and Criteria. Washington, D.C.: American Nurses Association, 1988.
Stern, T.A., et al. *The MGH Guide to Psychiatry in Primary Care.* New York: McGraw-Hill Book Co., 1998.

Addiction disorders

Central nervous system depressant–related disorders

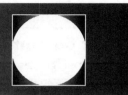

DSM-IV classifications

Sedative-, hypnotic-, anxiolytic-related disorders

Sedative, hypnotic, anxiolytic use disorders
304.10 Sedative, hypnotic, or anxiolytic dependence
305.40 Sedative, hypnotic, or anxiolytic abuse

Sedative-, hypnotic-, anxiolytic-induced disorders
292.89 Sedative, hypnotic, or anxiolytic intoxication
292.89 Sedative, hypnotic, or anxiolytic intoxication with delirium
292.89 Sedative-, hypnotic-, or anxiolytic-induced anxiety disorder
292.84 Sedative-, hypnotic-, or anxiolytic-induced mood disorder
292.82 Sedative-, hypnotic-, or anxiolytic-induced psychotic disorder
292.11 Sedative-, hypnotic-, or anxiolytic-induced psychotic disorder with delusions
292.12 Sedative-, hypnotic-, or anxiolytic-induced psychotic disorder with hallucinations
292.83 Sedative-, hypnotic-, or anxiolytic-induced persisting amnestic disorder
292.89 Sedative-, hypnotic-, or anxiolytic-induced sleep disorder
292.89 Sedative-, hypnotic- or anxiolytic-induced sexual dysfunction
292.89 Sedative-, hypnotic-, or anxiolytic intoxication
292.89 Sedative-, hypnotic-, or anxiolytic intoxication with delirium
292.00 Sedative, hypnotic or anxiolytic withdrawal
292.81 Sedative, hypnotic, or anxiolytic withdrawal with delirium
292.9 Sedative-, hypnotic-, or anxiolytic-related disorder not otherwise specified

Opioid-related disorders

Opioid use disorders
304.00 Opioid dependence
305.50 Opioid abuse

Opioid-induced disorders
292.89 Opioid intoxication
292.81 Opioid intoxication with delirium
292.11 Opioid-induced psychotic disorder, with delusions
292.12 Opioid-induced psychotic disorder, with hallucinations
292.84 Opioid-induced mood disorder
292.89 Opioid-induced sleep disorder
292.89 Opioid-induced sexual dysfunction
292.0 Opioid withdrawal
292.9 Opioid-related disorder not otherwise specified

Psychiatric nursing diagnostic class

Substance abuse

INTRODUCTION

The sedative, hypnotic, and anxiolytic (antianxiety) substances include the benzodiazepines, carbamates, barbiturates, and barbiturate-like hypnotics. *Sedative, hypnotic or anxiolytic dependence* is characterized by both physiologic tolerance and an identifiable withdrawal syndrome. In addition to being physiologically dependent, these individuals develop drug-seeking behaviors that gradually assume primary importance in their daily lives.

Sedative, hypnotic, or anxiolytic abuse can occur on its own or in combination with other substances. Often individuals use intoxicating doses of sedative, hypnotic, or anxiolytic agents to "come down" from central nervous system (CNS) stimulants, such as cocaine or amphetamines. Abusers may use these "downers" during high-risk or potentially hazardous situations.

Sedative, hypnotic, or anxiolytic intoxication involves a clinically significant and maladaptive pattern of behavioral and psychological changes. These behaviors can include inappropriate sexual or aggressive behavior, mood lability, impaired judgment, and impaired social and occupational performance. Slurred speech, ataxia, nystagmus, memory or attentional problems or both, along with decreased psychomotor function, may also occur, increasing the risk of accidents and injuries.

Sedative, hypnotic, anxiolytic withdrawal is marked by a syndrome that develops after the individual sharply curtails or stops taking the substance after several weeks of regular use. Symptoms of withdrawal include autonomic hyperactivity (increased heart rate, respiratory rate, blood pressure and temperature, and sweating); tremor of hands; insomnia; anxiety; nausea or agitation or both; and, possibly, seizures. (Refer to "Benzodiazepine withdrawal assessment," page 298, for information on how to assess and quantify benzodiazepine withdrawal syndrome.)

Sedative-, hypnotic-, anxiolytic-related disorder not otherwise specified comprises disorders associated with use of sedatives, hypnotics, or anxiolytics that are not classifiable under other sedative, hypnotic, anxiolytic-related diagnoses.

The opioids include natural opioids (morphine), semisynthetics (heroin) and synthetics with morphine-like action (codeine, hydromorphone, methadone, oxycodone, meperidine, fentanyl). Opioids are usually prescribed as analgesics, anesthetics, antidiarrheal agents, or cough suppressants.

Opioid dependence is marked by compulsive, prolonged self-administration of opioid substances. Individuals with opioid dependence develop regular patterns of compulsive drug use, and their daily activities revolve around obtaining and using the substance. The opioids may be obtained both legally and illegally. The individual may use polypharmacy (seeking prescriptions from multiple health care providers) or obtain the substance from an illegal dealer. An opioid-dependent health care provider may resort to diverting opioids from inhouse supplies, or directly from their clients.

Opioid abuse involves overuse or inappropriate use of opioids. Individuals who abuse opioids generally use these substances less often than those who experience opioid dependence. Typically, they do not develop tolerance or a withdrawal syndrome.

The essential feature of *opioid intoxication* is the presence of clinically significant maladaptive behavioral or psychological changes. Early symptoms include euphoria followed by apathy, dysphoria, or psychomotor retardation or agitation, impaired judgment, and impaired social and occupational functioning. Affected individuals may demonstrate inattention to their environment and may place themselves in hazardous or risky situations.

Opioid withdrawal involves the presence of a characteristic syndrome that develops after the individual suddenly reduces or stops taking the substance after frequent and prolonged use. Opioid withdrawal signs and symptoms include anxiety, restlessness, and an "achy feeling" that is generally located in the back and legs. These individuals also experience cravings and an increase in drug-seeking behavior, along with increased irritability and pain sensitivity.

Opioid-related disorder not otherwise specified comprises disorders associated with opioid usage that are not classifiable under existing opioid-related disorder criteria.

Etiology and precipitating factors
There is no single cause of sedative, hypnotic, or anxiolytic-related disorders, but many different factors are involved. Recent neurochemical research has demonstrated that substance use has specific effects on selected neurotransmitters (chemicals in the brain that transmit impulses from one nerve cell to the next). Certain drugs interfere with the effective work of neurotransmitters. CNS depressants act on GABA (gamma-aminobutyric acid) to potentiate the effects of GABA (anixiolytic and sedating). This is accomplished by facilitating the opening of a chloride ion channel. This effect helps explain the addictive and cross-tolerant ef-

fects that develop when alcohol is combined with barbiturates and benzodiazepines.

Psychological theories propose that a person uses substances to "feel better," and when this does occur, a beginning process of reinforcement is initiated. This occurs both at the biological and psychological level. Neurobiological studies suggest that CNS depressants, alcohol, and other drugs reinforce dependence by stimulating a "brain reward" mechanism located in the medial forebrain. This region is apparently served by axons associated with the mesotelencephalic dopamine system. Intoxication with CNS depressants or other drugs increases extracellular dopamine levels; the resulting dopamine related "high" becomes the reinforcement mechanism. The brain adjusts to the increased dopamine levels and causes a craving for increased amounts of the substance to reproduce the original pleasurable effect.

Potential complications
If left untreated, CNS depressant-related disorders can lead directly or indirectly to the following conditions: abscesses, osteomyelitis, acquired immunodeficiency syndrome (AIDS), amenorrhea, bacterial endocarditis, bronchitis, cardiac arrest, cellulitis, coma, dehydration, hepatitis, hypoglycemia, frequent infections, malnutrition, overdose, pulmonary emboli, renal failure, respiratory arrest, seizures, sepsis, sexually transmitted disease, tetanus, vascular disorders, or withdrawal states. (For details on managing an acute episode of depressant abuse, see appendix C, Managing acute substance abuse.)

ASSESSMENT GUIDELINES
Nursing history (functional health pattern findings)
Health perception–health management pattern
• Distorted pain perception
• Headache
• General discomfort
• Chronic pain or frequent emergency room visits for migraine headaches
• Depression or anxiety
• Numerous physical complaints
• Frequent viral or bacterial infections
• Inaccurate perception of health
Nutritional-metabolic pattern
• Inadequate food intake
• Lack of interest in food
• Abdominal pain
• Dental problems
• Altered skin integrity (including abscesses) and poor skin turgor
• Pale mucous membranes

Addiction disorders

- Weight loss
- Poor muscle tone

Elimination pattern
- GI cramps
- Diarrhea, nausea, or vomiting

Activity-exercise pattern
- Lethargy and fatigue
- Restlessness
- Inability to engage in physical activity
- Intolerance to activity secondary to decreased strength and endurance
- Decreased interest or participation in diversional activities
- Inability to complete normal daily activities

Sleep-rest pattern
- Difficulty falling asleep and remaining asleep
- Early morning awakenings and interrupted sleep
- Reversed normal sleep cycle
- Fatigue after sleep
- Anxiety about inability to sleep
- Use of additional prescribed sleep medications
- Increased dreaming that interrupts sleep

Cognitive-perceptual pattern
- Disorientation about people, places, and time
- Confusion
- Slowed information processing
- Hallucinations
- Short-term memory deficits
- Belief that quitting the drug is possible anytime
- Concentration difficulty
- Difficulty following directions
- Difficulty making decisions

Self-perception–self-concept pattern
- Difficulty acknowledging or accepting bodily changes
- Derogatory statements about self
- Feelings of inadequacy, guilt, and shame
- Anger over inability to control things or situations
- Self-destructive behaviors
- Feelings of hopelessness and powerlessness
- Feelings of grandiosity

Role-relationship pattern
- Difficulty with intimacy
- Changes in usual role responsibility and functioning
- Inability to express feelings
- Isolation or subculture existence
- Dysfunctional peer and family interactions
- Dysfunctional roles, rules, and rituals within the family

Sexual-reproductive pattern
- Actual or perceived sexual or reproductive limitations
- Decreased libido
- Difficulties achieving sexual satisfaction
- Concern about acquiring sexually transmitted diseases
- Disturbances in relationship with sexual partner

Coping–stress tolerance pattern
- Inability to cope
- Difficulty asking for help
- Projecting blame and responsibility for the disorder on others
- Refusal of health care attention
- Social withdrawal and isolation
- Presence of significant life stressors

Value-belief pattern
- Hopelessness about addiction and treatment outcome
- Anger with God or others for the disorder
- Inner conflict about beliefs
- Spiritual distress

Physical findings
Cardiovascular
- Anemia
- Bradycardia
- Cardiac arrest
- Cyanosis
- Diaphoresis
- Arrhythmias
- Elevated diastolic blood pressure
- Hemorrhage
- Hypotension
- Petechiae
- Shock
- Tachycardia

Respiratory
- Rapid or deep breathing
- Respiratory paralysis
- Slow or labored breathing
- Tachypnea

Gastrointestinal
- Abdominal pain
- Anorexia
- Bloody stools
- Colic
- Constipation
- Nausea and vomiting

Genitourinary
- Glycosuria
- Urinary tract infection
- Proteinuria
- Sexually transmitted disease

Integumentary
- Abrasions
- Abscesses
- Alopecia
- Bruises or hematoma
- Bullae
- Cyanosis
- Dermatitis
- Dryness
- Flushed complexion
- Hirsutism

- Jaundice
- Needle puncture marks
- Paleness
- Pruritis
- Urticaria

Musculoskeletal
- Dysarthria
- Old and healed fractures
- Hypotonia
- Muscle aches and pains
- Muscle rigidity and tension

Neurologic
- Acute delirium
- Anesthesia
- Ataxia
- Blurred vision
- Coma
- Confusion
- Depressed deep tendon reflexes
- Dizziness
- Auditory or visual hallucinations
- Headaches
- Hyperreflexia
- Hyperthermia
- Coordination loss
- Miosis

- Myoclonus
- "Nodding off"
- Horizontal or vertical nystagmus
- Paresthesia
- Pupil changes
- Seizures
- Sleepiness
- Spasms
- Stupor
- Tetanic rigidity
- Tinnitus
- Tremors, twitching

Psychological
- Agitation and anger
- Anxiety
- Depression or euphoria
- Floating feelings
- Hostility or irritability
- Manipulative behaviors
- Paradoxical excitement
- Restlessness
- Insomnia
- Violence

Nursing diagnosis

Ineffective denial related to feelings of low self-esteem

Nursing priority

Help the client accept responsibility for behavior and disease management and acknowledge the relationship between substance abuse and personal problems.

Patient outcome criteria

As treatment progresses, the client, family, or both should be able to:
- demonstrate a willingness to accept responsibility for behavior
- verbalize an understanding of the impact that the client's substance-abuse disorder has on their personal lives.

Addiction disorders

Interventions

1. Convey an accepting attitude to the client.

2. Educate the client to correct misinterpretations about substance use and abuse to alleviate negative feelings.

3. Confront the client's use of defense mechanisms, including rationalization and blaming.

4. Explore with the client significant events and situations that led to substance use as well as any consequential maladaptive behaviors resulting from drug use.

5. Reintroduce the client to facts about and the reality of the disorder if the client begins fantasizing about a lifestyle revolving around substance abuse or denying the negative impact on both his life and his family's ability to cope.

6. Schedule, encourage, and monitor the client's and family's participation in group and educational activities.

7. Provide the client with positive feedback whenever he recognizes connections between behaviors and substance abuse.

Rationales

1. An accepting attitude can promote feelings of dignity and self-worth.

2. Factual information, including the signs and symptoms of substance abuse or dependence, can help the client and family focus on their own behaviors and can decrease the ignorance of substance abuse that contributes to continued addiction.

3. These defense mechanisms can prolong the client's denial of his disorder. Exposing them is an important step toward recovery.

4. Helping the client to visualize the relationship between personal difficulties and substance abuse is an important first step in eliminating the client's denial of the disorder.

5. A realistic, yet supportive approach can facilitate the client's self-esteem and diminish the use of defense mechanisms.

6. The client may accept feedback more readily from peer groups than from the nurse or staff. A peer group setting also can decrease the client's feelings of uniqueness and isolation.

7. Positive reinforcement can increase the client's self-esteem and encourage healthy behaviors.

NURSING DIAGNOSIS

Knowledge deficit related to information about the risks involving substance abuse

Nursing priority

Teach the client about the effects of substance abuse on the body and help incorporate this knowledge into the client's daily life and family relationships.

Patient outcome criteria

As treatment progresses, the client, family, or both should be able to:
• identify substance abuse effects on bodily functions
• verbalize an understanding of the addiction disorder model.

Interventions

1. Assess the client's and family's knowledge of substance abuse, identifying any attitudes, misconceptions, and myths associated with the disorder.

2. Provide the client with factual information about substance abuse and dependence as well as addiction patterns. Also include information about how substance use affects pregnancy and the relationship between I.V. drug abuse and sexually transmitted diseases, as they apply to the client. (See *Medical consequences of parenteral drug use*, page 198.)

3. Use various teaching methods, including discussion groups, lectures, role playing, family sculpting, group exercises, audiovisual aids, and handouts.

4. Elicit the client's and family's interpretation of information and concepts covered in the teaching plan.

Rationales

1. Assessing the client's and family's knowledge can help the nurse to design and implement an appropriate educational plan based on standards of addictions nursing practice.

2. Comprehensive client and family education is essential to recovery. Include the following concepts: disorders associated with substance abuse and dependence, disorder model of addiction, the philosophy of support and self-help groups, family interactions and dynamics associated with addiction, nutritional effects of addiction, assertiveness and communication skills, specific treatment strategies, the disorder's impact on both the client's and family's lifestyles, adaptive coping strategies, relapse prevention, and prescription addiction.

3. These various teaching techniques can help ensure and reinforce client and family learning.

4. Having the client and family verbalize their understanding of the disorder can help the nurse evaluate the effectiveness of the teaching plan and identify points that need clarification.

NURSING DIAGNOSIS

Risk for infection related to compromised immunity, insufficient knowledge about disease, and participation in high-risk behaviors

Nursing priority

Help the client identify existing high-risk behaviors and develop an alternative lifestyle.

Patient outcome criteria

As treatment progresses, the client, family, or both should be able to:
• acknowledge the need for ongoing health assessments and treatment related to possible infection
• verbalize an awareness of resources for obtaining information about remaining infection free (AIDS-related safe sex, needle exchange program)
• report an understanding of community-based resources to assist with reduction of high-risk behaviors and maintain safety.

Addiction disorders

Interventions

1. Assess the client's existing risk factors, such as I.V. drug use, needle sharing, use of impure drugs, and malnutrition.

2. Develop and implement specific teaching plans related to the client's risk factors.

3. Monitor and review laboratory results with the client. Provide counseling before and after human immunodeficiency virus (HIV) screens are conducted.

4. Closely monitor the client's vital signs.

Rationales

1. Knowing the client's risk factors can help the nurse develop an appropriate care plan.

2. Increasing the client's knowledge of existing risk factors can promote behavioral change.

3. Laboratory results help the nurse to identify possible causes of infection and to initiate early counseling and outpatient support referrals should the client test HIV-positive.

4. An elevated temperature, heart rate, and respiratory rate may indicate infection, which can lead to sepsis.

Medical consequences of parenteral drug use

Infectious complications

- Brain abscesses
- Cellulitis
- Cutaneous abscesses
- Epidural abscess
- Endocarditis
- Gas gangrene
- Hepatitis A,B,C, and D viruses
- Human immunodeficiency virus (acquired immunodeficiency disease)
- Infected pseudoaneurysm
- Malaria
- Septic arthritis
- Subdural abscess
- Sexually transmitted diseases
- Tetanus
- Tuberculosis

Noninfectious complications

- Amenorrhea
- Arrhythmia
- Constipation with possible impaction
- Gastrointestinal motility disturbances
- Glomerulonephritis
- Mycotic aneurysm
- Myositis
- Necrotizing angiitis
- Needle embolus
- Nephrotic syndrome
- Overdose with possible coma and death
- Pneumomediastinum
- Pneumothorax
- Pulmonary edema (flash)
- Pulmonary fibrosis
- Pulmonary hypertension
- Renal failure (acute to chronic)
- Stroke (cerebrovascular accident)
- Talc granuloma (from talc used to cut illegal narcotics)
- Thrombocytopenia
- Trauma (unisystem or multisystem trauma from falls, jumps, burns, and vehicle crashes)

Adapted with permission from Miller, N.S. *The Principles and Practice of Addictions in Psychiatry.* Philadelphia: W.B. Saunders Co., 1997, p. 148.

Discharge criteria

Nursing documentation indicates that the client:
• understands about substance abuse and is aware of its impact on his life and the lives of family members
• has verbalized an understanding of the expected psychological, physiologic, and spiritual responses during the first year of recovery
• demonstrates an ability to use newly acquired coping strategies to facilitate recovery
• is aware of available medical and community resources, including HIV counseling and follow-up treatments.
• has scheduled the necessary follow-up appointments.
Nursing documentation also indicates that the family:
• has verbalized an understanding of the diagnosis, treatment, and expected outcomes
• has been referred to the appropriate community resources for ongoing family support
• has verbalized an understanding of when, why and how to contact appropriate health care professionals in case of a relapse or other emergency.

Selected references

Allen, K.M. *Nursing Care of the Addicted Client.* Philadelphia: Lippincott-Raven Pubs., 1996.

Boyd, M.A., and Nihart, M.A. *Psychiatric Nursing: Contemporary Practice.* Philadelphia: Lippincott-Raven Pubs., 1998.

Diagnostic and Statistical Manual of Mental Disorders, 4th ed. Washington, D.C.: American Psychiatric Association, 1994.

Gelenberg, A.J., and Bassuk, E.L. *The Practitioner's Guide to Psychoactive Drugs.* New York: Plenum Publishing Corp., 1997.

Lowinson, J.H., et al. *Substance Abuse: A Comprehensive Text,* 3rd ed. Baltimore: Williams & Wilkins Co., 1997.

Miller, N.S. *The Principles and Practice of Addictions in Psychiatry.* Philadelphia: W.B. Saunders Co., 1997.

Nathan, P.E., and Gorman, J.M. *A Guide to Treatments that Work.* New York: Oxford University Press, 1998.

Rundell, J.R., and Wise, M.G. *Textbook of Consultation Liaison Psychiatry.* Washington, D.C.: American Psychiatric Association, 1996.

Varcarolis, E.M. *Foundations of Psychiatric Mental Health Nursing,* 3rd ed. Philadelphia: W.B. Saunders Co., 1998.

Central nervous system stimulant–related disorders

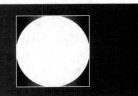

DSM-IV classifications

Amphetamine- (or amphetamine-like) related disorders

304.40 Amphetamine (or similarly acting sympatho-
        mimetic) dependence
305.70 Amphetamine abuse
292.89 Amphetamine intoxication
292.90 Amphetamine withdrawal
292.11 Amphetamine-induced psychotic disorder with
        delusions
292.12 Amphetamine-induced psychotic disorder with
        hallucinations
292.81 Amphetamine-intoxication with delirium
292.89 Amphetamine-induced anxiety disorder
292.89 Amphetamine-induced sexual disorder
292.89 Amphetamine-induced sleep disorder
292.89 Amphetamine intoxication
292.9 Amphetamine-related disorder not otherwise
        specified

Caffeine-related disorders

305.90 Caffeine intoxication
292.89 Caffeine-induced anxiety disorder
292.89 Caffeine-induced sleep disorder
292.2 Caffeine-related disorder not otherwise specified

Cocaine-related disorder

304.20 Cocaine dependence
305.60 Cocaine abuse
292.89 Cocaine intoxication
292.0 Cocaine withdrawal
292.11 Cocaine-induced psychotic disorder with delu-
        sions
292.12 Cocaine-induced psychotic disorder with hallu-
        cinations
292.81 Cocaine-intoxication with delirium
292.84 Cocaine-induced mood disorder
292.89 Cocaine-induced anxiety disorder
292.89 Cocaine-induced sexual dysfunction
292.89 Cocaine-induced sleep disorder
292.9 Cocaine-related disorder not otherwise specified

Nicotine-related disorders

305.10 Nicotine dependence
292.0 Nicotine withdrawal
292.9 Nicotine-related disorder not otherwise specified

Psychiatric nursing diagnostic class

Substance abuse

INTRODUCTION

Central nervous system (CNS) stimulants that are commonly used and abused include all forms of amphetamines, caffeine, cocaine, and nicotine. When these substances are ingested, inhaled, or injected, they commonly cause increased heart rate and blood pressure, appetite loss, and insomnia. Psychological symptoms commonly exhibited by the user include agitation, anxiety, mood swings, and paranoia. Dependence results as the user adapts physiologically to the continued use of the drug. Tolerance can occur rapidly.

Cocaine is the most potent CNS stimulant and is produced from the leaves of the coca plant. Caffeine and nicotine are the most prevalent and widely used stimulants. Amphetamines, nonamphetamine stimulants, and cocaine exert their effects by augmenting or potentiating the excitatory neurotransmitters dopamine, epinephrine, and norepinephrine. Caffeine and nicotine are considered stimulants and exert their actions directly, thereby increasing rates of cellular metabolism. Caffeine is a common ingredient in coffee, cola, chocolate, and tea. Nicotine is the primary psychoactive substance in all forms of tobacco products.

The CNS stimulant–related disorders have similar patterns of abuse, dependence, intoxication, and withdrawal. (For more information, see *Central nervous system stimulants: Clinical syndromes.*)

Etiology and precipitating factors

CNS stimulants produce an excitatory response by increasing production of dopamine, serotonin, norepinephrine, and acetylcholine. Hyperstimulation causes psychological effects, such as heightened energy, increased tolerance of pain, and improved intellectual performance. Tolerance requires increased amounts of the stimulant to obtain the desired effect; increasing the dosage, in turn, causes an overabundance of neurotransmitters and development of additional receptor sites. If the drug is suddenly stopped, neurotransmitter levels decrease, causing drug craving and withdrawal symptoms.

Potential complications

Identifying medical complications is the first priority. The client who is free from medical or psychiatric problems can more easily benefit from treatment. Complications may include seizures, cardiovascular shock, cardiac arrhythmias, destruction of the nasal septum, intracranial hemorrhage, and cardiac arrest.

Central nervous system stimulants: Clinical syndromes

Substance	Symptoms of abuse or intoxication	Symptoms of withdrawal
Amphetamines (long-acting) Dextroamphetamine (Dexedrine) Methamphetamine (Methadrine) Ice (synthesized for illicit use)	**Physiologic** Dilated pupils Elevated heart rate Elevated blood pressure Nausea/vomiting Twitching	Agitation Apathy Depression Disorientation Fatigue Lethargy Sleepiness
Cocaine, crack (short-acting) Injectable Nasal (snorted) Smokable	**Behavioral, Perceptual** Assaultive Elevated energy Euphoric or manic Grandiose Impaired judgment Impaired social function Impaired occupational function Violence	Anxiety Apathy Craving Depression Fatigue Use of CNS depressants to suppress anxiety and withdrawal
Nicotine Cigarettes Smokeless tobacco Nicotine gum Nicotine patch	**Physiologic** Anorexia Dilated pupils Elevated heart rate Insomnia	Anxiety Constipation Craving Decreased concentration ability Disruption in sleeping pattern Fatigue Gastrointestinal disturbances Headaches Increased eating (hyperphasia) Irritability "Nicotine fits"
Xanthines Caffeine	**Behavioral/Perceptual** Disturbed concentration Elation Grandiosity Impaired judgment Paranoid thinking Psychosis Resisting fatigue Violent, angry outburst No clear symptoms documented for nicotine intoxication **Physiologic** Arrhythmias Diuresis Excitement Flushed face GI complaints Nervousness Periods of being inexhaustible Psychomotor agitation Rambling speech Restlessness	No well-documented symptoms of a withdrawal state have been substantiated

Compiled from Miller, N.B., et al. *Manual of Therapeutics for Addictions.* New York: Wiley-Liss, 1997; and *Diagnostic and Statistical Manual of Mental Disorders,* 4th ed. Washington, D.C.: American Psychiatric Association, 1994.

Addiction disorders

ASSESSMENT GUIDELINES

Nursing history (functional health pattern findings)

Health perception–health management pattern
- Denial of medical or health care concerns
- Grandiose perception of health
- Preoccupation with physical complaints
- Overconcern with health issues
- General anxiety regarding personal well-being
- Inability to manage self-care
- Feelings of hopelessness and powerlessness about health
- Paranoia about health and fear of nonexistent illness
- Hypervigilance over health care
- Distorted body image
- Integumentary alterations, including abscesses and needle marks from I.V. drug use

Nutritional-metabolic pattern
- Chronic weight loss
- Malnourishment symptoms, including muscle wasting and altered skin and hair condition
- Denial of obvious nutritional needs
- Poor dentition and bruxism
- Increased or decreased appetite dependent on drug use
- Irregular eating patterns

Elimination pattern
- Heartburn, nausea, vomiting, or diarrhea
- Frequent urination

Activity-exercise pattern
- Mood swings
- Hyperactivity
- Chronic fatigue and apathy
- Lack of exercise or leisure activity
- Denial of normal activity disturbances
- Repetitive activities and psychomotor agitation

Sleep-rest pattern
- Insomnia
- Violent nightmares
- Disturbed sleep cycle
- Hypersomnia when not using drugs
- Need for sedative to aid sleep
- Racing thoughts that interfere with resting
- Sleep deprivation symptoms, including forgetfulness, emotional liability, and difficulty concentrating
- Denial of sleep needs
- Inability to stay awake

Cognitive-perceptual pattern
- Ongoing inappropriate paranoia and suspicion
- Racing thoughts, poor memory, fragmented thinking
- Delusional thought patterns
- Increased sensitivity
- Increased alertness

Self-perception–self-concept pattern
- Lack of control over drug use
- Poor self-esteem
- Feelings of grandiosity
- Denial of drug dependence
- Denial of feelings

Role-relationship pattern
- Alienation from family and close friends
- Shame or guilt concerning family or friends
- Denial of intimacy needs
- Problems with intimacy
- Extreme financial or emotional dependence on family and friends
- Absence of a productive social role

Sexual-reproductive pattern
- Hypersexuality
- Irregular menstrual cycle
- Promiscuity
- High-risk sexual practices (multiple partners and unprotected sex)
- Concerns about unsafe sexual practices
- Denial of unsafe sexual practices

Coping–stress tolerance pattern
- Hand tremors and bruxism
- Nervousness and impatience
- Compulsive activity
- Hyperalertness
- Feelings of not being in control
- Denial of obvious coping difficulties
- Violent outbursts or emotional immaturity

Value-belief pattern
- Breakdown of value system
- Denial of spirituality
- Heavy emphasis on drug use as a means of maintaining well-being
- Powerlessness over drug use
- Loss of trust in self and others

Physical findings

Cardiovascular
- Arrhythmias
- Endocarditis
- Cardiac depression
- Increased body temperature
- Increased blood pressure and heart rate
- Palpitations
- Sweating and chills

Respiratory
- Bronchitis
- Chest pain with deep inspiration
- Chronic productive cough
- Deviated nasal septum
- Dry, hacking cough
- Increased respiratory rate
- Nasal mucosa irritation

- Pulmonary congestion
- Respiratory depression
- Rhinitis
- Shortness of breath on exertion

Gastrointestinal
- Heartburn
- Increased gastric acidity
- Dry mouth
- Nausea or vomiting

Genitourinary
- Frequent urination

Musculoskeletal
- Ataxia
- Twitching
- Motor agitation
- Muscular rigidity
- Muscle wasting
- Tactile hallucinations

Neurologic
- Dilated pupils
- Headaches
- Inability to concentrate
- Intense agitation and irritability

- Tinnitus
- Seizures
- Insomnia

Psychological
- Aggression
- Delirium
- Depression
- Emotional liability
- Euphoria
- Exhaustion
- Mania
- Paranoia
- Violent outbursts
- Visual and auditory hallucinations

NURSING DIAGNOSIS

Altered health maintenance related to the effects of stimulant dependence on the client's self-esteem

Nursing priority

Help the client to acknowledge the need for improvements in maintaining health and to implement healthy self-care.

Patient outcome criteria

As treatment progresses, the client, family, or both should be able to:
- acknowledge health care deficits in their self-care
- report attention to health care maintenance (attending health care appointments, preventive care)
- demonstrate an awareness of factors that lead to infection and ways to control or prevent it.

Interventions

1. Maintain a nonjudgmental and caring attitude toward the client and his condition.

2. Establish a trusting relationship with the client.

3. Encourage the client to participate in normal activities of daily living.

4. Educate the client about positive health habits.

Rationales

1. Genuine concern and a nonjudgmental approach can enhance the client's self-esteem.

2. The client whose stimulant dependence may have caused paranoia and distrust can learn from the nurse's example how to trust again.

3. Participation in normal activities and personal care can enhance the client's self-worth and sense of control.

4. Learning positive health habits can enhance self-esteem.

Addiction disorders

5. Respond to the client's denial of stimulant dependence with genuine caring.

5. Denial can be a persistent defense mechanism for the stimulant-dependent client. By making the client face the reality of his condition in a sensitive and caring manner, the nurse can help to break down these defenses.

NURSING DIAGNOSIS

Altered nutrition: less than body requirements related to placing greater importance on drug use than on eating

Nursing priority

Help the client establish an adequate, nutritious diet and increase the client's body weight.

Patient outcome criteria

As treatment progresses, the client, family, or both should be able to:
• report and demonstrate improved dietary intake
• demonstrate weight gain or stabilization at optimal weight range.

Interventions

1. Provide the client with well-balanced meals.

2. Provide the client with nutritional supplements if prescribed.

3. Educate the client about proper nutrition.

Rationales

1. The stimulant-dependent client may be experiencing nutritional deficits from not eating during drug use, spending money on drugs rather than food, and eating junk food rather than well-balanced meals.

2. Nutritional supplements can help replenish vitamins and minerals that have been depleted by stimulant use.

3. Nutritional knowledge can help the client make appropriate dietary decisions.

NURSING DIAGNOSIS

Potential altered body temperature related to stimulant use

Nursing priority

Help the client maintain a normal body temperature.

Patient outcome criteria

As treatment progresses, the client, family, or both should be able to:
• demonstrate a restoration of normal thermoregulation function
• report decreased negative effects of increased temperature (discomfort, rigors, diaphoresis, increased metabolic rate).

Interventions

1. Monitor the client's body temperature

Rationales

1. Because stimulant abuse can severely elevate body temperature, the nurse should monitor for such temperature changes and institute appropriate actions, such as applying ice packs or a hypothermia blanket, as prescribed.

2. Administer antipyretics as necessary.

3. Monitor the client's fluid intake and output, and encourage the client to drink plenty of fluids.

2. Antipyretics will help lower the client's body temperature to a safe level.

3. Adequate fluid intake is needed to replace fluids lost because of elevated body temperatures and to aid in lowering the client's body temperature. Sufficient fluid intake also helps prevent dehydration.

Nursing diagnosis

Risk for impaired skin integrity related to changes in health maintenance

Nursing priority

Help the client maintain healthy skin integrity.

Patient outcome criteria

As treatment progresses, the client, family, or both should be able to:
• demonstrate no skin breakdown
• report decreased or no skin infections or abscesses from use of stimulants.

Interventions

1. Assess the client's integumentary system and explore any factors such as I.V. drug use that have led to skin breakdown.

2. Institute prescribed treatments and monitor the client's progress.

Rationales

1. I.V. drug use can lead to abscesses, skin breakdown, and infections. By assessing the client's integumentary system, the nurse can better plan appropriate interventions.

2. Proper treatment promotes healing. Monitoring helps prevent further complications.

Nursing diagnosis

Decreased cardiac output related to stimulant use

Nursing priority

Help the client maintain optimal cardiac function.

Patient outcome criteria

As treatment progresses, the client, family, or both should be able to:
• report improvement or stabilization in cardiac function
• report participation in cardiopulmonary exercise program (within functional limits).

Interventions

1. Assess and monitor the client's heart sounds, heart rate, and blood pressure.

2. Administer antihypertensives and antiarrythmics if prescribed.

3. Monitor the client's fluid intake and output.

Rationales

1. Stimulant abuse, especially cocaine abuse, increases the client's risk of cardiac arrest.

2. Cardiac output may be altered by stimulant use; various medications may effectively control and help prevent poor cardiac output.

3. An accurate measurement of fluid intake and output helps the nurse to monitor cardiac status.

NURSING DIAGNOSIS

Sleep pattern disturbance related to stimulant use

Nursing priority

Help the client establish and maintain a balanced sleep-awake cycle that enhances restfulness.

Patient outcome criteria

As treatment progresses, the client, family, or both should be able to:
• practice appropriate sleep-enhancement methods
• report improved sleep patterns, normal sensorium, and decreased paranoia.

Interventions

1. Provide the client with a comfortable sleeping environment.

2. Reassure the client that nightmares will diminish in time.

3. Encourage the client to take fewer naps during the day.

4. Encourage the client to engage in adequate exercise and other stimulating activities during the day.

5. Encourage the client to use nonpharmacologic sleep aids, such as drinking warm milk and practicing relaxation techniques, to promote sleep.

Rationales

1. Comfort and quiet will enhance the client's ability to obtain restful sleep.

2. Restless sleep and nightmares commonly occur with stimulant abuse and during withdrawal but tend to dissipate over time.

3. Avoiding daytime naps can help the client feel more fatigued at bedtime, facilitating a return to a normal sleep cycle.

4. Adequate exercise and activity can help the client return to a normal sleep cycle.

5. Warm milk and relaxation techniques both promote sleep. Because the chemically dependent client probably has used drugs to cope with most problems, he may benefit greatly from the nurse's encouragement in using nondrug solutions.

NURSING DIAGNOSIS

Sensory-perceptual alteration (visual, auditory, and kinesthetic) related to sensory overload from stimulant use

Nursing priority

Help the client establish a balanced sensorium and perception.

Patient outcome criteria

As treatment progresses, the client, family, or both should be able to:
• report and demonstrate a decrease in hallucinatory experiences
• report feeling safe
• demonstrate a reduction in paranoia
• demonstrate a decrease in irritability and agitation.

Interventions

1. Promote a quiet, nonthreatening atmosphere by decreasing environmental stimuli.

2. Explain all nursing procedures to the client before beginning them.

3. Observe the client for seizures, and administer prescribed medications, such as Valium or Librium, as needed.

4. Institute and maintain safety precautions.

Rationales

1. Decreasing environmental stimuli promotes relaxation and helps prevent potential complications such as seizures.

2. By sharing information, the nurse can help decrease the client's suspicion and paranoia.

3. The client withdrawing from stimulants may have seizures. Close monitoring by the nurse and administration of prescribed anticonvulsant medications can decrease the likelihood of seizures.

4. Because a client with a sensory disturbance is at risk for self-harm, the nurse should maintain a safe environment at all times. For example, remove articles from the room that the client can use to harm the self and restrain the client, if necessary.

NURSING DIAGNOSIS

Fear related to an altered thought process

Nursing priority

Establish a trusting and safe environment and help decrease the client's paranoia.

Patient outcome criteria

As treatment progresses, the client, family, or both should be able to:
• report decreased feelings of fear
• report decreased paranoia
• report feeling safe.

Interventions

1. Speak calmly and confidently to the client, thoroughly explaining all procedures.

2. Repeatedly orientate the client to people, places, time, and situations.

Rationales

1. By creating an honest, trusting relationship with the client, the nurse can decrease anxiety and enhance trust.

2. The nurse should keep the client oriented during drug withdrawal because he may be experiencing perceptual distortions.

NURSING DIAGNOSIS

Impaired social interactions related to isolation associated with drug use

Nursing priority

Promote the client's social interaction skills and self-esteem.

Patient outcome criteria

As treatment progresses, the client, family, or both should be able to:
• report increased social interaction
• demonstrate active participation in group activities, including therapy-focused groups
• report decrease anxiety or irritability in group and social interaction.

Interventions	Rationales
1. Arrange for the client to participate in an ongoing therapy group.	**1.** Group therapy provides the client with support and feedback from peers as well as opportunities for practicing social interaction skills.
2. Discourage the client from remaining isolated from others by limiting the client's time spent alone.	**2.** Limiting the client's time alone helps promote interaction with others.
3. Encourage the client to participate in group role-playing sessions.	**3.** Group role playing enables the client to rehearse newly learned social skills.

NURSING DIAGNOSIS

Risk for violence related to difficulty processing and interpreting thoughts and to sensory overload from stimulant use

Nursing priority

Help the client maintain a safe environment and decrease violent outbursts.

Patient outcome criteria

As treatment progresses, the client, family, or both should be able to:
• report a decrease or absence of violent outbursts
• acknowledge the relationship between CNS stimulant use and increased opportunity for violence.

Interventions	Rationales
1. Remove all harmful objects from the client's room, and provide necessary safety precautions.	**1.** The nurse should monitor closely the client at risk for violence and take necessary measures to prohibit the client's self-harm or harm of others, such as the use of soft restraints, one-to-one monitoring, and padding.
2. Administer prescribed sedatives when necessary.	**2.** Sedatives usually are provided for their calming effects during the initial stages of stimulant detoxification.
3. Provide a quiet, nonthreatening environment for the client.	**3.** By providing a quiet environment, the nurse can decrease sensory stimuli associated with stimulant withdrawal.

NURSING DIAGNOSIS

Ineffective family coping related to poor communication

Nursing priority

Help the client and family enhance their coping skills, thereby allowing for healthy communication.

Patient outcome criteria

As treatment progresses, the client, family, or both should be able to:
• verbalize an understanding of family dysfunction related to drug abuse
• demonstrate increased family support
• demonstrate a willingness to participate in family therapy and aftercare plans.

Interventions	Rationales
1. Provide or arrange for therapy sessions for the client's family	**1.** A family therapist can help sort out family dysfunction and communication problems. Through family therapy, the family can create a new system of healthy communication patterns and improved family functioning.
2. Educate the client's family regarding their dysfunction, and encourage them to attend self-help groups.	**2.** Self-help groups such as Cocaine Anonymous can provide support and assistance for the client's family.
3. Encourage the client and his family to participate in role-playing sessions.	**3.** Role playing enables the client and family to express their real needs and concerns within the safety of a therapeutic setting.
4. Refer the client and his family to outside support agencies as necessary.	**4.** Support and assistance resources can become an important part of the family's follow-up therapy.

NURSING DIAGNOSIS

Knowledge deficit related to denial of need for information

Nursing priority

Educate the client and family about addictions and when to seek help.

Patient outcome criteria

As treatment progresses, the client, family, or both should be able to:
• recognize triggers that can lead to the client's relapse
• identify and use relapse prevention.

Interventions	Rationales
1. Educate the client and family about addiction, including the physical effects of drug use, treatment, and aftercare.	**1.** Such knowledge allows the client and family to make informed decisions.
2. Instruct the client and family regarding signs of relapse, such as self-isolation, failure to follow aftercare plan, and stress.	**2.** Recognizing warning signs of relapse allows the client and family to seek assistance before relapse occurs.

Addiction disorders

DISCHARGE CRITERIA

Nursing documentation indicates that the client:
• has verbalized a knowledge of the addiction process and relapse triggers
• has demonstrated the ability to use relapse prevention
• has verbalized an understanding of the risk factors associated with stimulant use
• has demonstrated a willingness to participate in an appropriate self-help group such as Cocaine Anonymous
• is aware of the need for follow-up appointments
• has demonstrated an ability to use skills learned in treatment to maintain a drug-free lifestyle.

Nursing documentation also indicates that the family:
• is willing to participate in ongoing therapy
• has been referred to appropriate community resources for ongoing recovery and family support.

SELECTED REFERENCES

Allen, K. M. *Nursing Care of the Addicted Client.* Philadelphia: Lippincott-Raven Pubs., 1996.

Diagnostic and Statistical Manual of Mental Disorders, 4th ed. Washington, D.C.: American Psychiatric Association, 1994.

American Psychiatric Association. "Practice Guideline for the Treatment of Patients with Nicotine Dependence," *American Journal of Psychiatry* 153 (Suppl):1, 1996.

Fagerstom, K.O., and Sawe, U. "The Pathophysiology of Nicotine Dependence: Treatment Options and the Cardiovascular Safety of Nicotine," *Cardiovascular Risk Factors* 6:135-43, 1996.

Lowinson, J.H., et al. *Substance Abuse: A Comprehensive Text,* 3rd ed. Baltimore: Williams & Wilkins Co., 1997.

Mendelson, J.H., and Mellon, N.K. "Management of Cocaine Abuse and Dependence," *New England Journal of Medicine* 334: 965-72, 1996.

Miller, N.B., et al. *Manual of Therapeutics for Addictions.* New York: Wiley-Liss, 1997.

Hallucinogen or mind-altering drug–related disorders

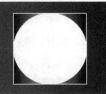

DSM-IV classifications
Cannabis
292.11 Cannabis-induced psychotic disorder with delusions

292.12 Cannabis-induced psychotic disorder with hallucinations

292.89 Cannabis intoxication

292.81 Cannabis intoxication with delirium

Hallucinogen
292.11 Hallucinogen-induced psychotic disorder with delusions

292.12 Hallucinogen-induced psychotic disorder with hallucinations

292.81 Hallucinogen-intoxication with delirium

292.89 Hallucinogen-induced anxiety disorder

292.84 Hallucinogen-induced mood disorder

292.89 Hallucinogen persisting perception disorder (flashbacks)

292.9 Hallucinogen-related disorder not otherwise specified

Phencyclidine (PCP) or similarly acting arylcyclohexylamine
304.90 PCP dependence

305.90 PCP abuse

292.89 PCP intoxication

292.11 PCP-induced psychotic disorder with delusions

292.12 PCP-induced psychotic disorder with hallucinations

292.81 PCP intoxication with delirium

292.84 PCP-induced mood disorder

292.89 PCP-related disorder not otherwise specified

Psychiatric nursing diagnostic class
Substance abuse

INTRODUCTION
Hallucinogens, also known as psychedelics or psychotomimetics, include naturally occurring plants, fungi, or roots as well as synthetically produced substances. Naturally occurring hallucinogens include mescaline (peyote), psilocybin (mushrooms), harmine, harmaline, dimethyltryptamine (barks and seeds), and ibogaine (root). Synthetic hallucinogens include lysergic acid diethylamide (LSD), diethyltryptamine (DET), dipropyltryptamine (DPT), 2,5-dimethoxy-4-methylamphetamine (DOM, STP), 2,5-dimethoxy-4-ethylamphetamine (DOET), and 3,4-methylenedioxymethamphetamine (MDMA, ADAM, ecstasy). Although each drug differs somewhat in its effects, their similarities are sufficient to consider them as a group.

Other substances can produce hallucinations. Cannabis, or tetrahydrocannabinoids (THCs [marijuana]), is a naturally occurring plant that may produce hallucinogenic experiences. Phencyclidine (PCP) and similarly acting arylcyclohexylamine (ketamine) are both anesthetic agents and can also cause hallucinations. PCP, which is inexpensive and easily synthesized, and other synthetic or designer drugs commonly contain toxic impurities that can cause various responses, including abscesses, infections, and possibly death.

Hallucinogen abuse and dependence is characterized by vivid and unusual changes in feelings, thoughts, and perceptions without delirium or severe generalized toxic physical effects. Such abuse and dependence can cause a wide range of psychological effects. An individual's experience is also influenced by their environment, personality, and expectations.

Etiology and precipitating factors
All the mind expansion and hallucinogen agents have complex agonist-antagonist activity at either the presynaptic or postsynaptic serotonin receptors; however, the exact mechanism of action of the hallucinogens remains unclear. They affect the electrical activity of neurons in the locus ceruleus and certain cortical regions, and at a systems level, theses effects could change how the brain handles sensory information and possibly alter cognitive and perceptual processing. Hallucinogenic drugs interact with several neurotransmitter systems; however, it appears that their ability to alter neurotransmission mediated by serotonin is of critical importance. The mechanism underlying postintoxication mood changes and flashbacks is not well understood at this time.

Potential complications
Hallucinogen dependence can lead to various complications, including decreased vital capacity, chromosomal damage, hypothermia, cardiovascular collapse, panic reaction, and drug-induced psychosis.

Assessment guidelines

Nursing history (functional health pattern findings)

Health perception–health management pattern
- Denial of health problems even when faced with physical evidence
- Use of mood-altering drugs or hallucinogens
- Decreased goal-directed activity
- Impaired social judgment
- Poor school or work performance
- Self-destructive behaviors or injury potential
- Apathy
- Compliance difficulties

Nutritional-metabolic pattern
- Increased salivation
- Erratic nutritional intake

Elimination pattern
- Nausea or vomiting

Activity-exercise pattern
- Unpredictable activity patterns
- Verbal or physical assaults on others
- Agitation

Sleep-rest pattern
- Fatigue
- Sleep deprivation
- Nightmares
- Daytime flashbacks

Cognitive-perceptual pattern
- Body image changes
- Visual and auditory distortions
- Illusions
- Feelings of depersonalization
- Paranoia
- Suspicion
- Fear of losing control
- Synesthesia (such as hearing colors or seeing sounds)
- Increased sense of color, sound, smell, and taste
- Time or space alterations

Self-perception–self-concept pattern
- Fearfulness
- Guilt and shame
- Denial of hallucinogen use

Role-relationship pattern
- Social, interpersonal, and economic problems
- Family history of substance abuse or dependence

Sexual-reproductive pattern
- Sperm abnormalities
- Sterility (in males)
- Anovulatory cycles
- Retarded sexual development (teenagers)
- Sexually transmitted diseases

Coping–stress tolerance pattern
- Anxiety or panic
- Fatigue or stress resulting in increased flashbacks
- History of psychiatric problems
- Substance abuse or dependence history
- Family history of psychiatric or substance use disorders

Value-belief pattern
- Religious or cultural belief systems that incorporate the drug use

Physical findings

Cardiovascular
- Coma or death from respiratory or cardiac failure (with PCP)
- Diaphoresis
- Hypertensive crisis (with PCP)
- Increased blood pressure
- Tachycardia or palpitations

Respiratory
- Asthma-like symptoms (with THC)
- Bronchitis (with THC)
- Lung cancer (with THC)
- Pneumonia (with THC)
- Sinusitis (with THC)

Gastrointestinal
- Increased salivation
- Nausea or vomiting

Genitourinary
- Decreased prostate and testes size
- Impaired sperm production and increased chromosomal breakage rate (with THC)

Musculoskeletal
- Muscle twitching

Neurologic
- Ataxia
- Confusion
- Quickened deep tendon reflexes with intoxication
- Delirium
- Dilated pupils
- Dizziness (with LSD)
- Headache (with LSD)
- Horizontal nystagmus (with PCP)
- Lack of coordination
- Muteness or catatonia
- Numbness or tingling of the lower extremities (with LSD)
- Piloerection
- Respiratory or cardiovascular depression with higher doses
- Restlessness
- Seizures
- Visual blurring

Psychological
- Altered time or space perceptions
- Anxiety or panic
- Depersonalization
- Distractibility
- Euphoria or calm
- Labile mood
- Suggestibility

NURSING DIAGNOSIS

Sensory or perceptual alterations (visual, auditory, kinesthetic, gustatory, tactile, or olfactory) related to decreased cognitive function resulting from hallucinogen intake

Nursing priority

Help the client respond appropriately to environment stimuli.

Patient outcome criteria

As treatment progresses, the client, family, or both should be able to:
• demonstrate focused and correct orientation to people, places, and time
• report a reduction or cessation of hallucinations.

Interventions	Rationales
1. Monitor the client's intoxication symptoms hourly.	**1.** Peak intoxication levels vary, so determining the last dosage time can be difficult. Hourly monitoring can help the nurse implement appropriate interventions.
2. Monitor and document hourly the client's orientation to people, places, and time.	**2.** Hallucinogens can cause misperceptions of time, place, and person. Accurate client orientation may indicate the alleviation of the drug's acute effects.
3. Document hourly the presence or absence of altered perceptions in the client.	**3.** Altered perceptions are a major symptom of acute hallucinogen intoxication.
4. Administer prescribed antianxiety or antipsychotic medications.	**4.** Benzodiazepines are indicated for extreme anxiety related to hallucinogen abuse. Haloperidol can diminish severe misperceptions.
5. Approach the client calmly and use care when touching the client.	**5.** Because the client may be experiencing visual and tactile alterations, the nurse should approach calmly and cautiously to avoid unnecessary agitation.
6. Encourage the client to keep his eyes open and to either sit up or walk in a quiet environment.	**6.** Because closed eyes can intensify altered perceptions, the nurse should keep the client focused on the current environment.

NURSING DIAGNOSIS

Risk for injury related to impaired judgment and disorientation

Nursing priority

Maintain the safety of the client and others.

Patient outcome criteria

As treatment progresses, the client, family, or both should be able to:
• report an absence of injury to himself or others.

Addiction disorders

Interventions

1. Search the client and the client's belongings upon admission to the unit.

2. Provide a safe, quiet environment for the client.

3. Use physical restraints on the client only after first trying psychological and chemical interventions.

4. If the client cannot comply with commands or requests, move the client to a calm environment.

5. Encourage the client to verbalize fears and harmful impulses.

Rationales

1. The client might be carrying illicit drugs. If self-administered, these drugs can complicate assessment and withdrawal.

2. Hallucinations can be frightening to the client and can foster self-aggression or aggression toward others. Decreasing the environmental stimuli can help prevent intensification of the hallucinations.

3. An actively hallucinating client will not perceive restraints as a calming experience. Rather, such a client will be more likely to physically resist the restraints, possibly increasing his anxiety level and become increasingly agitated.

4. Redirection and reorientation can help calm a hallucinating client, thereby promoting compliant behavior.

5. By encouraging the client to verbalize fears and harmful impulses, the nurse can begin to redirect and reorient the client.

NURSING DIAGNOSIS

Altered thought processes related to hallucinogen abuse and evidenced by auditory or visual hallucinations, inattentiveness, problem-solving inabilities, impaired memory, or inability to retain information

Nursing priority

Facilitate the client's ability to interpret reality appropriately.

Patient outcome criteria

As treatment progresses, the client, family, or both should be able to:
• report improved ability to interpret reality
• report a reduction or cessation of hallucinations
• demonstrate improved ability for problem solving.

Interventions

1. Assess the client for hallucinations or altered thought processes hourly.

2. Encourage the client to drink plenty of fluids, especially water and fruit juices.

3. Reorient the client to people, places, and time.

4. Monitor the client's laboratory values for electrolyte imbalances, arterial blood gas alterations, and urine pH levels.

Rationales

1. Hourly assessment provides the nurse with critical information about peak intoxication levels and about the duration of the drug's effects. This knowledge also can help the nurse to implement safe, appropriate interventions during detoxification.

2. An increased fluid intake helps flush the body of drugs. Fruit juice provides the client with both calories and vitamins.

3. Frequent reorientation can calm the client until the drug effects decrease and the client can regain and maintain baseline orientation.

4. Laboratory values provide a data base for determining drug effects as well as the effects of nursing or medical interventions.

5. Provide a safe, calm environment for the client by decreasing external stimulation.

5. Hallucinations can be frightening to the client and can foster self-aggression or aggression toward others. Decreasing the environmental stimuli can help prevent intensification of the hallucinations.

6. Collaborate with multidisciplinary team members to ensure comprehensive client management.

6. Multidisciplinary approaches can provide the client with the highest care quality during acute intoxication and withdrawal.

NURSING DIAGNOSIS

Sleep pattern disturbance related to hallucinogen abuse or intoxication as evidenced by verbal complaints of sleeping inability, nightmares, or interrupted sleep

Nursing priority

Ensure that the client receives at least 4 hours of uninterrupted sleep per day.

Patient outcome criteria

As treatment progresses, the client, family, or both should be able to:
• verbalize an understanding of how mood-altering substances interfere with sleep cycles
• demonstrate the ability to use nonmood-altering substances promote sleep.

Interventions

1. Determine the client's usual sleeping pattern and identify how exactly it has been altered.

2. Establish a daytime rest and activity schedule appropriate to the client's current detoxification status.

3. Educate the client and family about ways to promote normal sleep patterns.

4. Provide the client with a quiet environment.

Rationales

1. By identifying the client's usual sleeping pattern and the nature of the sleep disturbance, the nurse can more appropriately educate the client about hallucinogen abuse and dependence. Episodic disturbances may be directly related to the substance used, and it may be 6 months to 1 year before the client is able to return to a normal sleep pattern.

2. Such a schedule can foster a normal sleep cycle that provides adequate rest.

3. The nurse should encourage the use of natural relaxation measures without chemical use to improve the client's sleep pattern, such as decreasing caffeine intake, establishing consistent retiring and waking times, practicing relaxation techniques, decreasing environmental stimuli, drinking warm milk and eating snacks at bedtime, taking a warm bath before bedtime, and decreasing daytime napping. The client should avoid caffeine, a central nervous system stimulant.

4. A stimulating environment increases hypervigilance, thereby inhibiting the client from sleeping.

NURSING DIAGNOSIS

Risk for injury related to poisoning by use of adulterated street drugs

Nursing priority

Protect the client from the physical effects of adulterated drugs.

Addiction disorders

Patient outcome criteria

As treatment progresses, the client, family, or both should be able to:
• demonstrate an understanding of the relationship between adulterated drugs and the potential for localized or systemic health problems.

Interventions

1. Teach the client about the specific adulterated drugs and their effects.

2. Obtain a comprehensive toxicology screening of the client, and assess the client's risk for poisoning caused by adulterated drugs.

Rationales

1. Such knowledge can increase the client's understanding of the drug and encourage appropriate behavioral changes.

2. Toxicology screens provide the nurse with information about possible adulterated substances in the client's system. This allows the nurse to seek appropriate medical assistance to prevent life-threatening complications.

DISCHARGE CRITERIA

Nursing documentation indicates that the client:
• has verbalized an intent to maintain abstinence
• is maintaining vital signs within normal limits
• understands what occurs in hallucinogen abuse and dependence
• has demonstrated a willingness to participate in ongoing therapy
• has scheduled the necessary follow-up appointments.
Nursing documentation also indicates that the family:
• understands the client's diagnosis, treatment, and expected outcomes
• has been referred to the appropriate community and family resources
• has demonstrated a willingness to participate in a self-help group.
• understands when, why, and how to contact the appropriate health care professional in case of an emergency.

SELECTED REFERENCES

Allen, K.M. *Nursing Care of the Addicted Client.* Philadelphia: Lippincott-Raven Pubs., 1996.
Gelenberg, A.J., and Bassuk, E.L. *The Practitioner's Guide to Psychoactive Drugs.* New York: Plenum Publishing Corp., 1997.
Lowinson, J.H., et al. *Substance Abuse: A Comprehensive Text.* Baltimore: Williams & Wilkins Co., 1997.
Miller, N.S., et al. *Manual of Therapeutics for Addictions.* New York: Wiley-Liss, 1997.
Miller, N.S. *The Principles and Practice of Addictions in Psychiatry.* Philadelphia: W.B. Saunders Co., 1997.

Polysubstance-related disorder

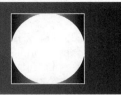

DSM-IV classification
304.80 Polysubstance dependence

Psychiatric nursing diagnostic class
Substance abuse

INTRODUCTION

Polysubstance dependence diagnosis is reserved for clients who use at least three different psychoactive substances (not including caffeine and nicotine) concurrently for more than 12 months. The substances used include any or all of the following: depressants (alcohol, sedatives, barbiturates, and benzodiazepines), stimulants (amphetamines, amphetamine-like substances, and cocaine), opioids (morphine, codeine, and heroin), and hallucinogens (marijuana or tetrahydrocannabinoids [THCs]; lysergic acid diethylamide [LSD]; 3,4-methylenedioxymethamphetamine [MDMA]; and phencyclidine [PCP]). Many clients with alcohol-related disorders also use marijuana or cocaine. Individuals on methadone maintenance have been found to use cocaine intravenously.

Individuals with polysubstance dependence expose themselves not only to the serious physical consequences of chronic involving several substances but also to diseases resulting from poor diet and poor personal hygiene. Furthermore, cocaine use can cause sudden death from cardiac arrhythmia, cerebrovascular accident, myocardial infarction, or respiratory arrest. Using and sharing contaminated needles for I.V. administration of amphetamines, cocaine, or heroin exposes users to various infections, including human immunodeficiency virus (HIV) and its related disorders. Additionally, it is not uncommon for individuals who are under the influence of several substances to have unprotected sex or not be able to recall if they practiced safe sex, which places them at risk for sexually transmitted diseases (including HIV).

Like other psychoactive substance use disorders, polysubstance dependence is characterized by intoxication; interference with work, family life, and social relationships; withdrawal symptoms; and physical diseases caused by the toxic effects of the drugs. Addicted individuals typically rely on the drugs to produce desired states and believe that they need the drugs to cope with life. Additionally they need the drugs to avoid withdrawal symptoms. As a result, they develop strong defense mechanisms to protect their substance-abuse dependence and to avoid anxiety.

Etiology and precipitating factors
Research suggests that many polysubstance-dependent individuals use alcohol and psychoactive substances to relieve anxiety, stress, or depression. Depressants may be combined with stimulants to alter moods and assist with sleep or relaxation. Narcotics may be used to produce a euphoria that alleviates irritability, anger, aggression, and rage. Alcohol may be used to decrease or intensify the effects of other drugs, to modify withdrawal symptoms, or to substitute for an unavailable drug. Individuals vulnerable to this kind of polysubstance abuse typically have low self-esteem, poor coping skills, and an inability to control or master their environment.

Biological research suggests that a genetic vulnerability to addiction may play a part in polysubstance dependence. Neurologic changes, which follow prolonged drug exposure and which cause alterations in mood and drive, may further reinforce the addiction tendency.

Psychological research suggests that polysubstance use is associated with an increased incidence of behavior and conduct problems, psychiatric disorders (including depression), attention deficit hyperactivity disorder, and anxiety disorder.

Potential complications
Polysubstance dependence can lead to various complications, including acquired immunodeficiency syndrome (AIDS), alcoholic hepatitis, anxiety, aspiration pneumonia, cardiac arrest, cardiomyopathy, cerebellar degeneration, cerebral hemorrhage, child abuse or neglect, cirrhosis, death from asphyxiation, dementia, fetal alcohol syndrome, hyperpyrexia, immunosuppression, legal problems, marital discord and family problems, nasal septum perforation, nose and throat cancer, acute or chronic pancreatitis, psychosis, pulmonary emboli, reduced testosterone and sperm count, respiratory depression and arrest, learning difficulties, sexual dysfunction, and Korsakoff's syndrome.

ASSESSMENT GUIDELINES
Nursing history (functional health pattern findings)
Health perception–health management pattern
- Denial of treatment need
- Minimizing of addiction problems
- Concern about alcohol or certain drug while denying substance use
- Underestimation of daily alcohol consumption

- Overestimation of or bragging about functional abilities while under alcohol or drug influence
- Exaggeration of drug use
- Resistance to treatment
- Hostility and defensiveness when questioned about drug use
- Belief that drinking or drug use can be stopped at any time

Nutritional-metabolic pattern
- Weight gain or loss
- Lack of interest in nutritious foods and beverages
- Tendency to buy drugs and alcohol rather than food
- Overconsumption of junk food

Elimination pattern
- Concern over GI disturbances (pain, diarrhea, nausea, constipation, vomiting, bleeding)
- Frequent urination or urine retention

Activity-exercise pattern
- Mobility problems related to automobile accidents, falls, or traumatic injuries
- Hyperactivity or lethargy
- Unexplained syncope and dizziness
- Unsteady gait

Sleep-rest pattern
- Insomnia or excessive sleep

Cognitive-perceptual pattern
- Difficulty concentrating
- Difficulty with decoding sensory input
- Worry over inability to think clearly
- Distorted perceptions
- Grandiose thinking

Self-perception–self-concept pattern
- Lack of eye contact
- Isolation
- Difficulty accepting positive reinforcement
- Feelings of hopelessness and worthlessness
- Excessive criticism of self and others
- Anxiety about entering hospital for treatment
- Little or no family support
- Suicidal ideation or suicidal gestures
- Blame of drug use on external sources
- Description of self as dependent and controlled by psychoactive substances or as superior and in control of lifestyle

Role-relationship pattern
- Concern about relationships with family and loved ones
- Alienation from others
- Job performance difficulties or frequent job changes

Sexual-reproductive pattern
- Difficulties with intimacy
- Reliance on chemicals to perform sexually
- Sexual dysfunction
- Concern about participation in high-risk sexual activity in conjunction with I.V. drug use

Coping-stress tolerance pattern
- Denial of present anxiety
- Feelings of being out of control
- Fear of entering the hospital and of having to give up alcohol or other drugs
- Reliance on chemicals to feel good
- Inability to meet basic daily needs
- Maladaptive defenses (such as denial, rationalization, and projection)
- Hostility when questioned
- Low frustration tolerance

Value-belief pattern
- Feeling powerless to achieve life goals
- Lack of interest in anything
- Guilt and shame
- Diminished sense of spirituality

Physical findings
Cardiovascular
- Elevated or low blood pressure
- Flushed face
- Spider nevi or angioma
- Orthostatic hypotension
- Arrhythmias
- Cold, clammy skin
- Edema
- Increased or decreased heart rate
- Heart failure
- Dehydration and electrolyte imbalance

Respiratory
- Respiratory depression or failure

Gastrointestinal
- Emaciation
- Hepatomegaly
- Nausea and vomiting
- Splenomegaly

Genitourinary
- Gynecomastia
- Small testes

Integumentary
- Cigarette stains or burns on fingers
- Many scars or tattoos
- Poor personal hygiene
- Unexplained bruises, abrasion, or cuts

Musculoskeletal
- Muscle weakness

Neurologic
- Agitated behavior
- Dizziness
- Lack of coordination
- Nystagmus
- Parotid gland enlargement

- Seizures
- Slurred speech
- Staggered gait
- Tremulousness

Psychological
- Anxiety
- Irritability
- Sleep disturbances

NURSING DIAGNOSIS

Sensory and perceptual alterations related to multiple psychoactive substance withdrawal

Nursing priority

Help the client achieve detoxification with minimum psychological and physiologic effects.

Patient outcome criteria

As treatment progresses, the client, family, or both should be able to:
- report the absence of psychoactive substance withdrawal symptoms
- exhibit no evidence of physical injury obtained during detoxification.

Interventions

1. Compile a history of the client's alcohol and drug use.

2. Determine the client's intoxication or withdrawal stage, assessing for orientation, hallucinations, speech pattern, and need for safety measures.

3. Monitor the client's response to medications given for withdrawal symptoms. (The use of objective quantification assessment tools is recommended. See "Benzodiazepine withdrawal assessment," page 298.)

4. Provide the client with a safe, calm environment with minimal stimuli.

5. Monitor the client's vital signs at least four times daily for the first 72 hours after admission.

Rationales

1. By thoroughly assessing and documenting the client's drug and alcohol use, the nurse can better distinguish the withdrawal symptoms from other symptoms and behavior.

2. The nurse should complete a comprehensive assessment upon admission and continuously assess the client during the course of treatment. This allows the nurse to determine if the client is experiencing complications caused by intoxication (signs of impending shock) or by the withdrawal of the drug

3. The nurse's observations help determine how much medication the client needs to relieve withdrawal symptoms and prevent severe physical or psychological complications.

4. Providing a safe environment helps the nurse prevent the client from harming himself or anyone else during withdrawal. A calm environment prevents unnecessary agitation.

5. Vital signs provide the most reliable information about the client's condition during acute detoxification.

NURSING DIAGNOSIS

Ineffective individual coping related to maladaptive reliance on alcohol and other drugs

Nursing priority

Help the client develop positive coping skills.

Addiction disorders

Patient outcome criteria

As treatment progresses, the client, family, or both should be able to:
• identify ineffective coping behaviors and their negative consequences
• demonstrate an ability to cope with stress constructively.

Interventions	Rationales
1. Establish a trusting relationship with client by being honest, keeping appointments, and being available.	**1.** Establishing trust is the first step in convincing the client to develop more appropriate, positive behaviors.
2. Encourage the client to verbalize feelings, fears, and anxieties.	**2.** Verbalizing feelings in a nonthreatening environment can help the client recognize and begin to resolve many uncomfortable feelings that may have led to polysubstance dependence.
3. Provide the client with opportunities to rehearse problem-solving strategies within the treatment milieu.	**3.** Such rehearsals can improve the client's ability to use effective, healthy means to solve problems.
4. Teach the client positive long-term coping strategies that focus on assertiveness, sharing thoughts and feelings with others, and relaxing.	**4.** These strategies can help the client learn to cope with feelings and stress in a more constructive way.
5. Set limits on the client's manipulative and irresponsible behavior.	**5.** Limiting and enforcing the consequences of irresponsible behaviors can help the client learn more appropriate behaviors.
6. Examine specific problems to help the client identify how substance abuse is causing problems in his life.	**6.** Acknowledging the relationship between substance abuse and problems can assist in decreasing the client's defenses and develop positive coping methods.
7. Positively reinforce the client's efforts to solve problems constructively.	**7.** Reinforcement enhances self-esteem and encourages the client to adopt acceptable behaviors.
8. Encourage the client to become involved in support groups.	**8.** The client will probably need long-term support for effective coping; suggest groups such as Alcoholics Anonymous or Narcotics Anonymous.

NURSING DIAGNOSIS

Self-esteem disturbance related to perceived failures and lack of positive feedback

Nursing priority

Help the client develop and maintain feelings of increased self-worth.

Patient outcome criteria

As treatment progresses, the client, family, or both should be able to:
• verbalize awareness of anxiety and low self-esteem
• acknowledge that polysubstance abuse is a problem
• demonstrate improved problem-solving skills
• verbalize positive personal traits.

Interventions

1. Communicate acceptance of the client and his condition.

2. Spend scheduled time with the client.

3. Work with the client to identify and focus on personal strengths and accomplishments.

4. Encourage the client to participate in group and family therapy sessions.

5. Encourage the client to participate in treatment-related decisions and to accept responsibility for his condition.

6. Reinforce the client's belief in the ability to change.

7. Help the client to explore both positive and negative traits and behaviors.

Rationales

1. By conveying an accepting attitude, the nurse can enhance the client's feelings of self-worth.

2. Time scheduled with the client provides the nurse with opportunities to convey acceptance and to enhance the client's feelings of self-worth.

3. Doing so can help the client develop a more positive outlook.

4. Positive feedback and support from others can enhance the client's feelings of self-worth. Group and family therapies allow the client to develop open and honest communication.

5. Such participation promotes an attitude of self-care and encourages the client to adopt positive behaviors.

6. Reinforcing the client's belief in self-change can instill an attitude of hope and self-control over drug dependence.

7. The client may be using drugs to deny the existence of such traits and behaviors. Encouraging discussions and exploration of feelings will help to validate the client's feelings and enhance the client's self-worth.

NURSING DIAGNOSIS

Powerlessness related to lack of control over psychoactive substance use

Nursing priority

Help the client develop values and skills that will enable him to regain a sense of control and meaning in life.

Patient outcome criterion

As treatment progresses, the client, family, or both should be able to:
• demonstrate acceptance of responsibility for self-care.

Interventions

1. Help the client to identify feelings of powerlessness.

2. Encourage the client to make choices and establish goals.

3. Help the client to differentiate situations that can be changed from those that cannot.

Rationales

1. The client probably has been coping with feelings, including intense cravings and resentment about the substance dependency, through denial and drug use and must now begin to recognize and resolve feelings in more positive ways.

2. By actively participating in decision-making activities and establishing short-term and long-term goals, the client can regain a sense of control over his condition and work toward a more productive life.

3. By identifying what the client does and does not have control over, the client can learn to direct his energies productively.

4. Encourage the client to accept the spiritual dimension of 12-step treatments.

4. Twelve-step groups such as Alcoholics Anonymous stress reliance on a higher power, which is said to provide relief from anxiety caused by feelings of powerlessness.

DISCHARGE CRITERIA

Nursing documentation indicates that the client:
• has verbalized an understanding of how polysubstance abuse affects health
• has demonstrated an improved self-concept and an increased feeling of control
• uses positive coping skills to control cravings and anxiety
• has verbalized an understanding of situations that trigger polysubstance use
• has verbalized an awareness of the relationship between high-risk behaviors (I.V. drug use, unprotected sex, and AIDS)
• has demonstrated an awareness of safe sex practices that decrease the risk of spreading HIV
• has verbalized an intent to participate in ongoing outpatient therapy and peer support through a 12-step group in the community
• is aware of available community support services
• has expressed a willingness to participate in an ongoing treatment program.
Nursing documentation also indicates that the family:
• has been referred to the appropriate community and family support resources.

SELECTED REFERENCES

Allen, K.M. *Nursing Care of the Addicted Client.* Philadelphia: Lippincott-Raven Pubs., 1996.

Diagnostic and Statistical Manual of Mental Disorders, 4th ed. Washington, D.C.: American Psychiatric Association, 1994.

Boyd, M.A., and Nihart, M.A. *Psychiatric Nursing: Contemporary Practice.* Philadelphia: Lippincott-Raven Pubs., 1998.

Kinney, J. *Clinical Manual of Substance Abuse,* 2nd ed. St. Louis: Mosby–Year Book, Inc., 1996.

Lowinson, J.H., et al. *Substance Abuse: A Comprehensive Text,* 3rd ed. Baltimore: Williams & Wilkins Co., 1997.

Miller, N.S. *The Principles and Practice of Addictions in Psychiatry.* Philadelphia: W.B. Saunders Co., 1997.

Part 9

Eating disorders

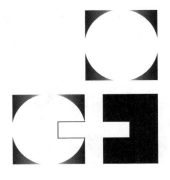

Anorexia nervosa and bulimia nervosa

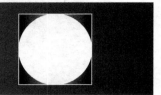

DSM-IV classifications
307.10 Anorexia nervosa
307.51 Bulimia nervosa
307.50 Eating disorder not otherwise specified

Psychiatric nursing diagnostic class
Disordered eating pattern

INTRODUCTION

Eating disorders are characterized by severe disturbances in eating behavior. Individuals with these disorders tend to alternate between anorexia nervosa and bulimia nervosa, or between bulimia nervosa and obesity. A disturbance in perception of body shape and size is an essential feature of both disorders.

Anorexia nervosa is characterized by a refusal to maintain a minimally normal body weight. The individual is intensely fearful of gaining weight and exhibits significant disturbance in the perception of body size, shape, or both. Postmenarcheal females with this disorder are typically amenorrheic.

Bulimia nervosa is characterized by repeated episodes of binge eating followed by inappropriate compensatory behaviors, such as self-induced vomiting; misuse of laxatives, diuretics, or other medications; fasting; or excessive exercise. A binge episode is also accompanied by a sense of being out of control and feeling frenzied. There are two subtypes of bulimia nervosa: purging and nonpurging. The purging subtype involves an individual who engages in self-inflicted vomiting and abuses diuretics, laxatives, or enemas. The nonpurging subtype involves an individual who fasts or uses excessive exercise to maintain body weight

Although simple obesity is coded as a general medical condition, it is not recognized as a mental disorder by *DSM-IV* at this time because it has not been consistently associated with a psychological or behavioral syndrome.

Etiology and precipitating factors

The causes of eating disorders are not completely understood, but clinicians and researchers agree that numerous biopsychosocial factors are involved. Biochemical evidence points to potential disruptions of the nuclei in the hypothalamus. There are specific CNS nuclei in the lateral hypothalamus that are associated with many aspects of hunger and satiety. Disruption in these nuclei may be the result of extreme weight loss and starvation. Deficits (decreases or alterations) in the lateral hypothalamus result in decreased eating, decreased response to sensory stimuli, decreased arousal, and other behaviors related to eating.

Norepinephrine, serotonin, dopamine, and several neuropeptides may all interact to initiate eating behavior or decrease food intake. Additionally, norepinephrine and serotonin have an important role in mood regulation and mood states.

No single gene or genetic trait has yet been found specific to eating disorders. Work continues in this area, but it has been difficult to separate potential genetic contributions from the influences of family patterns and behavior.

Psychological theories have focused on the maternal-child relationship as the foundation of eating disorders. Developmental theorists, influenced by feminist perspectives, have attempted to understand how mothers and daughters share vulnerabilities to eating disorders that may be associated with female sex role socialization. Additional research is targeted at conflict around separation and individuation processes, gender identity, self-image, body image, and sexuality in any interpersonal relationships

According to family theorists, individuals with eating disorders typically come from families with rigid rules and roles, blurred or nonexistent boundaries, and overprotective parents. Typically, the family might have rules against talking, expressing feelings, and discussing sexuality. Perfectionism is usually a family expectation. These stressors and vulnerabilities occur in our societal context, which has established and overvalued an idealization of thinness. (See *Potential risk factors for eating disorders.*)

Potential complications

Eating disorders have numerous medical consequences and severe complications. The most life-threatening complications include cardiac arrhythmias, coronary artery disease, dehydration, gastrointestinal bleeding, hypokalemia, hypothermia, metabolic acidosis, pancreatic dysfunction, pulmonary insufficiency, substance abuse or dependence, an undiagnosed affective disorder, or sudden death.

Potential risk factors for eating disorders

• Age of onset is early childhood to adolescence (ages 9 to 13)
• Concurrent psychiatric disorders in self and family members
• Consistent presence of self-esteem issues
• Denial of disturbance in eating or any emotional problems
• Disturbed family system relationships in which rigidity and perfectionism are characteristic family themes
• Duration of illness is longer
• Persistently low weight
• Premorbid history of weight issues (obesity)
• Sexual abuse history
• Predisposing emotional and psychological factors include black-and-white thinking (all or none), fear of losing control, self-esteem that is other-oriented (dependent on what others think of them), and a sense of helplessness or powerlessnes

Adapted with permission from Boyd, M.A., and Nihart, M.A. *Psychiatric Nursing: Contemporary Practice.* Philadelphia: Lippincott-Raven Pubs., 1998, p. 679.

ASSESSMENT GUIDELINES

Nursing history (functional health pattern findings)

Health perception–health management pattern
• Inability to control feelings
• Denial of health problems even when confronted with concrete evidence indicating physical problems
• Hypervigilance about weight and body shape
• Use of alcohol, caffeine, nicotine, or other drugs

Nutritional-metabolic pattern
• Restricted daily food intake
• Binge eating
• Purging behaviors (vomiting, intense exercise, fasting)
• Use of diuretics, cathartics, and diet pills
• Obsession with counting calories
• Hiding and hoarding food
• Frequent weight fluctuations
• Being underweight (at least 15% of ideal body weight)
• Increased incidence of dental problems, including caries
• Hair loss
• Dry or yellowish skin

Elimination pattern
• Constipation or diarrhea
• Use of cathartics and diuretics
• Rebound water retention after purging
• Bowel obstruction

Activity-exercise pattern
• Compulsive exercise
• Sedentary lifestyle
• Normal daily activity disruptions

Sleep-rest pattern
• Inability to sleep without interruption

Cognitive-perceptual pattern
• Difficulty concentrating
• Distorted perception of body image

Self-perception–self-concept pattern
• Perception of eating as a problematic behavior
• Preoccupation with food
• Description of self as fat even when emaciated
• Overconcern with and intense fear of gaining weight
• Guilt and shame
• Negative self-concept
• Obsession with body image and appearance
• Feelings of powerlessness

Role-relationship pattern
• Overprotective family system
• High and unrealistic family expectations
• Role reversal, characterized by feeling responsible for nurturing parents
• Avoidance of intimate relationships

Sexual-reproductive pattern
• History of amenorrhea
• Breast atrophy
• Confusion or anxiety over sexual role
• Promiscuity
• Significantly delayed psychosexual development
• Decreased libido

Coping–stress tolerance pattern
• Use of food and eating behaviors as primary coping mechanisms
• Inability to identify and name feelings
• Anxiety
• Depression
• Difficulties with impulse control
• Sexual abuse or incest
• Low self-esteem
• Substance use or abuse

Value-belief pattern
• Inability to achieve goals
• Belief that perfection is unattainable
• Difficulty trusting others

Physical findings

Cardiovascular
• Anemia
• Arrhythmias
• Cyanosis of extremities
• Dehydration
• Peripheral edema
• Emetic-induced cardiomyopathy
• Orthostatic hypotension
• Hypertension (with obesity)
• Hypochloremia, hyponatremia, or hypokalemia

- Rebound water retention after purging
Respiratory
- Aspiration pneumonia
- Pulmonary insufficiency (with obesity)
Gastrointestinal
- Parotid gland swelling
- Bleeding gums
- Bloating secondary to delayed gastric emptying
- Cachexia
- Constipation
- Caries
- Diarrhea
- Emaciation
- Esophagitis
- Gastric rupture
- Hematemesis
- Mouth sores
- Rectal bleeding
- Rectal prolapse
Genitourinary
- Amenorrhea
- Vaginal mucosa atrophy

- Dyspareunia
- Irregular menses
- Renal calculi
Musculoskeletal
- Muscle weakness
- Osteoporosis
Neurologic
- Dizziness or faintness
- Light-headedness
- Reduced attention and concentration
Psychological
- Apathy
- Anxiety
- Depression
- Guilt
- Irritability
- Mood lability
- Obsession with body image and thinness
- Shame
- Sleep disturbances
- Social withdrawal

NURSING DIAGNOSIS

Altered nutrition: less than body requirements, related to refusal to eat, purging activities, or excessive physical exercise

Nursing priority

Help the client reduce the incidence of food restriction and purging behaviors.

Patient outcome criterion

As the treatment progresses, the client and family should be able to:
- report a decrease in or absence of binge eating or purging.

Interventions

1. Collaborate with the client and multidisciplinary team to identify a target weight range (about 90% of the client's ideal body weight), and determine the calories necessary to provide adequate nutrition and achieve the targeted weight.

2. Establish a weight gain range and make a contract with the client for attaining this goal.

3. Explain to the client the benefits of compliance and the consequences of noncompliance with the established behavioral program.

Rationales

1. Including both the care team and the client in such decisions can enhance the client's sense of self-control and offers reassurance that staff members are not plotting to make the client overweight.

2. A weight range can help the client learn to accept small weight fluctuations as normal. A contract enhances the client's sense of self-control.

3. The client should understand that when body weight falls to 15% below ideal body weight (IBW) and body fat levels are 10% below ideal levels, weight restoration treatment becomes a priority. If the client fails to demonstrate appropriate meal patterns and weight restoration after several weeks, an inpatient hospital setting becomes necessary for the client's physical well-being.

4. Establish and monitor a behavioral program appropriate to the client's condition.

4. A complete, well-defined behavioral modification program typically is prescribed on inpatient psychiatric units to enhance the client's compliance with treatment. Parameters might include some or all of the following:
• weighing the client daily to three times per week
• using the same scale and maintaining a consistent weighing schedule
• having the client wear the same amount of clothing for each weighing
• inspecting the client's clothing for objects or weights that would artificially increase weight
• monitoring and limiting the client's fluid intake to not more than 500 ml at one time
• directly observing the client at mealtime for food hoarding and hiding
• establishing a defined time for finishing meals (approximately 30 minutes)
• arranging specific times for prescribed and monitored physical activity
• monitoring the client's vital signs and intake and output
• establishing a primary nurse or case manager system
• incorporating behavioral and social rewards for appropriate eating.
Privileges should be granted or restricted based on compliance and weight restoration.

5. Assure the client that a quick weight gain is not desirable and that a slow, regulated weight gain is the goal.

5. This can allay any client anxiety over rapid weight gain.

6. Begin exploring the client's fear of gaining weight as the nutritional status stabilizes and normal eating behaviors become established. Have the client take an eating attitudes test to help identify specific problem areas.

6. The client must begin identifying and acknowledging underlying emotional issues if maladaptive responses are to be changed.

7. Check the client's belongings for laxatives, diuretics, and diet medications upon admission and when the client returns from therapeutic passes and off-unit activities.

7. The client may seek out and conceal such substances if compulsive purging needs are not met or addressed in a therapeutic atmosphere.

8. Encourage the client to participate in group sessions and to ask for feedback about food intake and activity.

8. Group feedback provides the client with support during attempts to establish an appropriate balance between food intake and amount of physical activity; many anorexics also exercise compulsively.

9. For the client in an outpatient setting, establish specific behavioral criteria that would signal a need for inpatient care.

9. Criteria for inpatient care might include a life-threatening weight loss or medical complication, suicidal ideation or attempts, uncontrolled purging, and concomitant chemical dependency. Negotiating a contract with the client about potential inpatient care can facilitate a trusting relationship between the client and nurse and promote client safety.

NURSING DIAGNOSIS

Altered nutrition: potential for less than body requirements related to binge eating and purging

Nursing priority

Help the client to demonstrate a reduction in signs and symptoms of binge eating and purging.

Patient outcome criterion

As the treatment progresses, the client and family should be able to:
• obtain and maintain an appropriate healthy food intake.

Interventions

1. Sit with the client during meals.

2. Teach the client delay and distraction measures to use when faced with the urge to binge.

3. Once nutritional status has improved, explore the client's feelings associated with weight gain.

4. Help the client identify high-risk times for binge eating and purging, such as when bored or feeling lonely.

Rationales

1. This provides support for the client and permits observation of intake.

2. Distraction measures can help the client learn to differentiate an emotional response from hunger. Measures might include speaking with a staff member, calling a friend, attending a support group meeting, calling a sponsor, or using relaxation techniques. These measures also can help the client to learn the relationship between mood changes and the eating disorder.

3. Emotional issues need to be resolved if the client is to refrain from maladaptive eating behavior.

4. This allows the nurse and the client to explore better ways to deal with those times, such as by calling a friend, taking a bath, or going for a walk instead of eating.

NURSING DIAGNOSIS

Body image disturbance related to the client's misperceived physical appearance

Nursing priority

Help the client verbalize misperceptions of body image, including those of shape and size.

Patient outcome criterion

As the treatment progresses, the client and family should be able to:
• verbalize a realistic body image.

Interventions

1. Ask the client to define an ideal body shape and size, then determine the client's perception of meeting that standard. Point out the client's positive physical attributes.

Rationales

1. Identifying positive physical attributes can enhance the client's self-worth and self-esteem.

2. Provide the client with positive reinforcement and factual feedback, but do not argue or challenge the client's distorted perceptions. Encourage the client to seek community or group feedback.

3. Refer the client to art and movement therapies that will provide objective information about body image.

4. Acknowledge and discuss the client's cultural and family values, beliefs, and stereotypes, especially those related to thinness and attractiveness.

5. Limit the client's discussions and comments about actual weight gain.

2. Positive reinforcement and factual feedback can enhance the client's self-esteem and provide opportunities for initiating and practicing independent functioning. Arguments or power struggles will only increase the client's underlying need to control.

3. External, objective feedback can help the client begin to recognize that his perceptions of body image are unrealistic and unhealthy.

4. Such information can help the client realize how family and cultural factors have fostered an unrealistic body image.

5. Any attention on actual weight gain may escalate the client's anxiety, thereby increasing phobic behaviors.

NURSING DIAGNOSIS

Knowledge deficit about nutrition and eating disorders

Nursing priority

Teach the client about nutrition and about eating disorders and their influence on physical and emotional well-being.

Patient outcome criteria

As the treatment progresses, the client, family, or both should be able to:
• demonstrate knowledge about the causes and effects of the eating disorder
• demonstrate an increased knowledge of nutrition.

Interventions

1. Collaborate with the dietitian to teach the client and family about nutrition, calories, food values, a balanced dietary plan, and foods that promote normal bowel function.

2. Arrange for the client to attend meal-planning classes, and encourage the client's participation in helping to plan a unit meal.

Rationales

1. Factual nutrition information can help the client challenge myths, fantasies, and misperceptions about food. Maintaining normal bowel function by diet may encourage the client to reduce laxative and cathartic use.

2. Participation in unit activities can enhance the client's sense of sharing and self-control and can decrease the client's sense of isolation.

NURSING DIAGNOSIS

Risk for injury related to excessive exercise or potentially harmful behaviors

Nursing priority

Help the client maintain personal safety.

Patient outcome criterion

As the treatment progresses, the client, family, or both should be able to:
• demonstrate an increased knowledge of nutrition.

Interventions

1. Explain to the client the physiologic impact of excessive exercise.

2. Collaborate with the client and multidisciplinary team to establish an appropriate activity schedule. Observe and monitor the client during private time.

3. Help the client to develop specific diversionary activities that can be used when he feels a need to exercise.

Rationales

1. The client should learn that excessive exercise can cause significant shifts in hormonal and metabolic functioning. This can result in amenorrhea, ketosis, and vitamin deficiency.

2. Collaborating in the care plan can enhance the client's sense of control; initially, however, the client may need protection from compulsive behaviors and possibly from escalating anxiety, guilt, and shame, which can precipitate a relapse into injurious compulsive exercising.

3. Diversionary activities can serve as concrete options to exercising. During a crisis, these activities can decrease the client's overwhelming anxiety and compulsive behaviors.

NURSING DIAGNOSIS

Altered family processes related to a dysfunctional family system as evidenced by a pervasive sense of perfectionism, overprotectiveness, or chaos

Nursing priority

Help the client and family identify roles, rules, and rituals that impede autonomous, differentiated functioning among family members and contribute to the client's eating disorder.

Patient outcome criterion

As the treatment progresses, the client and family should be able to:
• demonstrate the ability to establish appropriate boundaries and autonomy within the family.

Interventions

1. Explore the degree of dependency and enmeshment within the client's family.

2. Teach the client and family about family functions, roles, boundaries, and messages. Explore family patterns that reinforce the client's compulsive behavior.

3. Teach the client to develop problem-solving skills and rehearse ways in which to use them.

4. Encourage the client and family to participate in multiple family psychodrama or family sculpting sessions.

5. Initiate family therapy or refer the family to an appropriate therapist within the community.

Rationales

1. Dependency and enmeshment impede the normal separation process and the development of autonomy within the family.

2. Group educational sessions enable the client and family members to identify and validate feelings in a supportive, safe environment.

3. The client needs to develop skills and strategies that decrease the overinvolvement of family in the client's life. Such skills can increase the client's sense of self-control.

4. Family psychodrama and sculpting can help the client and family to clarify dysfunctional roles and messages in a safe, therapeutic environment.

5. The nurse can help the client and family identify alternative ways to meet their present and future needs.

NURSING DIAGNOSIS

Ineffective denial related to a lack of knowledge about real or potential dangers associated with eating disorders

Nursing priority

Challenge the client's denial and facilitate the client's participation in a treatment plan.

Patient outcome criterion

As the treatment progresses, the client, family, or both should be able to:
• demonstrate a willingness to participate in treatment.

Interventions

1. Ask the client's family and peers to encourage the client to seek treatment. Allow the client to express any anger or fears about being involved in treatment.

2. Collaborate with the client to identify problems and to establish mutually determined priorities.

Rationales

1. The client may require some pressure from others into starting treatment. Allowing the client to express anger and fear about treatment can foster a trusting nurse-client relationship.

2. Allowing the client to participate in the plan of care can enhance feelings of self-control and decrease anxiety.

NURSING DIAGNOSIS

Impaired social interaction related to withdrawal from peer group, fear of rejection, and preoccupation with eating behaviors or rituals

Nursing priority

Help the client develop positive strategies that facilitate socialization.

Patient outcome criterion

As the treatment progresses, the client, family, or both should be able to:
• demonstrate increased socialization skills.

Interventions

1. Individually or in a group, instruct and rehearse with the client interpersonal communication, socialization, and assertiveness skills. Use didactic and role-playing methods to reinforce learning.

2. Identify leisure activities that require minimal productivity from the client, and teach the client relaxation techniques for use during leisure time.

3. Arrange for the client to attend a self-help or support group.

Rationales

1. Social withdrawal may result from feelings of inadequacy in social situations and interpersonal relationships. Learning strategies for dealing with these feelings can draw the client out of isolation.

2. The client should learn to enjoy leisure activities as a counterbalance to a probably too-rigid need to be productive and successful.

3. Participation in support groups, such as Overeaters Anonymous or Anorexics and Bulimics Anonymous, can diminish the client's sense of social isolation and foster feelings of hope for recovery.

DISCHARGE CRITERIA

Nursing documentation indicates that the client:
• has demonstrated an increased ability to recognize signs and symptoms of eating disorders
• can use newly learned skills for managing anxiety, guilt, shame, and triggers that induce compulsive eating
• can identify appropriate internal and external support resources
• can use alternate coping skills
• has verbalized a desire to participate in an ongoing treatment program.

Nursing documentation also indicates that the family:
• has verbalized a knowledge of the client's diagnosis, treatment, and expected outcomes
• has been referred to the appropriate family and community resources
• has expressed a willingness to participate in an ongoing therapy program
• understands when, why, and how to contact the appropriate health care professional in case of an emergency.

SELECTED REFERENCES

Diagnostic and Statistical Manual of Mental Disorders, 4th ed. Washington, D.C.: American Psychiatric Association, 1994.

Boyd, M.A., and Nihart, M.A. *Psychiatric Nursing: Contemporary Practice.* Philadelphia: Lippincott-Raven Pubs., 1998.

Garner, D.M., and Garfinkel, P.E., eds. *Handbook of Treatment for Eating Disorders.* New York: Guilford Press, 1997.

McGowan, A., and Whitbread, J. "Out of Control! The Most Effective Way to Help the Binge-Eating Patient," *Journal of Psychosocial Nursing* 34(1):30-37, 1996.

Nathan, P.E., and Gorman, J.M. *A Guide to Treatments that Work.* New York: Oxford University Press, 1998.

Varcarolis, E.M. *Psychiatric-Mental Health Nursing,* 3rd ed. Philadelphia: W.B. Saunders Co., 1998.

Part 10

Psychophysiologic disorders

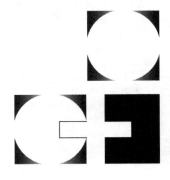

Somatoform and factitious disorders

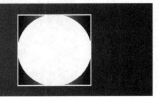

DSM-IV classifications

Somatoform disorders

300.11	Conversion disorder
300.7	Hypochondriasis
300.7	Body dysmorphic disorder
307.80	Pain disorder
300.81	Somatization disorder
300.81	Undifferentiated somatoform disorder
300.81	Somatoform disorder not otherwise specified

Factitious disorder

300.16 Factitious disorder with predominantly psychological symptoms

300.19 Factitious disorder with predominantly physical symptoms

300.19 Factitious disorder with combined psychological and physical symptoms

300.19 Factitious disorder not otherwise specified

Psychiatric nursing diagnostic class

Psychophysiologic response

INTRODUCTION

Somatoform disorders

The common feature of somatoform disorders is the presence of physical symptoms that suggest a general medical condition; however, the symptoms are not fully explained by a general medical condition, by the direct effects of substance abuse, or by any other mental disorder. The symptoms must produce clinically significant distress or problems in social or occupational functioning. The essential feature of *somatization disorder* is a pattern of recurring, multiple, clinically significant somatic complaints. Individuals with somatization disorder usually describe their complaints in colorful, often exaggerated terms; however, focused and factual information is often absent.

Conversion disorder is characterized by a lost or altered physical function without the presence of any physiologic disorder.

Hypochondriasis involves a preoccupation with the fear of developing or having a serious disease or disorder. This unwarranted fear, which typically is accompanied by physical signs or sensations, usually persists even after a comprehensive evaluation has eliminated physical causes.

Body dysmorphic disorder is characterized by a preoccupation with an imagined physical appearance defect. The most common complaints involve facial flaws.

The individual with *pain disorder* has a preoccupation with pain, which usually cannot be explained by physical findings. Psychological factors have a key role in its onset, severity, exacerbation, or maintenance. The pain causes significant distress or impairment in social, occupational, or other important areas of functioning.

Undifferentiated somatoform disorder is characterized by unexplained physical complaints lasting at least 6 months. These symptoms are below the threshold for a diagnosis of somatization disorder. The most common complaints are chronic fatigue, loss of appetite, and GI or genitourinary symptoms.

Somatoform disorder not otherwise specified comprises somatoform symptoms that do not meet the criteria for any of the specified somatoform disorders.

Factitious disorders

Factitious disorders are characterized by physical or psychological symptoms, or both, that are intentionally produced or feigned by the client who wishes to assume the sick role. The judgment that a particular symptom is intentionally produced is substantiated by direct evidence and by exclusion of other possible causes of the symptom. It is important to remember that the presence of factitious symptoms does not preclude the coexistence of true physical or psychological symptoms. Factitious disorder has three discrete subtypes, delineated by the predominant symptoms: *factitious disorder with predominantly psychological symptoms, factitious disorder with predominantly physical symptoms,* or *factitious disorder with combined psychological and physical symptoms.*

Factitious disorder not otherwise specified is a category that includes a disorder with factitious symptoms that do not meet the criteria for factitious disorder. An example is factitious disorder by proxy, which is the feigning of physical or psychological symptoms in another person who is under the individual's care for the purpose of indirectly assuming the sick role.

Etiology and precipitating factors

The exact cause of somatoform disorders is unknown, but neurobiological evidence suggests a left hemisphere dysfunction related to somatization disorder. EEG studies hint at abnormalities in cortical function, especially in the frontal region. Biochemical research focuses on possible involvement of the hypothalamic-pituitary-gonadal axis, which regulates estrogen and testosterone secretion and its impact on developing somatization disorder. Genetic research suggests an increased risk of somatization disorder in first-degree family relatives.

Psychological theories focus on somatization as a form of social or emotional communication. The physiologic symptoms express emotions that the individual has difficulty verbalizing. Over a period of time, physical symptoms develop in response to any perceived threat.

The etiology of factitious disorder may be psychodynamically based. Theorists propose that clients experiencing factitious disorder have been abused in childhood and only experienced nurturance when they were physically ill. They then try to recapture this nurturance by recreating the illness or injury to receive attention and love.

Potential complications

The most common complications of somatoform and factitious disorders include extensive and repetitive hospital admissions, repetitive or unnecessary surgical procedures, drug dependence, marital and family conflict or divorce, and suicide attempts. Contractures or disuse atrophy from paralysis related to prolonged functional loss may accompany *conversion disorder.* Numerous attempts to obtain medical validation for multiple symptoms may cause an individual with *hypochondriasis* to overlook a real physical problem.

ASSESSMENT GUIDELINES

Nursing history (functional health pattern findings)

Health perception–health management pattern
• Extreme worry over general health
• Obsessive interest in body processes, concerns, or diseases
• Preoccupation with an imagined appearance defect
• Physical symptoms involving one or several body systems
• Severe and prolonged pain as primary symptom
• Inability to use a specific body part or system
• Intense fear of a serious disease
• Numerous, comprehensive evaluations for physical symptoms
• Overuse of health care system to ease physical symptoms
• Annoyance with or failure to follow through on psychiatric mental health referrals

Nutritional-metabolic pattern
• Weight gain or loss
• Rigorous monitoring of reactions to dietary intake
• Concern about hair, nails, skin, or glands

• Hypervigilance about small wounds or bruises
• Concern about infection
• Extreme concern about dentition

Elimination pattern
• Numerous GI symptoms
• Frequent urination
• Concern over sweating or cold, clammy skin
• Intense worry about bowel elimination patterns

Activity-exercise pattern
• Decreased ability to engage in occupation due to physical symptoms
• Decreased interest in leisure activity
• Concern about becoming easily fatigued following activity
• Concern about life changes due to restricted activity caused by physical symptoms

Sleep-rest pattern
• Sleep disturbance
• Fatigue after sleep
• Sleep aid use, not always reported

Cognitive-perceptual pattern
• Sudden inability to hear or see
• Hearing loss
• Concern about hearing one's own heartbeat
• Memory difficulties

Self-perception–self-concept pattern
• Perception of self as not feeling good
• Difficulty describing feelings
• Denial of anger, anxiety, frustration, or fear
• Perception of self as dependent
• Concern over body image, self-esteem, or self-worth

Role-relationship pattern
• Concern about physical symptom impact on family
• Fear about inability to function at job
• Needing loved one's presence during testing, examinations, procedures, or explanations of treatment options
• Concern about being socially isolated or alienated
• Family system that does not discuss or resolve problems

Sexual-reproductive pattern
• Lack of satisfaction or interest in sexual relations
• Menstruation problems
• Sexual functioning problems

Coping–stress tolerance pattern
• Denial as a coping mechanism
• Significant lifestyle changes that may contribute to physical symptoms
• Difficulty identifying anyone to discuss and assist with feelings or problems
• Excessive analgesic use with minimal pain relief

Value-belief pattern
• Feeling powerless to achieve life goals

Physical findings

Cardiovascular
- Chest pain
- Palpitations

Respiratory
- Shortness of breath
- Smothering sensation

Gastrointestinal
- Abdominal pain
- Bloating
- Burning sensation in rectum
- Diarrhea
- Food intolerance
- Nausea or vomiting

Genitourinary
- Impotence
- Painful intercourse
- Painful, irregular, or excessive menstruation
- Painful urination
- Pseudocyesis
- Urine retention or difficulty urinating

Musculoskeletal
- Aches or pains
- Muscle spasms
- Muscle weakness

Neurologic
- Akinesia or dyskinesia
- Amnesia
- Anesthesia or paresthesia
- Anosmia
- Aphonia
- Blindness
- Blurred or double vision
- Coordination disturbances
- Deafness
- Dizziness or fainting
- Dysphagia
- Loss of consciousness
- Seizures
- Back or joint pain
- Pain in extremities

Psychological
- Anhedonia
- Anxiety
- Denial of feelings
- Dependency
- Depression
- Insomnia
- Sleep disturbances

NURSING DIAGNOSIS

Body image disturbance related to low self-esteem evidenced by preoccupation with real or imagined altered body structure or function

Nursing priority

Help the client to realize that the perceived body changes are exaggerated.

Patient outcome criteria

As treatment progresses, the client, family, or both should be able to:
- demonstrate a realistic perception and self-acceptance of body appearance or function.

Interventions

1. Assess the body change with which the client is preoccupied. If the client's normal appearance or functioning has changed, help the client to explore his feelings about the change.

2. Collaborate with the client to identify misperceptions regarding body image. Provide accurate feedback in a direct, nonthreatening manner.

3. Encourage the client to participate in body-image group activities and movement therapy activities.

Rationales

1. By exploring and expressing feelings about a real change, the client can begin to resolve those feelings. Doing so also can help the client to identify which feelings are appropriate and which are exaggerated.

2. Collaborating with the client in a nonjudgmental, nonthreatening manner can help establish a trusting nurse-client relationship.

3. Group activities, including a judicious and therapeutic use of touch, can help the client to feel accepted by others and diminish fears of being rejected because of body structure or function changes.

4. Encourage and reinforce the client's independent, self-care activities, participating or assisting only when necessary.

5. Encourage the client to use cognitive restructuring strategies.

4. Active participation in self-care activities can enhance the client's self-esteem and provide opportunities for confronting body functions realistically.

5. Cognitive restructuring strategies, such as saying "Okay, just because I made a mistake doesn't mean I'm stupid," instead of "That was a stupid thing to do," can enhance the client's self-esteem and help the client develop new thinking patterns and diminish negative messages about the self.

NURSING DIAGNOSIS

Chronic pain related to unmet dependency needs or repressed anxiety as demonstrated by verbal complaints with no pathophysiologic validation

Nursing priority

Help the client to recognize and understand the relationship between pain and psychological problems.

Patient outcome criterion

As treatment progresses, the client, family, or both should be able to:
• demonstrate the ability to complete daily activities without pain interference.

Interventions

1. Review the client's past and present medical records and monitor any laboratory studies and reports. Assist the multidisciplinary team in developing a thorough diagnosis.

2. Observe and record the duration, location, and intensity of the client's pain. Collaborate with the client to identify factors that precipitate and help to diminish the pain.

3. Acknowledge the client's pain perception as a real event.

4. Collaborate with the client, multidisciplinary team, and a chronic pain specialist (if one is available) to determine appropriate treatment, such as the client's participation in a chronic pain program. Provide the client with pain medication as prescribed.

5. Collaborate with the client to identify additional strategies that can produce comfort.

Rationales

1. A comprehensive assessment can help ascertain the presence or absence of an organic condition or problem.

2. A comprehensive pain assessment can enable the nurse, client, and multidisciplinary team to develop a more effective plan of care.

3. Denying or challenging the client's pain perception will only heighten the client's need to convince the health care team of the pain, thus draining the client of energy.

4. Including a chronic pain specialist in the multidisciplinary team can facilitate skill building among staff members while providing quality client care.

5. Strategies that may be physically comforting to the client include massage therapy, warm baths or showers, applications of heating pads or ice packs, splinting, Therapeutic Touch, and use of a transcutaneous electrical nerve stimulation (TENS) unit.

Psychophysiologic disorders

6. Encourage the client to begin to identify and use alternate coping strategies to manage stress.

6. Using alternate coping strategies may diminish the client's reliance on physical pain as a primary coping response to stress.

7. Teach the client pain-cycle disrupting strategies to use when stress symptoms begin. Encourage family member participation.

7. Disrupting the pain cycle can help diminish the client's need to use pain as a response to stress. Useful strategies include visual and auditory distractions, breathing exercises, guided imagery and visualization, therapeutic massage, relaxation techniques, and cold and heat application.

8. Encourage the client to verbalize feelings about pain, to connect pain to increased anxiety, and to identify specific anxiety-causing situations.

8. Encouraging the client to verbalize feelings in a supportive environment can facilitate expression, problem solving, and the resolution of disturbing issues.

9. Help the client's family to develop a positive reinforcement program. Encourage family members to participate in family sessions and provide referrals for outpatient family therapy.

9. By reinforcing and encouraging client self-control, family members can decrease the amount of time they spend attending to the client's pain behaviors.

NURSING DIAGNOSIS

Ineffective individual coping related to the client's inability to manage emotional conflict, extreme need for approval and acceptance, unmet dependency needs, or low self-esteem

Nursing priority

Help the client to acquire and use adaptive coping strategies that manage conflict while reducing reliance on physical symptoms.

Outcome criterion

As treatment progresses, the client, family, or both should be able to:
• demonstrate the ability to use specific strategies that manage stress responses and avoid exacerbating physical symptoms.

Interventions

1. Use a time-line chart to determine when the client's somatic symptoms first appeared and what social, financial, emotional, familial, and occupational events were transpiring. Also, note any symptom flare-ups, treatments, and hospitalizations that occurred. With the client, determine what roles the need for attention and distraction from problems play in the disorder.

2. Help the client to identify and determine the causes of any anger or resentment he might feel.

3. Teach and rehearse with the client methods for directly expressing feelings. Positively reinforce the client's use of adaptive coping strategies.

Rationales

1. Such a history can help the nurse to develop a more appropriate plan of care and may illuminate some connections between crises or conflicts and the emergence of the disorder's symptoms.

2. The time-line chart can help the client target the source of the anger or resentment. Identifying and exploring these feelings can help decrease the maladaptive use of physical symptoms to express emotions.

3. Role modeling and rehearsing alternate behaviors can increase the client's ability to use and modify new behaviors. Reinforcement encourages the client to continue desired behaviors.

4. Collaborate with the multidisciplinary treatment team to develop a comprehensive, consistent approach to the client's somatic complaints.

5. Teach the client assertiveness skills and incorporate these skills in role-playing sessions.

6. Collaborate with the client to identify positive personal characteristics. Encourage the client to use personal affirmations based on these characteristics.

7. Teach the client how to ask for attention, nurturing, and support.

4. A coordinated treatment team can limit the client from trying to persuade staff members to side with them against other staff members about their condition. A consistent approach of setting limits and feedback can enhance behavioral change.

5. Learning assertiveness skills can help the client communicate more openly and honestly and can decrease conflict avoidance.

6. Building the client's self-esteem can help decrease his excessive dependency needs.

7. Learning to communicate needs directly can help to decrease the client's reliance upon physical complaints as a means of getting emotional needs met.

NURSING DIAGNOSIS

Knowledge deficit related to denial, intense repressed anxiety level, preoccupation with self and pain, or lack of interest in learning

Nursing priority

Help the client to understand the psychological foundation of physical symptoms.

Patient outcome criteria

As treatment progresses, the client, family, or both should be able to:
• verbalize an understanding of the relationship between emotional conflicts, problems, and physiologic or psychological symptoms.

Interventions

1. Assess the client's knowledge about psychological problems and their effects on physiologic functioning.

2. Assess the client's overt and covert anxiety level and his ability to participate in educational sessions.

3. Consult with occupational, physical, recreational, and movement therapists to establish appropriate treatment plans and to determine adaptive coping strategies.

Rationales

1. Identifying knowledge deficits and misperceptions can enable the nurse to develop an appropriate care plan to confront the client's denial system.

2. Intense anxiety can inhibit the client's ability to learn and retain information.

3. Comprehensive team consultations can provide individualized and specialized techniques for identifying and dealing with stressors. Techniques might include decision making and problem solving, art therapy, horticultural therapy, leisure time management, pet therapy, movement therapy, and psychodrama.

NURSING DIAGNOSIS

Ineffective family coping, compromised, related to struggles for control and power

Nursing priority

Help the client's family to develop and use positive coping strategies that can decrease the reliance on physical symptoms as a means of coping.

Patient outcome criterion

As treatment progresses, the client, family, or both should be able to:
• demonstrate the ability to use specific strategies to effectively manage family-related stressors that may exacerbate symptoms.

Interventions	**Rationales**
1. Explore specific family member roles and ways in which the client's disorder has changed the family organization.	**1.** Family perceptions may have prevented the client from being identified as the family member with a disorder. Understanding the family's perspective of their roles can help the nurse understand the family's dynamics.
2. Identify underlying situations that inhibit the family's ability to provide the client with needed assistance, support, or nurturing. Encourage family members to verbalize feelings.	**2.** Doing so can help the family to reestablish appropriate boundaries and to express feelings honestly.
3. Discuss with the client and family how they get needs met within and outside the family. Explore with family members the issues of power and control within their system.	**3.** By learning and using an inclusive and participative family process, the client and family can decrease the use of illness as a tool or method of communication to express emotional conflict.
4. Provide the family with referrals for ongoing family therapy after discharge.	**4.** Ongoing therapy can promote progress in behavioral changes within the family and provide an additional avenue for managing family stress.

NURSING DIAGNOSIS

Self-care deficit related to activity intolerance, neuromuscular or musculoskeletal impairment, pain, discomfort, or perceptual or cognitive impairment

Nursing priority

Help the client to regain the ability to perform normal daily functions.

Patient outcome criteria

As treatment progresses, the client, family, or both should be able to:
• demonstrate increased independence in self-care.

Interventions	**Rationales**
1. Assess the client's impairment in relation to feeding, bathing and hygiene, dressing and grooming, and toileting. Document strengths and inabilities.	**1.** This information can enable the nurse to develop an adequate plan of care.
2. Modify the client's environment to enable him to perform normal daily functions at his ability level.	**2.** Environmental adjustments can increase the client's chances of successfully performing daily functions, thereby increasing his self-esteem and promoting self-care.
3. Allow the client enough time to perform daily functions and positively reinforce successful performance. Be available to help the client if symptoms interfere with his ability to function independently.	**3.** Positive reinforcement enhances client self-esteem and encourages repetition of desired behaviors.

4. Consult occupational and physical therapists when appropriate.

5. Encourage the client to participate in group therapy to discuss feelings about his disability or impairment and the dependency need it produces.

4. Teaching by occupational and physical therapists can facilitate optimal client functioning.

5. As the client becomes able to explore his feelings about his impairment and dependency needs, he can begin to address unresolved conflicts.

NURSING DIAGNOSIS

Sensory-perceptual alteration evidenced by lost or altered physical functioning suggesting a physical disorder but without evidence of organic pathology

Nursing priority

Help the client and family to recognize relationship between emotional conflict and altered physical functioning.

Patient outcome criteria

As treatment progresses, the client, family, or both should be able to:
• verbalize an understanding of the relationship between emotional conflicts and problems and physical symptoms

Interventions

1. Encourage client and family participation in education sessions describing stress responses and psychophysiologic conditions.

2. Offer only limited attention to the client's preoccupation with his disability or impairment and encourage independence within the client's physical limits.

3. Have the client keep a daily log of feelings, thoughts, and symptoms. Regularly review the log with the client.

4. Encourage the client to participate in scheduled therapeutic activities. Do not permit the client to avoid participation because of his disability or impairment; withdraw attention when he pursues this as rationale.

Rationales

1. Education can help the client and family to understand the relationship between emotional stress and physical symptoms.

2. Attention given to the client's preoccupation with his disability can reinforce the continued use of the maladaptive response to fulfill dependency needs. Support and encouragement for achievements can foster repetition of desired behaviors.

3. A daily log can provide the client the opportunity to discover the links between conflicts and physical symptoms.

4. Participating in scheduled therapeutic activities can enhance the client's self-esteem and reinforce positive behaviors.

NURSING DIAGNOSIS

Social isolation related to physical symptoms or disability

Nursing priority

Provide the client with opportunities for increased socialization.

Patient outcome criteria

As treatment progresses, the client, family, or both should be able to:
• verbalize an awareness of support and ongoing therapy needs
• report and demonstrate increased involvement in activities within any functional limitations.

Interventions

1. Collaborate with the client and multidisciplinary team to determine appropriate diversionary and expressive therapies.

2. Work with the client to identify concrete ways to increase social contacts within physical limitations.

3. Identify and discuss community resources, self-help groups, and volunteer groups that may benefit the client.

Rationales

1. Structuring the client's day with different activities, such as occupational, recreational, art, movement, music, and pet therapies, can decrease preoccupation with physical symptoms.

2. Broadening the client's social contacts can increase his support sources.

3. Engaging in group activities can begin to alleviate the client's social isolation.

Discharge criteria

Nursing documentation indicates that the client:
• has recognized and acknowledged psychological reasons for physical symptoms
• has demonstrated the ability to use newly learned skills to manage emotional conflict
• has demonstrated the ability to use appropriate internal and external support sources.
Nursing documentation indicates that the client and family:
• have verbalized an understanding of the diagnosis, treatment, and expected outcomes
• have verbalized a willingness to participate in ongoing therapy
• have verbalized an awareness of community support groups and programs, such as chronic pain management programs and vocational retraining programs, and their referrals
• have verbalized an understanding of when, why, how, and whom to contact in case of an emergency.

Selected references

Artingstall, K. *Practical Aspects of Munchausen by Proxy and Munchausen Syndrome Investigation.* Boca Raton, Fla.: CRC Press, 1998.

Boyd, M.A., and Nihart, M.A. *Psychiatric Nursing: Contemporary Practice.* Philadelphia: Lippincott-Raven Pubs., 1998.

Diagnostic and Statistical Manual of Mental Disorders, 4th ed. Washington, D.C.: American Psychiatric Association, 1994.

Feldman, M., and Eisendarth, S. *The Spectrum of Factitious Disorders.* Washington, D.C.: American Psychiatric Association, 1996.

Keefe, F., and Goli, V. "A Practical Guide to Behavioral Assessment and Treatment of Chronic Pain," *Journal of Practical Psychiatry and Behavioral Health* 5:151, 1996.

Phillips, K.A. *The Broken Mirror: Understanding and Treating Body Dysmorphic Disorder.* New York: Oxford University Press, 1996.

Pope, H.G., et al. "Muscle Dysmorphia: An Underrecognized Form of Body Dysmorphic Disorder," *Psychosomatics* 38(6): 548-57, 1997.

Rundell, J.R., and Wise, M.G. *Textbook of Consultation Liaison Psychiatry.* Washington, D.C.: American Psychiatric Association, 1996.

Varcarolis, E.M. *Foundations of Psychiatric-Mental Health Nursing.* Philadelphia: W.B. Saunders Co., 1998.

Watkins, A. *Mind-Body Medicine: A Clinician's Guide to Psychoneuroimmunology.* New York: Churchill Livingstone, Inc., 1997.

Woodman, C.L., et al. "The Relationship Between Irritable Bowel Syndrome and Psychiatric Illness: A Family Study," *Psychosomatics* 39(1):45-54, 1997.

Part 11

Sleep disorders

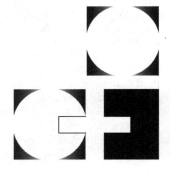

Sleep disorders

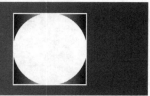

DSM-IV classifications
Primary sleep disorders
Dyssomnias
307.42   Primary insomnia
307.44   Primary hypersomnia
347   Narcolepsy
780.59   Breathing-related sleep disorder
307.45   Circadian rhythm sleep disorder
307.47   Dyssomnia not otherwise specified
Parasomnias
307.47   Nightmare disorder
307.46   Sleep terror disorder
307.46   Sleepwalking disorder
307.40   Parasomnia not otherwise specified
Secondary sleep disorders
Sleep disorders related to another mental disorder
307.42   Insomnia related to (indicate Axis I or II disorder)
307.44   Hypersomnia related to (indicate Axis I or II disorder)
Other sleep disorders
780.xx   Sleep disorder due to (indicate general medical condition)
780.52   Insomnia type
780.54   Hypersomnia type
780.59   Parasomnia type
780.59   Mixed type
xxx.xx   Substance-induced sleep disorder (refer to substance-related disorders for specific codes)

Psychiatric nursing diagnostic class
Sleep disturbance

INTRODUCTION

Sleep disorders can develop when an individual's usual cycle of sleep and wakefulness becomes altered. These disorders are divided into two major categories: primary and secondary. The primary sleep disorders include dyssomnias and parasomnias. The *dyssomnias* are disorders of initiating or maintaining the sleep state or of excessive sleepiness. They are characterized by disturbances in the amount, quality, or timing of sleep

Insomnia refers to difficulty falling asleep, trouble maintaining sleep, or nonrestorative sleep. *Primary insomnia* is the most prevalent, with estimates ranging from 30% to 35%. *Primary hypersomnia* is excessive sleepiness for at least 1 month demonstrated by either daytime sleep episodes or sleeping for extended periods at night. These individuals exhibit excessive daytime sleepiness, along with poor concentration and impaired memory.

Narcolepsy is an overwhelming urge to sleep, which occurs at anytime of the day regardless of the amount of sleep the person has had over a 24-hour interval. Falling asleep occurs at inappropriate and often embarrassing times. The sleep episodes are usually short, lasting 5 to 20 minutes.

Narcolepsy is distinguished by a group of symptoms termed the "narcolepsy tetrad": daytime sleepiness, cataplexy, hypnagogic hallucinations, and sleep paralysis. Daytime sleepiness occurs in all individuals with narcolepsy, whereas incidence of the other three symptoms varies. Cataplexy is the bilateral loss of muscle tone triggered by a strong emotion. The frequency and severity gradually increases with sleep deprivation. Approximately 70% of individuals with narcolepsy report cataplexy. Hypnagogic hallucinations are intense dreamlike images that occur as an individual is falling asleep. Usually the hallucinations are visual, but some individuals experience auditory and kinetic-type hallucinations. Hypnagogic hallucinations are reported by 20% to 40% of individuals diagnosed with narcolepsy. In sleep paralysis, the individual cannot speak or move when falling asleep or awakening. This muscle atonia is usually described as terrifying and is accompanied by a sensation of struggling to speak or move.

Breathing-related sleep disorder is a broad and diverse class of sleep disorders that includes obstructive sleep apnea (OSA) syndrome, central sleep apnea (CSA) syndrome, and central alveolar hyperventilation syndrome. OSA syndrome is the most frequently diagnosed breathing-related sleep disorder. It is characterized by excessive snoring during sleep and episodes of sleep apnea (breathing cessation) that disrupt sleep and cause daytime sleepiness. Snoring may be loud and disruptive to the bed partner. Children with OSA syndrome have more subtle symptoms. They may not snore, but they may have unusual sleep postures along with agitated arousals. Although they may not appear sleepy, they do experience poor attention span and deteriorating school performance.

CSA syndrome is characterized by episodes where there is no effort to breathe. Unlike OSA syndrome, there is no airway obstruction and no chest wall and abdominal breathing movements during the apnea episode. Snoring is either absent or mild. CSA syndrome is typically seen at sleep onset, and difficulty falling asleep is the most common presenting complaint.

Circadian rhythm sleep disorder represents a mismatch between the individual's internal sleep-awake circadian rhythm and their timing and duration of sleep. The diagnosis is reserved for individuals who present with marked sleep disturbance or significant social or occupational impairment. Individuals with this disorder report insomnia and excessive sleepiness. Circadian rhythm sleep disorder includes several subtypes, including delayed sleep phase type, jet lag type, shift work type, and unspecified type.

Parasomnias are characterized by abnormal physiological behavior that occurs in relationship to sleep and specific sleep stages or at transition from sleep to arousal and wakefulness. Individuals often complain of unusual behavior during sleep. There are three identified types of parasomnias: nightmare disorder, sleep terror disorder, and sleep-walking disorder. The individual with nightmare disorder has repeated occurrences of frightening dreams that cause the individual to rapidly awaken. Typically, the individual can recall details of the dream that involve physical danger. The individual experiences a persistent sense of anxiety or fear after full awakening.

The characteristic feature of sleep terror disorder is the repetition of episodes of sleep terrors that produce clinical distress and impairment of social, occupational, or other functions. Additional diagnostic considerations may include the potential for injury to self or others. An episode is characterized by screaming, fear and panic with increased heart rate, increased respiratory rate, dilated pupils, and flushed skin.

Sleep-walking disorder, also referred to as somnambulism, is an arousal disorder. It occurs when an individual is partially awake and partially asleep and is an interruption of the normal arousal process. The characteristic feature is the complex motor behavior during sleep and can entail episodes from simply getting out of bed to complex actions such as walking around outside or driving an automobile.

Secondary sleep disorders are related to another mental disorder (depression, illness, posttraumatic stress disorder, anxiety disorder), general medical condition or substance-induced disorder. The essential feature of a sleep disorder from a general medical condition is a prominent disturbance in sleep that is significant enough to warrant independent clinical care and is caused by a general medical condition, such as heart disease, chronic obstructive pulmonary disease, or chronic pain disorder.

Substance-induced sleep disorder is a prominent sleep disturbance that is significant enough to require independent clinical treatment and has been determined to be from the direct physiologic effects of a substance such as a prescribed medication, an over-the-counter drug, an illicit drug, or a toxin.

Etiology and precipitating factors

Individuals at risk for developing primary insomnia often describe themselves as "light sleepers" before their sleep problems developed. They typically report a tendency to be more easily aroused physiologically or psychologically at night. While the insomnia may be precipitated by stressful situations and tension, it persists after the stressful situation resolves.

The cause of narcolepsy is still unknown, but it is believed to involve many environmental and genetic factors. Some workers suggest that genetically predisposed individuals become actively symptomatic after an injury to the central nervous system. In addition, there is some evidence of a narcolepsy susceptibility gene located on chromosome 6, in the class II human leukocyte antigen.

An obstruction or collapse of the airway causes apnea (cessation of breathing). The obstruction occurs in the pharyngeal area in most cases. In individuals with OSA syndrome, the pharyngeal portion of their airway is smaller and is often compromised by enlarged tonsils, the tongue, the soft palate, and uvula. Vibration of these soft and pliable tissues located in the pharyngeal portion of the airway causes the snoring sounds that occur during breathing. Snoring is worsened by alcohol ingestion, sleeping in a supine position, and previous sleep deprivation.

Instability in the respiratory control system causes CSA syndrome. Many conditions can create this instability, including heart failure, cerebrovascular accident, myasthenia gravis, encephalitis, or autonomic dysfunction in Shy-Drager syndrome.

The disconnection of the internal circadian pacemaker and conventional time frames causes circadian rhythm sleep disorders. The cause may be intrinsic (delayed sleep phase) or extrinsic (jet lag or shift work).

The most important factor in the etiology of sleep terror disorder is a genetic predisposition. Individuals often report a family history of either sleep terrors or sleep-walking. However, the exact mode of the inheritance is not known. Additionally, fever and sleep deprivation can increase the frequency of episodes. There also appears to be a genetic predisposition to sleep-walking. Internal stimuli, such as a full bladder or pain, or external stimuli, such as noise or heat, can precipitate an episode. Fever, sleep deprivation, and stress may increase the chance of an episode.

Technological advances have provided clinicians and researchers with the means to identify and measure the electrophysiologic characteristics of sleep, changes in muscle tone, and incidence of rapid eye movements. Sleep technology has demonstrated that sleep is a cycle of discrete phases. (See *Stages of sleep*, page 246.)

Potential complications

If left untreated, sleep disorders can lead to cognitive impairment, confusional state delirium, impaired occu-

Stages of sleep

This chart indicates the physiologic changes that occur during the stages of sleep.

Stage	Description	Physiologic changes
Awake-alert	Normal daytime wakefulness	Normal vital signs
Stage 1 nonrapid eye movement (NREM)	Drowsiness; decreased reactivity to external stimuli; thinking no longer reality based	Decreased body temperature, heart rate, blood pressure, and respiratory rate
Stage 2 NREM	Light sleep	Decreased body temperature, heart rate, and blood pressure; slow, regular respiration
Stages 3 and 4 NREM	Deep sleep	Decreased body temperature, heart rate, and blood pressure; few body movements; release of growth hormone; markedly slow and regular respiration
Rapid eye movement	Rapid movement of eyes; dream state	Reduced muscle tone; bursts of eye movements and muscle twitching; decreased autonomic heart rate and blood pressure control; thermoregulation respiration; vivid dreaming; penile erection; increased blood flow to brain

pational and social functioning, self-injury, sleep terror disorder, and perceptual or memory deficits.

Various psychiatric and medical conditions can produce symptoms associated with sleep disorders; if left untreated, these disorders can cause serious, even life-threatening problems. (For a list of specific conditions, see *Disorders that cause sleep disturbances.*)

ASSESSMENT GUIDELINES

Nursing history (functional health pattern findings)

Health perception–health management pattern
- Frequent colds, viruses
- General lack of well-being

Nutritional-metabolic pattern
- Significant daily caffeine intake
- Obesity
- Weight gain or loss

Elimination pattern
- Gastric pain or discomfort
- Nocturnal bowel irritability or diarrhea
- Nocturnal urination
- Night sweats

Activity-exercise pattern
- Decreased interest in recreation activities
- Decreased exercise

Sleep-rest pattern
- Difficulty initiating sleep
- Early morning awakening
- Inability to sleep at desired time
- Inability to remain asleep
- Daytime sleepiness
- Nightmares or terrors
- Reliance on sleep aids
- Increased dreaming
- Not feeling rested or refreshed after sleep

Cognitive-perceptual pattern
- Decreased alertness
- Memory deficits
- Difficulty concentrating
- Distorted perceptions
- Experiencing pain
- Incomplete pain relief

Self-perception–self-concept pattern
- Perception of self as anxious or depressed
- Perception of self as inadequate or overwhelmed

Role-relationship pattern
- Distressful family situation
- Stressful work environment
- Isolation

Sexual-reproductive pattern
- Decreased libido
- Difficulty with intimacy

Coping–stress tolerance pattern
- Mood lability

Disorders that cause sleep disturbances

Certain psychiatric and medical disorders can produce various sleep disturbances, particularly insomnia and excessive daytime sleepiness. This chart includes some of the most common disorders associated with both insomnia and daytime sleepiness.

Sleep disturbance	Psychiatric disorders	Medical disorders
Insomnia	• Adjustment disorder • Bipolar disorder • Cyclothymic disorder • Dysthymic disorder • Generalized anxiety disorder • Hypomania • Major depression • Masked depression (undiagnosed) • Obsessive-compulsive disorder • Panic disorder • Posttraumatic stress disorder • Psychoactive substance abuse disorder • Schizophrenia • Somatoform disorders	• Addison's disease • Anorexia nervosa • Arthritis • Asthma • Chronic headache, neoplasms, head trauma, postencephalitic subdural hematoma • Cushing's syndrome • Cystic fibrosis • Diabetes • Epstein-Barr virus • Heart failure • Human immunodeficiency virus–related disorders, including acquired immunodeficiency syndrome (AIDS) • Myocardial infarction • Neurosyphilis • Overeating, esophageal reflux, hiatal hernia, chronic inflammatory bowel disease, peptic ulcer • Parkinson's disease
Excessive daytime sleepiness	• Seasonal affective disorders associated with physiologic changes • Major depression • Masked depression (undiagnosed)	• Asthma • Chronic obstructive pulmonary disease • Sleep apnea

• Irritability
• Tearfulness
• Feeling vulnerable
• Diminished coping ability after period of sleep disturbance

Value-belief pattern
• Feeling powerless to achieve life goals
• Spiritual distress or conflict

Physical findings
General appearance
• Dark circles under eyes
• Eyelid ptosis
Cardiovascular
• Cardiac arrhythmias
• Chest pain
• Coexisting cardiovascular disorders
• Increased or decreased blood pressure (sleep stage–dependent)
• Increased or decreased heart rate (sleep stage–dependent)

Respiratory
• Apnea
• Decreased respiratory rate
• Snoring
Gastrointestinal
• Abdominal discomfort
• Nausea or diarrhea
• Abdominal pain
• Dry mouth or oral mucus membranes
Genitourinary
• Nocturnal penile erection
Musculoskeletal
• Posture changes
• Increased fatigue
• Muscle aches, pain, soreness, or tension
• Restless legs
Neurologic
• Confusion
• Delirium
• Frequent yawning
• Mild hand tremors
• Fleeting nystagmus

Sleep disorders

- Restlessness
- Thick speech with mispronunciation and incorrect word use

Psychological
- Agitation
- Concentration problems
- Irritability
- Lethargic mood lability

NURSING DIAGNOSIS

Sleep pattern disturbance related to medical illness, pain, psychological stress, or external factors, such as hospital routines, environmental noise, and changing work shifts

Nursing priority

Facilitate a normal sleep pattern that enables the client to fall asleep within 30 minutes of retiring and to sleep at least 6 to 8 hours per day.

Patient outcome criteria

As treatment progresses, the client, family, or both should be able to:
- verbalize an understanding of sleep disorders
- identify specific sleep-inducing measures
- adjust lifestyle and daily schedule to accommodate chronobiological rhythms
- report an improved sleep pattern
- report feeling rested
- report less excessive daytime sleepiness
- verbalize an awareness of the possible need for a comprehensive sleep disorder evaluation.

Interventions

1. Assess the client's current sleep pattern and take a complete sleep history. (See *Sleep history assessment.*)

2. Identify both internal and external factors that are inhibiting the client's sleep.

3. Ascertain the client's sleep-related routines and rituals. Encourage the client to use sleep-promoting methods. (See *Sleep-enhancement strategies,* page 250.)

4. Encourage the client to maintain a sleep diary or chart and to make a practice of using sleep strategies. Inform the client that improvements may not occur for 4 to 5 weeks.

5. Provide comfort measures, such as back rubs, comfortable night clothes, and prescribed pain medications.

Rationales

1. A comprehensive assessment can help the nurse more accurately identify the client's sleep disorder.

2. By identifying sleep-inhibiting factors, such as pain, itching, depression, metabolic disorders, noise, heat, and light, the nurse can develop an appropriate, effective plan of care for the client.

3. The client may have ineffective sleep patterns and, consequently, may need to learn specific planning strategies for managing sleep. Many sleep-enhancement strategies are natural sedative measures that can promote sleep.

4. The client should know that the sleep disorder will not be corrected quickly. Offering encouragement and support can help the client stay with a specific program.

5. Increasing the client's comfort can facilitate sleep.

Sleep history assessment

An accurate sleep history is of utmost importance in evaluating a client's sleep disorder. The sleep history provides an assessment of the complaint in relation to environmental, familial, and medical factors and helps the nurse to determine the origin of the sleep disturbance. Typically, a thorough sleep history explores the client's daytime or awake behaviors, sleep patterns, sleep hygiene, and medical, psychological, and pharmacologic history. The form below includes appropriate questions to ask when assessing a client's sleep pattern.

1.a. When did these symptoms begin?

_____

b. Which pattern best describes the frequency of the symptoms?

Occur persistently   Yes ❏   No ❏
Wax and wane   Yes ❏   No ❏
Occur seasonally   Yes ❏   No ❏

2.a. Are these symptoms associated with any of the following factors?

Medical problems   Yes ❏   No ❏
Job pressure   Yes ❏   No ❏
Stress   Yes ❏   No ❏

b. If yes, how long have the factors persisted?

_____

c. Do these factors relate to the intensity of symptoms?
Yes ❏   No ❏

3.a. Does anything seem to alleviate these symptoms?
Yes ❏   No ❏

b. If yes, what makes them better?

_____

c. What makes them worse?

_____

d. What happens on a vacation (for example, do they improve, worsen, or persist)?

_____

4. How has this sleep disturbance made an impact on your life?

_____

5. What is your typical daily schedule?

_____

6. Describe your usual sleep hygiene (sleep routines and rituals).

_____

7.a. Do any other family members complain of sleep difficulties?   Yes ❏   No ❏
If yes, who?

_____

b. Are the complaints similar to yours?   Yes ❏   No ❏
If dissimilar, characterize the complaints.

_____

8.a. Which sleep remedies or treatments have you tried so far?

_____

b. How effective have these treatments been?

_____

9.a. Which drugs have you used in the past?

Prescribed   Yes ❏   No ❏

Over-the-counter   Yes ❏   No ❏
Illicit   Yes ❏   No ❏

b. Which drugs are you currently using?

_____

Prescribed   Yes ❏   No ❏
Over-the-counter   Yes ❏   No ❏
Illicit   Yes ❏   No ❏

c. Do you smoke?   Yes ❏   No ❏
Frequency: _____

d. Do you ingest caffeine-containing foods or beverages (such as coffee, tea, chocolate, or soda)?   Yes ❏   No ❏
Frequency:_____

10.a. Do you drink alcohol?   Yes ❏   No ❏

b. If yes, how often?_____

c. In what quantity?_____

11.a. Do you ever have any unusual sleep time experiences?
Yes ❏   No ❏

b. If yes, describe them.

_____

_____

12. What is your usual sleep time?_____

13. What is your usual awakening time?_____

14. How long do you usually take to fall asleep?_____

15.a. Do you awaken during sleep time?   Yes ❏   No ❏

b. If yes, why? _____

c. Are you able to go back to sleep?   Yes ❏   No ❏

16. Do you have a history of any of the following?

Bruxism (teeth grinding)   Yes ❏   No ❏
Kicking during sleep   Yes ❏   No ❏
Restless leg syndrome   Yes ❏   No ❏
Sleep talking   Yes ❏   No ❏
Sleep walking   Yes ❏   No ❏
Snoring   Yes ❏   No ❏

17. Do you feel rested and refreshed after sleeping?
Yes ❏   No ❏

18. What is the condition of your bed linens after sleeping?

_____

19.a. Do you experience daytime sleepiness?   Yes ❏   No ❏

b. Do you experience daytime fatigue?   Yes ❏   No ❏

20.a. Can you provide any additional information that may be related to your sleep disturbance? If yes, describe.

_____

_____

Sleep disorders

6. Arrange the timing of nursing care to provide at least a 4-hour block of uninterrupted time before sleep.

6. Providing uninterrupted time by clustering care, treatments, medications, and other nursing procedures can decrease the number of awakenings and facilitate a normal sleep pattern.

7. Assess the amount and types of psychoactive drugs the client is taking. Administer medications at bedtime if doing so is not contraindicated.

7. Some psychoactive drugs interfere with normal sleep. A bedtime dosing schedule can facilitate sleep, especially if the drug has a sedative effect.

8. Collaborate with multidisciplinary team members to discuss the client's sleep history and sleep log. Consider referring the client to a sleep disorder assessment center or a sleep-related breathing disorder center.

8. The client may require a comprehensive evaluation that is best accomplished in a sleep disorder assessment center. A sleep-related breathing disorders center can be helpful if the client has sleep apnea syndrome or a related disorder.

9. If appropriate and needed, refer the client to a chronotherapy unit.

9. Participating in chronobiological therapy may help reset the body's sleep clock, especially if the client has delayed sleep onset insomnia.

10. Teach the client and family about common sleep disturbances and methods of assessing and treating them.

10. Such instruction can enhance the client's and family's level of awareness and decrease the use of ineffective home sleep remedies, such as drinking a glass of wine or taking benzodiazepines before bed.

Sleep-enhancement strategies

If your client has difficulty falling asleep, suggest the following sleep-promoting techniques.

Activity-exercise strategies
- Maintain a balance between rest, activity, and exercise.
- Engage in various social activities during the day.
- Exercise regularly in the late afternoon or early evening.
- Avoid daytime napping.
- Maintain a normal daily schedule even if fatigued.

Bedtime schedule and presleep "ritual" strategies
- Establish a regular time for going to bed.
- Schedule "worry time" and "thinking time" separate from in-bed hours.
- Avoid oversleeping.
- Schedule "wind down" time before bed; activities that promote relaxation include selecting clothes for the next day, reading a book, or taking a warm bath or shower.
- Go to bed when tired.

Fluid restriction and chemical reduction strategies
- Restrict alcohol, coffee, tea, and caffeinated soft-drink intake.
- Restrict or discontinue nicotine intake.

Mindfulness-relaxation strategies
- Use relaxation techniques.

Sleep environment strategies
- Establish and maintain a quiet sleeping environment.
- Use dark shades or eye covers if needed.
- Adjust the room temperature to a comfortable level.
- Establish a regular time for rising in the morning.
- Determine how sleeping with a bed partner (spouse, loved one, or pet) affects sleep.
- Reduce external stimuli, such as a television or radio, in the bedroom.

11. Monitor the effects of the client's medication regimen, including the effects of methylphenidate (Ritalin, prescribed for narcolepsy) and pain medications.

11. Monitoring is necessary to determine the possible effects of medications on the client's sleep.

DISCHARGE CRITERIA

Nursing documentation indicates that the client:
• has displayed the ability to recognize the symptoms of an altered sleep pattern
• has displayed the ability to use newly learned strategies that facilitate a normal sleep pattern
• understands that further assessment and treatment may be necessary
• is aware of available social and family resources
• has scheduled any necessary follow-up treatments.
Nursing documentation also indicates that the family:
• understands the diagnosis, treatment, and expected outcomes
• has been referred to the appropriate community resources
• has demonstrated a willingness to schedule follow-up appointments and participate in ongoing psychotherapy if needed.

SELECTED REFERENCES

Ancoli-Israel, S. *All I Want Is a Good Night's Sleep.* St. Louis: Mosby–Year Book, Inc., 1996.

Arendt, J., and Deacon, S. "Treatment of Circadian Rhythm Disorders—Melatonin," *Chronobiology International* 14(2):185-204, 1997.

Blumenthal, S., and Fine, T. "Sleep Abnormalities Associated with Mental and Addictive Disorders: Implications for Research and Clinical Practice," *Journal of Practical Psychiatry and Behavioral Health* 3:67, 1996.

Buysse, D.J., and Perlis, M.E. "The Evaluation and Treatment of Insomnia," *Journal of Practical Psychiatry and Behavioral Health* 3:80, 1996.

Costo, G. "The Problem: Shift Work," *Chronobiology International* 14(2):89-98, 1997.

Diagnostic and Statistical Manual of Mental Disorders, 4th ed. Washington, D.C.: American Psychiatric Association, 1994.

Ganguli, M., et al. "Prevalence and Persistence of Sleep Complaints in a Rural Older Community Sample: The MOVIES Project," *Journal of the American Geriatric Association* 44(7):778-84, 1996.

Goldberg, J.R., ed. *The Pharmacological Management of Insomnia: A White Paper of the National Sleep Foundation.* Washington, D.C.: National Sleep Foundation, 1996.

Rundell, J.R., and Wise, M.C. *Textbook of Consultation Liaison Psychiatry.* Washington, D.C.: American Psychiatric Association, 1996.

Sleep disorders

Part 12

Sex-related disorders

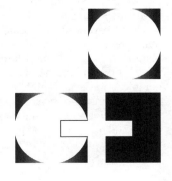

Gender identity disorders

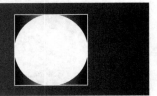

DSM-IV classifications
302.60 Gender identity disorder of childhood
302.85 Gender identity disorder of adolescence or
        adulthood
302.9   Gender identity disorder not otherwise speci-
        fied

Psychiatric nursing diagnostic class
Sexual response variations

INTRODUCTION

Gender identity disorders occur when gender identity — a person's sense of being male or female — does not correspond to his or her sexual anatomy. Individuals with gender identity disorders usually experience persistent and intense distress about their biological sex and wish to be the other sex. They even may insist that they are the other sex. Such individuals may be averse to wearing the stereotypical clothing of their sex, choosing rather to dress, or cross-dress, in the clothes of the other sex. Some gender identity disorders are only mildly disturbing to the individual, whereas others may produce severe anxiety and personal dysfunction. Furthermore, behaviors that deviate from sexual norms imposed by society and culture are commonly harshly judged. Such judgments are a potential source of guilt and shame for the nonconforming individual.

Among children referred for treatment, gender identity disorder occurs in a ratio of five boys to each girl. The ratio is less pronounced among adults, two to three men to each woman.

Etiology and precipitating factors
The etiology of gender identity disorder is not yet well defined. Research carried out over the last 10 years into such areas as cognitive abilities, sibling sex ratio, birth order, temperament, and physical attractiveness, or on a deeper level into endocrinologic or chromosomal abnormalities, have not provided definitive evidence.

Recent psychosocial research with children proposes that parents' marital conflicts set the stage for insecure relationships with their children. In such an environment, children become insecure, temperamentally vulnerable, and develop high levels of anxiety. A boy experiences an insecure relationship with the mother, while a girl perceives the marital conflict as a situation in which the mother is unable to defend herself. This creates intense anxiety about the child's own self. Addi-

tionally, mothers of girls with gender identity disorder often feel acutely "put down" by their spouses, and the fathers tend to see females as less competent.

Potential complications
Unresolved gender identify conflicts can lead to anxiety, depression, alcoholism, or drug abuse and possibly suicide.

ASSESSMENT GUIDELINES

Nursing history (functional health pattern findings)
Health perception–health management pattern
• Anxiety or depression
Self-perception–self-concept pattern
• Belief that gender is incongruent with anatomy
• Concern or confusion about personal identity
• Discomfort with gender identity and expected sex-role behaviors
• Cross-dressing
• Severe anxiety over homosexual feelings
Role-relationship pattern
• Disturbed interpersonal relationships
• Discomfort with assigned sex roles
• Dissatisfaction or confusion about sexual preference
• Inability to establish satisfying sexual relationship
• Dressing or lifestyle reflective of gender identity rather than anatomical sex
Sexual-reproductive pattern
• Lack of interest in sex
• Unsatisfactory sexual experiences
• Sexual dysfunction or disorder
• Desire to be the opposite sex
• Discomfort over preferred means of sexual expression
Coping–stress tolerance pattern
• Extreme anxiety about sex or sexuality
• Use of sexual behavior to cope with anxiety
Value-belief pattern
• Belief that sexual activity is wrong

Physical findings
A complete physical examination and comprehensive sexual history are necessary for an accurate diagnosis of the client's condition. Psychological findings may include depression and anxiety. (See *Sexual history.*)

Sexual history

The goal of the sexual history is to determine a client's level of sexual health and sexual functioning. Obtaining a sexual history, in addition to gathering data for assessment, may also be therapeutic by promoting the client's sexuality and sexual function as legitimate aspects of health and well-being.

Sexual history formats include the brief sexual history, the comprehensive sexual history, and the sexual problem history. The brief sexual history can be part of a total health history or nursing assessment. The comprehensive sexual history supplements the brief sexual history and can be used in the context of sexual counseling. If a brief or comprehensive sexual history indicates that the client may have a sexual dysfunction disorder, a health care professional with expertise in sexual counseling or therapy needs to conduct a thorough history of the sexual problem and plan-focused interventions.

Brief sexual history

1. Has anything (such as illness, pregnancy, or surgery) interfered with your roles and relationships as a spouse or parent?
Yes ❑   No ❑

2. Has anything (such as illness, surgery, hospitalization, injury, or medical treatment) changed the way you feel about yourself as a man or woman?   Yes ❑   No ❑

3. Has anything (such as surgery, medication, illness, or medical treatment) changed your ability to function sexually?
Yes ❑   No ❑

4. Are you currently sexually active?   Yes ❑   No ❑

a. If no, does this make you uncomfortable?   Yes ❑   No ❑

If yes, are you satisfied with your sexual activity in terms of:

1. Frequency?   Yes ❑   No ❑
2. Arousal?   Yes ❑   No ❑
3. Ability to attain erection?   Yes ❑   No ❑
4. Orgasm?   Yes ❑   No ❑
5. Comfort during intercourse?   Yes ❑   No ❑

(If the client answers no to any of the five items, conduct a comprehensive sexual history.)

5. Do you have any questions or concerns that you would like to discuss at this time?   Yes ❑   No ❑

If yes, please describe:_____

_____

Comprehensive sexual history (Use information obtained from "Brief sexual history" above.)

General information

1.a. When you were growing up, from whom did you learn about sex?

_____

_____

b. What did you learn?

_____

_____

c. When was your first sexual encounter?

_____

_____

d. Was your first sexual encounter:

What you expected?   Yes ❑   No ❑
Satisfying?   Yes ❑   No ❑
Mutually desired?   Yes ❑   No ❑
Safe?   Yes ❑   No ❑

If you answered no to any of these items, please explain:

_____

_____

2. If you are currently sexually active, are you taking birth control measures?   Yes ❑   No ❑

3. Do you experience any physical or emotional discomfort during sexual activity?   Yes ❑   No ❑

4. Have you ever had or been exposed to a sexually transmitted disease?   Yes ❑   No ❑

Desire for sexual activity

5. Has your desire for sexual activity:

Increased?   _____

Decreased?_____

Fluctuated?_____

6. Do you have concerns about your sexual performance?
Yes ❑   No ❑

7. Please describe any specific feelings (positive or negative) about your body image and how it affects your desire for sexual activity:

Sexual interaction with partner

8. Describe your usual "preliminaries" to lovemaking in terms of initiation and degree of communication:

_____

_____

9. Describe usual characteristics of "love play" in terms of:

a. Behaviors that enhance the overall encounter:

_____

_____

b. Behaviors that detract from the overall encounter:

_____

_____

c. Sexual norms within the relationship:

_____

d. Extracoital alternatives:

_____

_____

10. Do you think your partner is satisfied with your sexual relationship?   Yes ❑   No ❑

11. Have you or are you engaged in an extramarital relationship? If yes, describe the frequency and duration of these relationships:
Yes ❑   No ❑

_____

(continued)

Sex-related disorders

Sexual history *(continued)*

12. Have you engaged in any high-risk sexual activities, such as:

Multiple sexual partners?   Yes ❑   No ❑

Unprotected sexual intercourse?   Yes ❑   No ❑

Sexual intercourse when under the influence of alcohol or drugs?   Yes ❑   No ❑

Sexual intercourse with an unknown partner?   Yes ❑ No ❑

Male-specific questions

1.a. Please describe:

Quality of erections:

_____

_____

Situations that interfere with erection:

_____

_____

Satisfaction with penis size:

_____

_____

2.a. Please describe:

Frequency of orgasm or climax: _____

How you achieve orgasm or climax:

Vaginal penetration   Yes ❑   No ❑

By hand   Yes ❑   No ❑

Orally   Yes ❑   No ❑

Anally   Yes ❑   No ❑

b. Has there been any change in the quality of orgasm?
Yes ❑   No ❑

c. Do you experience any discomfort or pain with orgasm?
Yes ❑   No ❑

d. Are your concerned with your partner achieving an orgasm?
Yes ❑   No ❑

e. Does this concern interfere with your experience?
Yes ❑   No ❑

3. Do you use the same position during intercourse?
Yes ❑   No ❑

Female-specific questions

1.a. Do you have enough time for vaginal lubrication before intercourse?   Yes ❑   No ❑

b. Please describe how long it takes you to become adequately lubricated:

Has this time increased or decreased?_____

2. Do you ever experience pain during intercourse?

If yes, please describe: Yes ❑   No ❑

3.a. Do you usually achieve orgasm? Yes ❑   No ❑

b. How do you achieve orgasm?

Masturbation   Yes ❑   No ❑

Orally   Yes ❑   No ❑

Manipulation by partner   Yes ❑   No ❑

c. How often do you achieve orgasm?_____

d. Please describe situations that interfere with orgasm:

_____

NURSING DIAGNOSIS

Personal identity disturbance related to conflict between anatomical sex and gender identity

Nursing priority

Help the client to develop self-affirming social and psychological supports that can enhance a positive self-image.

Patient outcome criteria

As treatment progresses, the client, family, or both should be able to:
• demonstrate evidence of improved self-esteem
• identify and participate in available resources such as support groups.

Interventions

1. Assess the client's knowledge and beliefs about sexuality.

2. Provide the client with accurate information about sexuality in an open, nonjudgmental manner.

3. Assess the degree to which the client's occupational, social, and interpersonal functioning have been affected by the condition.

4. Assess the effectiveness of social and psychological supports available to the client.

5. Assess the client's history of drug and alcohol use.

6. Whenever possible and with client approval, include the client's family in education sessions.

7. Inform the client of available community counseling and treatment resources.

Rationales

1. Such assessment can reveal conflicts concerning the client's sexual experiences and expectations.

2. By educating the client about sexuality, the nurse can correct misinformation and help the client see himself or herself in a wider, more realistic context of sexual behaviors.

3. Gender confusion and transsexual behaviors can cause extreme social isolation and limit occupational choices, sometimes to prostitution.

4. Because the client may be isolated or estranged from the family, social and emotional supports are often limited, manipulative, or exploitative. As a result, the client may have been forced to choose social environments that reinforce maladaptive behaviors.

5. The client's social environments and relationships as well as anxiety about the disorder may contribute to drug and alcohol use as the client tries to deal with anxiety and depression.

6. Because of ignorance of or misunderstandings about gender identity disorders, family members may have rejected the client. By educating everyone involved, the nurse can help rebuild disturbed family relationships.

7. Knowing available options and resources, such as hormonal or sex therapies, sexual reassignment, and support groups, can enhance the client's sense of self-control.

NURSING DIAGNOSIS

Anxiety related to conflict between desires and expected sex role behavior

Nursing priority

Decrease the client's anxiety and promote self-acceptance.

Patient outcome criteria

As treatment progresses, the client, family, or both should be able to:
• verbalize an increased knowledge of human sexuality
• demonstrate decreased anxiety.

Interventions

1. Convey to the client unconditional caring and positive regard.

2. Assess the degree to which the client is agitated and threatened by sexual impulses.

Rationales

1. Acceptance can enhance self-esteem and help the client overcome fears of rejection.

2. The client's sexual impulses can produce agitated and aggressive gender behavior (macho or ultrafeminine) as a way of enhancing self-image and self-esteem. Recognizing these inappropriate responses is an important step toward developing positive behaviors.

Sex-related disorders

3. Assess the client's history for possible sexual abuse with a same-sex adult.

4. Provide a safe, nonthreatening, and nonjudgmental environment in which the client can discuss sexual feelings and impulses

5. Educate the client about human sexuality and sexual responses.

6. Encourage the client to verbalize personal values, beliefs, and attitudes about sexuality and sexual preference.

7. Inform the client of available follow-up care or treatment alternatives.

3. Conflict and ambivalence over homosexual activity can generate considerable anxiety. Identifying such feelings can help the nurse develop a more appropriate plan of care.

4. A nonjudgmental environment can help the client express frightening and overwhelming feelings or thoughts.

5. Sex education can help alleviate the client's guilt over having experienced pleasure from homosexual or other sexual behaviors.

6. Talking about sexuality can help the client identify causes of anxiety and conflict.

7. Therapy that focuses on sexuality can help the client resolve, adapt to, and be comfortable with chosen sexual preferences.

Discharge criteria

Nursing documentation indicates that the client:
• has demonstrated increased self-acceptance
• has verbalized an increased knowledge of human sexuality and sexual responses
• has reported decreased anxiety when dealing with sexuality
• has verbalized a knowledge of available support and treatment resources.
Nursing documentation also indicates that the family:
• has demonstrated a knowledge and understanding of the client's condition
• has been referred to available community and family resources.

Selected references

Beemer, B. "Gender Dysmorphia Update," *Journal of Psychosocial Nursing* 34(4):12, 1996.

Boyd, M.A., and Nihart, M.A. *Psychiatric Nursing: Contemporary Practice.* Philadelphia: Lippincott-Raven Pubs., 1998.

Diagnostic and Statistical Manual of Mental Disorders, 4th ed. Washington, D.C.: American Psychiatric Association, 1994.

Varcarolis, E.M. *Foundations of Psychiatric Nursing,* 3rd ed. Philadelphia: W.B. Saunders Co., 1998.

Sexual disorders

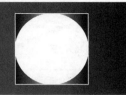

Psychiatric nursing diagnostic class

Sexual response variations

INTRODUCTION

Sexual disorders are characterized primarily as paraphilias and sexual dysfunctions. The *paraphilias* involve different means of arousal. The means of arousal may be an object not normally considered sexually stimulating (fetish), an act involving humiliation or control (sadism or masochism), an act involving lack of another's awareness or consent (frotteurism, exhibitionism, voyeurism), or contact with children (pedophilia). These behaviors cause clinically significant impairment or distress in social or occupational functioning. (For a more complete list of paraphilias, see *Paraphilias*, page 260.) *Sexual dysfunctions* are characterized by a disturbed or disrupted ability to experience the complete sexual response cycle, the phases of which are desire, arousal, orgasm, and resolution. These disorders can cause significant distress and interpersonal difficulty.

Etiology and precipitating factors

Behavioral theorists propose that paraphilias can be acquired through conditioning, in which an initial pairing of an object is associated with, and then becomes necessary for, sexual release. The need then becomes generalized to other situations that are related to anxiety. Biological theories suggest that abnormal hormonal activity and genetic predisposition interacts with social and family factors to influence the development of fantasies and sexual acts. These behaviors may occur in normal sexual activity, but when they become the primary source of sexual satisfaction, they may cause problems for the individual or significant others.

Sexual arousal dysfunctions have biological and psychological factors. Erectile dysfunction may result from normal aging processes, heavy cigarette smoking, genital trauma, hormonal deficiencies, diabetes, vascular insufficiency, multiple sclerosis and Parkinson's disease. Psychosocial factors include fear of failure, relationship stress, and fear of rejection.

Orgasmic dysfunction, can be caused by any local genital or pelvic pathology, surgery, or trauma that produces painful intercourse or impaired response to sexual stimulation. Disorders that damage the spinal cord and interfere with the transmission of any sexual stimuli may also impair orgasm. Many systemic diseases interfere with sexual response due to pain, decreased functional capacity, or side effects of treatments. (See

Paraphilias

The paraphilias classified in *DSM-IV* as sexual disorders are recurrent, intense, sexually arousing fantasies; sexual urges or behaviors involving nonhuman objects; and suffering and humiliation of self or partner, children, or another nonconsenting person. Diagnosis considers the frequency of the behavior and its interference with function. Some paraphilias that violate social mores or norms are considered sex offenses or sex crimes. Everyone has sexual fantasies, and sexual behavior between two consenting adults that's not physically or psychologically harmful should not be considered a paraphilia.

Type of paraphilia	Source of sexual arousal
Exhibitionism	Exposure of genitals in public
Fetishism	Use of clothing, such as leather or shoes for erotic pleasure
Frotteurism	Sexual gratification received by rubbing against clothing of a person of the opposite sex
Necrophilia	Sexual activity with a corpse
Pedophilia	Sexual activity with children; may be homosexual, heterosexual, or incestuous
Sexual masochism	Being humiliated, beaten, bound, or otherwise made to suffer
Sexual sadism	Inflicting physical/mental pain on sexual partner
Transvestic fetishism	Recurrent and persistent cross-dressing by a heterosexual male
Voyeurism	Watching others engaged in sexual activity or undressing
Zoophilia	Sexual activity with animals

Medical and surgical conditions associated with sexual dysfunctions.) Many drugs produce sexual adverse effects, and it is important to discuss this with the patient and significant others before initiating the particular medication. (See appendix C, Commonly prescribed medications associated with adverse sexual effects and dysfunction.)

Orgasmic function is directly affected by specific emotions such as guilt, anger, or hostility toward the partner, sexual anxiety, and depressive or intrusive thoughts. Lack of information and misinformation can be a cause of orgasmic inhibiting states. Finally, social, religious, and cultural prohibitions influence an individual's view of their sexuality and can foster guilt and shame for moving outside those boundaries.

Potential complications

A complete physical examination is essential to elicit organic causes for sexual dysfunction, many of which can be treated or reversed. Without proper treatment, individuals with these disorders may become depressed and develop feelings of worthlessness and hopelessness, which can progress to suicidal ideation. Paraphilias may lead to physical abuse or violence against nonconsenting adults or children, requiring arrest and incarceration.

ASSESSMENT GUIDELINES

Nursing history (functional health pattern findings)

Health perception–health management pattern
• History of physical or emotional illness
• Insistence that dysfunction is related to physical change

Self-perception–self-concept pattern
• Poor self-image and self-esteem
• Discomfort with sex role
• Feelings of inadequacy or undesirability
• Fear of sexual performance failure

Role-relationship pattern
• Disturbed personal relationships
• Fear of rejection
• Inability to establish sexual relationships
• Fear of intimacy

Sexual-reproductive pattern
• Lack of interest in sex

Medical and surgical conditions associated with sexual dysfunctions

Condition	Sexual dysfunction
Endocrine disorders	
Adrenal dysfunction	Impotence
Diabetes mellitus	Early impotence
Hypogonadism	Decreased vaginal lubrication
Hypothyroidism	Decreased libido
Local genital disease	
Male	
Hydrocele, Peyronie's disease, priapism, prostatitis, urethritis	Decreased libido, impotence
Female	
Endometriosis	Decreased arousal
Imperforate hymen	Vaginismus
Pelvic inflammatory disease	Decreased libido
Vaginitis	Dyspareunia
Neurologic disorders	
Alcoholic neuropathy	Decreased libido
Diabetic neuropathy	Impaired orgasm
Herniated disc disorder	Decreased libido
Multiple sclerosis	Decreased or increased libido
Spinal cord injury	Impotence
Temporal lobe epilepsy	Decreased or increased libido
Postoperative-surgical conditions	
Female	
Episiotomy	Dyspareunia
Oophorectomy	Decreased lubrication
Vaginal repair of prolapse	Vaginismus
Male	
Abdominal-perineal bowel resection	Ejaculatory dysfunction
Prostatectomy (perineal-radical)	Impotence
Both sexes	
Amputation (lower limb)	Structural (mechanical difficulties in sexual acts)
Ostomies (colostomy, ileostomy)	Body image disturbance, avoidance of sex, fear of odor or accidental spill
Systemic-chronic disease	
Hepatic, infections, malignancies, pulmonary, renal	Decreased arousal, decreased libido, impotence
Vascular disease	
Atherosclerosis, cerebrovascular accident, hypertension, sickle cell anemia, and venous insufficiency	Impotence

- Guilt or shame about sex
- Distress about sexual expression
- Fear of unwanted pregnancy
- Fear of sexually transmitted diseases
- History of unsatisfying or difficult sexual experiences
- History of sexual assault or violence
- Compulsive sexual activity
- High-risk sexual practices, including unprotected sex

Coping–stress tolerance pattern
- Extreme anxiety about sex or sexuality
- Use of sexual behavior to cope with anxiety

Value-belief pattern
- Belief that sexual activity is wrong

Physical findings
Cardiovascular
- Angina
- Heart failure
- Arrhythmias
- Hypertension
- Myocardial infarction
- Palpitations

Respiratory
- Chronic obstructive pulmonary disease
- Cystic fibrosis
- Lung cancer

Sex-related disorders

Gastrointestinal
- Abdominal pain
- Colitis, especially with colostomy

Genitourinary
- Benign prostatic hypertrophy
- Bladder cancer
- Cystitis
- End-stage renal disease
- Erectile dysfunction
- Penile, prostate, or testicular cancer
- Peyronie's disease (distorted erection)
- Priapism
- Prostatism
- Urinary incontinence

Gynecologic
- Benign uterine tumors
- Cervical cancer
- Dysmenorrhea
- Endometrial cancer
- Endometriosis
- Hysterectomy
- Menopause
- Ovarian tumors
- Pelvic exenteration

- Vaginal infections
- Vaginal or vulvar tumors
- Vulvectomy

Musculoskeletal
- Ankylosing spondylitis
- Fatigue
- Lupus erythematosus
- Muscular dystrophies
- Pain
- Rheumatoid arthritis or osteoarthritis
- Stiffness or weakness

Neurologic
- Central nervous system tumors
- Closed head injury
- Neuroendocrine disorders

Psychological
- Conversion disorder
- Eating disorders
- History of incest or sexual assault
- Mood disorders
- Psychoactive substance abuse disorders
- Schizophrenia
- Rape trauma syndrome
- Somatization disorder

NURSING DIAGNOSIS

Altered sexuality patterns related to inability to achieve sexual satisfaction in socially acceptable ways

Nursing priority

Help the client to develop alternative methods of achieving sexual satisfaction

Patient outcome criteria

As treatment progresses, the client, family, or both should be able to:
- verbalize an understanding of sexual disorders
- acknowledge the need for ongoing treatment
- demonstrate the ability to use adaptive coping methods
- identify the effects of disruptive behavior
- demonstrate improved self-esteem.

Interventions

1. Obtain a complete medical, social, and sexual history from the client.

2. Assess the client's anxiety or discomfort about the disorder.

3. Remain nonjudgmental, and avoid seeming curious about or repulsed by the client's behavior.

Rationales

1. A complete history can help the nurse to identify causes of or precipitating factors for the client's disorder or dysfunction.

2. Anxiety can indicate that the client wants to change or learn about the disorder.

3. Both curiosity and repulsion can diminish the client's self-esteem. A nonjudgmental approach can both enhance client self-esteem and establish trust between the client and nurse.

4. Assess the client's knowledge of sexuality and sexual response patterns. Provide information and correct misinformation.

5. Inform the client of treatment options, including different kinds of sex therapies, and offer referrals.

6. When possible, provide education and support for the client's family or loved ones.

4. Many people's knowledge about sexuality consists of myth and misinformation. Correct and accurate information can enable the client to understand and make informed choices.

5. Learning about the disorder as well as treatment options can help alleviate the client's anxiety.

6. Family members and loved ones also are affected by sexual disorders. Their participation in treatment can enhance the client's compliance.

DISCHARGE CRITERIA

Nursing documentation indicates that the client:
• has demonstrated an understanding of the condition and of human sexual responses
• has demonstrated the ability to identify alternative methods of achieving sexual satisfaction
• has demonstrated an improved self-esteem
• has verbalized an awareness of the need for further treatment.

SELECTED REFERENCES

Boyd, M.A., and Nihart, M.A. *Psychiatric Nursing: Contemporary Practice.* Philadelphia: Lippincott-Raven Pubs. 1998.

Crensahw, I., and Goldberg, J. *Sexual Pharmacology: Drugs That Affect Sexual Function.* New York: W.W. Norton & Co., 1996.

Diagnostic and Statistical Manual of Mental Disorders, 4th ed. Washington, D.C.: American Psychiatric Association, 1994.

Finger, W.W., et al. "Medications That May Contribute to Sexual Disorders: A Guide to Assessment and Treatment in Family Practice," *Journal of Family Practice* 44(1):33-43, 1997.

Wincze, J.P., and Barlow, D. *Enhancing Sexuality: A Problem-Solving Approach: Client Workbook.* New York: Psychological Corporation, 1996.

Sex-related disorders

Part 13

Disorders associated with violence

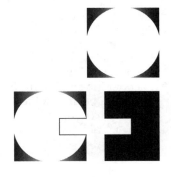

Interpersonal abuse and violence

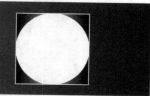

DSM-IV classifications
Victim/survivor focused
995.52   Neglect of child
995.53   Sexual abuse of child
995.54   Physical abuse of child
995.81   Physical abuse of adult
995.83   Sexual abuse of adult
Perpetrator focused
V61.21   Neglect, physical or sexual abuse of child
V61.12   Physical or sexual abuse of adult by partner
V62.83   Physical or sexual abuse of adult by person other than partner

Psychiatric nursing diagnostic class
Violence

INTRODUCTION

Interpersonal violence occurs at staggering rates in American society—some health care professionals describe it as an epidemic. Violent behavior is not limited to isolated populations. It crosses all social, ethnic, economic, and cultural boundaries. Today our children as well as adults are bombarded with scenes of interpersonal violence on television and in movies. Violence is woven into the fabric of our society. Failure to respond to violent behavior may passively condone it and perpetuate the cycle of violence.

Nurses in every practice setting face the challenge of caring for both the victims and perpetrators of violent behavior. Developing an understanding of the causes and effects of violent and abusive behavior enable the nurse to intervene in a therapeutic manner and provide comprehensive care. When treating and caring for the victims of violence, maintain objectivity and a systems perspective. Remember that the psychological and emotional consequences of violence may be more severe and long lasting than the physical injuries. Developing an understanding of victimization can help the nurse to care for those caught in the cycle of violence. The first step comes in being able to identify and assess victims of violence. (See *Identifying and assessing victims of interpersonal violence.*) Once a general assessment has been completed and there is clear evidence that interpersonal violence is involved in the health care situation, it is important to obtain additional information. (See *Abuse assessment screen.*)

When dealing with the perpetrator of violence, assess for a history of violent behavior, including the type of

violence and the situational and interactional factors associated with it. Aggressive behavior as a means of coping is not limited to persons with a diagnosed psychiatric disorder. Aggression may manifest itself as abusive, neglectful, or violent behavior, including child neglect and physical and sexual abuse, spousal abuse, elder abuse and neglect, rape, and sexual assault.

Etiology and precipitating factors
Nurses in all practice settings must become more proficient at identifying and treating victims of sexual assault. Although many people assume that rape follows a

Abuse assessment screen

The abuse assessment screen was developed by the Nursing Research Consortium on Violence and Abuse (1989).

1. Have you ever been emotionally or physically abused by your partner or someone important to you?
Yes ❑   No ❑
If yes, by whom: _____
How many times: _____

2. Within the past year, have you been hit, slapped, kicked, or otherwise physically hurt by someone?
Yes ❑   No ❑
If yes, by whom: _____
How many times: _____

3. Since you have been pregnant, have you been hit, slapped, kicked, or otherwise physically hurt by someone?
Yes ❑   No ❑
If yes, by whom: _____
How many times: _____

4. Within the past year, has anyone forced you to have sexual activities?
Yes ❑   No ❑
If yes, by whom: _____
How many times: _____

5. Are you afraid of your partner or anyone listed above?
Yes ❑   No ❑

Identifying and assessing victims of interpersonal violence

The chart below describes nursing interventions and rationales appropriate when assessing possible victims of interpersonal violence.

Interventions	Rationales
• When assessing the client, determine whether the injury is consistent with the report of how it occurred (injury coincides with mechanism of injury reported).	• Most victims of abuse will not volunteer that someone harmed them, but instead will blame the action on an accident or their own clumsiness.
• Include questions about abuse, such as "This kind of injury can be caused by someone else. Has someone hurt you?"	• When asked directly, most victims will answer honestly. Victims of abuse are usually relieved when someone brings up the subject so that they can talk about it.
• Provide privacy and safety for the client when performing the assessment.	• The perpetrator of violence will usually insist that the victim not be left alone with the nurse. This should raise a red flag. Without privacy, fear of repercussions and further abuse will prevent the victim from telling the truth.
• Be alert for behavioral signs and symptoms common in victims of abuse, such as hypervigilance, anxiety, apprehension or fear about answering questions, evasiveness, and difficulty making decisions.	• Victims of abuse may appear nervous or apprehensive in the presence of perceived authority. They also tend to place others' needs ahead of their own.
• Determine from hospital records or the client interview if the client has a history of previous injury (especially injury that is inconsistent with mechanism reported).	• Although many victims of abuse may seek treatment from several different health care facilities, making tracking difficult, they will eventually revisit the same facility. A history of injuries attributed to accidents or clumsiness can signal abuse.
• Be alert for clients who repeatedly report vague, unfounded somatic complaints.	• Some victims develop GI or neurologic symptoms. For these people, a physical complaint is more acceptable than admitting to abuse. This is not attention-seeking behavior; it is a call for help.
• If a child shows any sign of physical, sexual, or emotional abuse or neglect, report it to the appropriate agency, such as the state's department of youth or protective services for elders.	• Health care workers are required to report all instances of confirmed or suspected child abuse. As mandated reporters, health care workers cannot be sued if their suspicions are unfounded.
• If the victim is an adult, share your suspicions and offer resources for help, such as shelters, hotlines, and support groups.	• Telling the client about suspicions and offering options can help the client acknowledge the problem.
• Do not force the client to accept help immediately. Let the client think about the available options.	• The dynamics of abusive relationships can be so complex that the client may have difficulty sorting out the next action. Leaving an abusive relationship may be more frightening than staying. Accept this and support the client in making the decision that best meets personal needs.
• Maintain a supportive, nonjudgmental approach even if the client is hesitant in accepting help or making changes.	• A victim who chooses to return to an abusive situation can be extremely frustrating for the nurse. Responding with anger will only alienate the victim and reinforce feelings of low self-esteem and victimization.
• Assess the client for signs and symptoms of acute stress disorder or posttraumatic stress disorder.	• Victims of abuse are at risk for these disorders. Adult survivors of untreated or unresolved childhood abuse are prone to behavior that reenacts the trauma or facilitates repeated victimization. Such behavior represents serious psychological problems requiring treatment beyond that for the current abusive situation.
• Understand that treating an abused client is a long-term process. Do not expect to treat or resolve the issue in a short-term encounter. Remember that engaging in a discussion and offering referral is important to the victim of interpersonal violence and abuse.	• Nurses who feel they must resolve all problems they identify are setting themselves up for failure and a sense of futility. To keep their perspective, nurses must realize that starting the healing process is a great step.
• Be aware of the impact of absorbing the trauma of others. Seek out support and opportunities for personal ventilation and discussion.	• By virtue of their closeness to the trauma of others, nurses are susceptible to a phenomenon known as vicarious trauma. By being aware of their susceptibility and taking preventive measures, nurses can help maintain their mental health.

Sexual behavior: The force continuum

Sexual consent and participation can be conceptualized across a continuum demonstrating degrees of coercion described in this overview.

Freely consenting. Partners with equal power mutually choosing sexual activity. Equal power means each partner has equal status, knowledge, and ability to consent. This includes one partner agreeing to engage in sexual activity, even if not interested, as an expression of love and caring for the other person.

Economic partnership. One person agrees to sexual activity as part of an economic agreement. The type of sexual behaviors permitted are mutually determined as part of the economic agreement.

Seduction. One party attempts to persuade the other to engage in sexual activities.

Psychic rape. Assault to another person's dignity and self-respect, such as verbal abuse, street harassment, or the portrayal of violence or pornography in the media.

Bribery or coercion. The use of emotional or psychological force to persuade another to take part in sexual activities. This includes situations of unequal power between the individuals, especially when one person is in a position of authority.

Acquaintance rape. Sexual assault occurring when one party abuses the trust of a relationship and forces another into sexual activities.

Fear rape. When one party engages in sexual activities out of fear of potential violence.

Violent rape. When violence is threatened or occurs. This includes forced sexual activity between spouses, acquaintances, or strangers.

From Stuart, G.W., and Laraia, M.T. *Principles and Practice of Psychiatric Nursing*, 6th ed. St. Louis: Mosby–Year Book, Inc., 1998; 835. Used with permission.

---

surprise attack by a stranger in an isolated setting (blitz or fear rape), statistics indicate that victims typically are raped by someone they know (confidence or acquaintance rape). More attention is now paid to date rape, but marital rape is not widely discussed.

Violence involves force, including verbal and physical force, threats, and intimidation, which the victim is either unable to resist or complies with out of fear. The force involved in sexual violence can be described on a continuum ranging from free consent to violent rape. (See *Sexual behavior: The force continuum*.) This distinction is made to highlight the need for sensitive intervention with these victims.

While the long-term consequences of either blitz or confidence rape can include acute stress disorder and eventually posttraumatic stress disorder, the immediate response to confidence rape can be more emotionally devastating. Victims of blitz rape may question personal judgment about where they were or what they did to make themselves vulnerable to attack and may even blame themselves for the rape. Victims of confidence rape are forced to question trust in others and examine personal responsibility for provoking the assault. The sense of betrayal and devastation is compounded by the fact that most assailants in confidence rape do not believe they have committed a crime, leaving the victim to question and doubt interpretations of the event.

Although most victims of sexual assault are female, males also are sexually assaulted. Contrary to common beliefs, sexual assaults on males do not only occur in the absence of a suitable or preferred partner (such as in prison situations). As with females, assaults on males are acts of violence. Information about these assaults is minimal because of the shame and embarrassment of being victimized and because of the stigma of homosexuality.

What is known is that male victims respond to rape in much the same way as women. The prevailing myth that the rape victim somehow "wanted it" also applies to men, which then implies homosexuality or unfulfilled homosexual desires. If the victim is homosexual, he may fear the response of others. As with females, the male victim may feel that he may have done something to provoke or deserve the assault or that others will feel this way. Such fears and perceptions may be a significant factor in the low numbers of male rapes reported. Treatment of the male victim should proceed as for a female victim.

Potential complications

Complications of rape may include disfigurement, physical injury, posttraumatic stress disorder, substance abuse, death from physical injuries, and suicide. (Refer to "Stress-related anxiety disorders," and "Dissociative disorders," for more information.)

ASSESSMENT GUIDELINES
Nursing history (functional health pattern findings)

Assessment findings may be similar to those found in anxiety disorder, especially generalized anxiety disorder, posttraumatic stress disorder, or dissociative disorders. Signs and symptoms may vary depending on the amount of time between the event and health care interventions.

Health perception–health management pattern
• Denies severity of rape's impact
• Expresses disbelief
• Reports symptoms of anxiety or panic
• Reports or show signs of substance abuse

Activity-exercise pattern
• Reports or shows evidence of restlessness or trembling

Sleep-rest pattern
• Reports difficulty falling asleep or staying asleep

- Reports nightmares

Cognitive-perceptual pattern
- Reports or demonstrates difficulty concentrating
- Reports or demonstrates impaired recall of the rape
- Reports or demonstrates a sense of depersonalization
- Appears hypervigilant

Self-perception–self-concept pattern
- Reports or exhibits feelings of shame, humiliation, helplessness, guilt, or diminished self-esteem
- Expresses concerns about body image or self-concept
- Expresses feelings of responsibility for the rape

Role-relationship pattern
- Expresses concern about changes in relationships
- Expresses concern about other's responses to the rape
- Expresses fears about future intimacy with others

Sexual-reproductive pattern
- Expresses concerns about future sexual activity
- Expresses concerns about sexually transmitted diseases

Coping-stress tolerance pattern
- Exhibits physical tension
- Experiences labile mood
- Reports intrusive memories of the rape
- Exhibits or reports psychological numbing

Value-belief pattern
- Reports or exhibits feelings of powerlessness
- Uses such defense mechanisms as denial, intellectualization, or rationalization

Physical findings

A comprehensive physical examination is conducted to assess the client for evidence of physical trauma. Findings from the physical examination must be carefully and completely documented because they will be an important part of the evidence used in any legal proceedings. Physical evidence is collected during the examination, and may include taking photographs of injuries, swabbing orifices for semen, and assessing for sexually transmitted diseases. Other evidence may be collected, such as fingernail scrapings, blood and saliva samples, clothing, and pubic hair. Awareness of institutional and municipal requirements for the proper collection and preservation of evidence is extremely important.

Specific physical findings may include cuts, bruises, fractures, and dislocations. Such injuries can appear anywhere on the body. Pay close attention to the head and neck for evidence of choking or attempted strangulation, and assess for loss of consciousness, which may indicate potentially serious head trauma.

NURSING DIAGNOSIS

Posttrauma response related to physical neglect or abuse, sexual abuse or assault, or interpersonal violence

Nursing priority

Help the client to achieve optional adjustment to the interpersonal violence and maintain his or her safety.

Patient outcome criteria

As treatment progresses, the client, family, or both should be able to:
- state that the traumatizing event produces less anxiety
- demonstrate age-appropriate ability to manage emotional reactions
- demonstrate appropriate lifestyle changes and actively pursue support from other family members
- express a sense of control over the present situation
- identify effective coping methods for eliminating negative self-perception
- verbalize an increased sense of self-esteem and hope
- develop and use a safety (escape) plan when they perceive a threat to their safety

Interventions

1. Assess for physical trauma.

Rationales

1. Sexual assault may cause physical injury that is not readily apparent.

Maintaining your safety in a violent situation

Please remember that your safety is important. Follow these suggestions and plan ahead for the next episode of family violence.

• Ask a friend or neighbor to call the police when they hear loud arguments or screaming.

• Develop a signaling system with a friend or neighbor so that they know to call the police.

• Collect and store away from home the following: money, clothes (for you and any children), extra set of car and house keys.

• Plan to take any valued pets with you (store food for pets with your belongings).

• Remove all weapons.

• Make sure you have the following documents (originals or copies) readily accessible to you: birth certificates, driver's license, social security cards, medical insurance cards, bank account numbers, rent or mortgage receipts, insurance policy, marriage license. Also consider important pictures, keepsakes, jewelry.

Remember: Plan ahead! Individuals have been harmed, even killed, going back for a pet or something else important to them. Pack it before or go with police protection. Your life is important!

---

2. Establish a safe, trusting, empathetic, nonjudgmental environment in which the client can discuss the rape.

3. Explain the legal obligation to report the crime to the proper authorities and describe the client's rights.

4. Provide privacy for the client during the interview and physical examination.

5. Encourage the client to verbalize feelings and talk about the violent act.

6. Identify adaptive and maladaptive coping skills. Educate the client about safety and develop with them an escape or safety plan. (See *Maintaining your safety in a violent situation*.)

7. Do not challenge the client's coping style. Instead, provide education about violence and explain how people usually respond to this form of assault.

8. Help the client identify and mobilize resources and support systems.

9. Educate the family and loved ones about emotional responses to violence and involve them in prevention programs.

2. Because of a sense of violation, shame, and guilt, the client may have difficulty recounting the event. The clinician's objectivity and empathy are essential in helping the client regain self-esteem, self-confidence, and a sense of trust.

3. Most victims of interpersonal violence are unable to make decisions immediately after the event and may not report the crime. By acknowledging this obligation, the nurse can alleviate the client's ambivalence about reporting the rape. The client also needs to know about personal rights and appropriate legal recourse.

4. Lack of privacy during the client's description of the violent attack can increase the sense of shame, guilt, and vulnerability.

5. Verbalization provides an opportunity to dispel myths about rape and to help the client develop an accurate perception of the event.

6. Victims of violence may express considerable self-doubt and recrimination, which can hinder recovery. Denial, repression, rationalization, and intellectualization may all be evident. Due to these protective defense mechanisms, they need assistance with having a concrete plan for safety or escape if a perceived or actual threat of violence occurs.

7. Education can help the client understand victimization and respond to it. Challenging the coping style will only undermine the client's damaged ego and may increase self-doubt and feelings of responsibility for the event.

8. Emotional consequences of violence may make victims reluctant to tell others, including the police and loved ones, about the event. Support will enhance the client's sense of safety and control.

9. Preparing the family and loved ones for the client's emotional responses helps gain their ability to offer understanding and support.

10. Refer the client to mental health personnel or an appropriate agency for victim of violence counseling. With the client's permission, contact the Sexual Assault Nurse Examiner (SANE) if this is a sexual assault situation.

11. If the victim is a child:
• Consult with a therapist with expertise in childhood sexual assault.

• Assess the child's level of knowledge about anatomy and sex.

• Identify the child's vocabulary for body parts and genitals, then use these words to ensure clear communication.
• Be consistent, honest, and reliable.

• Use visual aids when needed, such as anatomically correct dolls, pictures, or puppets, to help the child describe what happened.

• Explain all procedures. Allow the child to look at the examination room and touch equipment before the physical examination.

• Provide emotional support for and enlist the help of the child's caretaker (unless that is the perpetrator) during the examination.

• Educate the caretaker about the sexual assault and abuse of children. Dispel myths that hold the child responsible or that suggest the child fabricated the event.

10. Recovery from violence takes time. Emotional support, counseling, and therapy can foster client and family adjustment and recovery.

11. Not all victims of violence are adults.
• Children have special needs when dealing with the psychological aftermath of violent assaults.

• When dealing with children, related to sexual assault, some special issues arise. Most children lack the knowledge of anatomy, sexuality, and vocabulary usually involved in the assessment and care of victims of sexual assault. Gaining knowledge about the child's level of understanding can help the nurse to gather accurate information, avoid misunderstandings, and prevent misinterpretation of information.
• Clinical terms may confuse or frighten the child, making data collection difficult.

• Fear, mistrust, and anger toward strangers and adults are common responses for child victims of violent assaults. Feelings toward the abuser may be generalized to all adults.
• A child's lack of knowledge and understanding about sex and sexuality can complicate the telling of what happened. Visual aids can make the child's explanations clearer.
• For children, the physical examination can be more traumatic emotionally than the sexual assault. Developing as much trust and rapport as possible lessens the negative consequences and difficulties inherent in such an examination.
• The primary caretaker may feel guilt, shame, and anger or may express disbelief. Avoid alienating this person; support and praise the caretaker for bringing the child for examination and treatment.
• Children rarely make up stories about sexual assault. Sexual assault and abuse is the responsibility of the perpetrator, not the victim.

DISCHARGE CRITERIA

Nursing documentation indicates that the client:
• has demonstrated an increased ability to recognize the impact of the rape and to use age-appropriate strategies that diminish that impact
• can effectively use age-appropriate strategies that diminish feelings of powerlessness
• has demonstrated a willingness to participate in the plan of care and decision making
• can use alternative coping skills
• is aware of available support resources.

SELECTED REFERENCES

Diagnostic and Statistical Manual of Mental Disorders, 4th ed. Washington, D.C.: American Psychiatric Association, 1994.

Farrell, M. "Healing: A Qualitative Study of Women Recovering from Abusive Relationships with Men," *Perspectives of Psychiatric Care* 32:23, 1996.

Feiring, C., et al. "Social Supports and Children's and Adolescents' Adaptation to Sexual Abuse," *Journal of Interpersonal Violence* 13(2):240-60, 1998.

Kaplan, S., ed. *Family Violence: A Clinical and Legal Guide.* Washington, D.C.: American Psychiatric Association, 1996.

Kaufman-Kantor, G., and Jasinki, J. *Out of the Darkness: Contemporary Perspectives on Family Violence.* Thousand Oaks, Calif.: Sage, 1997.

Rhea, M., et al. "The Silent Victims of Domestic Violence: Who Will Speak?" *Journal of Child and Adolescent Psychiatric Nursing* 9:7, 1996.

Russell, D.E.H. *Dangerous Relationships: Pornography, Misogyny and Rape.* Thousand Oaks, Calif.: Sage, 1998.

Salmon, P., and Calderbank, E. "The Relationship of Childhood and Physical and Sexual Abuse to Adult Illness Behavior," *Journal of Psychosomatic Research* 40:329-36, 1996.

Silverman, A.B., et al. "The Long-Term Sequelae of Child and Adolescent Abuse: A Longitudinal Community Study," *Child Abuse and Neglect* 20:709-23, 1996.

Stuart, G.W., and Laraia, M.T. *Principles and Practice of Psychiatric Nursing,* 6th ed. St. Louis: Mosby—Year Book, Inc., 1998.

Tardiff, K., et al. *Concise Guide to Assessment and Management of Violent Patients.* Washington, D.C.: American Psychiatric Association, 1996.

Ullman, S. "Does Offender Violence Escalate When Rape Victims Fight Back?" *Journal of Interpersonal Violence* 13(2):179-92, 1998.

Wiehe, V.R. *Working with Child Abuse and Neglect: A Primer.* Thousand Oaks, Calif.: Sage, 1996.

Wilt, S., and Olson, S. "Prevalence of Domestic Violence in the U.S.," *Journal of American Medical Women's Association* 51(3):77-82, 1996.

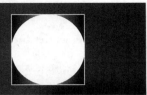

Vicarious traumatization

INTRODUCTION

Vicarious traumatization refers to the cumulative and transformative effect upon a health care provider of working with survivors of traumatic life events. Although this discussion focuses on the effects on health care providers, the phenomenon is relevant to all types of trauma-related workers, including prehospital emergency service personnel, disaster management and relief personnel, firefighters, police, criminal defense lawyers, protective and homeless shelter staff members, crisis hotline workers, and sexual assault workers as well as clergy and other individuals who engage in an empathetic relationship with survivors and victims of traumatic and often life-changing events.

Traumatic events involve some type of traumatic loss, and after the trauma nothing is ever the same. This loss of the familiar is the hallmark of trauma. Health care providers are faced with this reality on a daily basis; therefore, actively engaging in trauma therapy assaults our own self-protective beliefs regarding control, attachment, predictability, and overall safety.

Vicarious traumatization is a developing process, not a solitary event. The process involves our affective responses and self-protective defenses. It involves our strong emotional reactions of grief, rage, and moral outrage that develop over time in response to repeated exposure to the torture, humiliation, and betrayal that individuals perpetuate against others. Additionally, this process involves our responses of sorrow, emotional numbing, and a profound sense of loss.

Etiology and precipitating factors

Health care professionals who have been exposed to the detailed and painful experiences of trauma victims are at risk for vicarious traumatization. Such exposure creates a sense of vulnerability and fragility; it also can awaken old memories and unresolved pain related to trauma in the health care professional's personal life.

Potential complications

Unacknowledged or untreated vicarious traumatization can lead to posttrauma response, acute stress disorder or posttraumatic stress disorder. It also may result in negative coping strategies, such as substance abuse or dependence, aggressive or violent behavior, an inability to function in the workplace, cynicism, and an inability to be compassionate.

ASSESSMENT GUIDELINES

Nursing history (functional health pattern findings)

Health perception–health management pattern
- Possible extreme concern about "going crazy"
- Inattentiveness to medical and dental problems

Nutritional-metabolic pattern
- Possible concern over eating behaviors, such as using food to suppress feelings
- Weight fluctuations

Elimination pattern
- GI system disturbances, such as pain, flatulence, diarrhea, nausea, constipation, vomiting, and intestinal bleeding
- Frequent urination
- Increased sweating and cold, clammy skin

Activity-exercise pattern
- Agitation and restlessness
- Fluctuations in energy and activity levels
- Decreasing interest in participation in leisure and social activities

Sleep-rest pattern
- Possible fatigue after sleep
- Dreams or nightmares about traumatic events happening to others
- Inability to fall asleep or stay asleep or problems with early morning awakening
- Possible use or dependence on aids (such as drugs or alcohol) to facilitate sleep

Cognitive-perceptual pattern
- Memory impairment
- Difficulty concentrating
- Acute or chronic pain
- Difficulty learning

Self-perception–self-concept pattern
- Self-described anxiety or sense of inadequacy
- Feeling detached or estranged from others

Role-relationship pattern
- Inability to maintain relationships with family or significant others
- Disillusionment with job
- Inability to sustain job performance
- "Compassion fatigue" or inability to care about others
- Feeling alone and uninvolved with environment

Sexual-reproductive pattern
- Decreased sexual desire
- Difficulties in sexual performance or satisfaction

Coping–stress tolerance pattern
- High levels in anxiety
- Feelings of tenseness most of the time
- Flashbacks or recurrences of own traumatic events
- Significant stress or number of stressful events during the last year
- Feelings of "going crazy" or being unable to cope
- Feelings of high vulnerability and fragility

Value-belief pattern
- Increasing cynicism
- Spiritual distress
- Inability to achieve life goals

Physical findings

Cardiovascular
- Excessive perspiration
- Fatigue
- Increased heart rate
- Increased blood pressure

Gastrointestinal
- Abdominal distress or pain
- Diarrhea
- Nausea
- Ulcers

Musculoskeletal
- Muscle aches
- Muscle tension
- Restlessness
- Trembling

Neurologic
- Headaches
- Hyperalertness
- Hypervigilance
- Memory impairment
- Sleep disturbance
- Startle reaction
- Tremors or tics

Psychological
- Anger
- Constricted affect
- Diminished interest
- Feelings of detachment or estrangement
- High anxiety
- Illusions
- Intrusive thoughts of events that happened to others
- Nightmares
- Numbing of responsiveness to environment
- Process-behavioral addiction (such as compulsive gambling, spending, or working)
- Recurrent dreams of traumatic events
- Recurrent thoughts of own traumatic events
- Significant irritability
- Social withdrawal
- Substance abuse or dependence
- Sudden acting out or feeling as though traumatic event is recurring
- Survivor guilt

Respiratory
- Hyperventilation
- Increased respiratory rate

NURSING DIAGNOSIS

Posttrauma response related to the subjective experience of single or multiple traumatic events through repeated exposure to trauma victims (vicarious traumatization)

Nursing priorities

Assess the effect of secondary trauma on the health care professional and evaluate the degree of perceived threat and minimize its impact.

Patient outcome criteria

As treatment progresses, the health care professional will be able to:
- verbalize a reduction in feelings of anxiety or fear when intrusive thoughts emerge
- demonstrate the ability to manage emotional reactions effectively
- use individual clinical supervision to manage countertransference issues and to obtain support
- participate in group clinical supervision with peers
- identify feelings and effective methods to cope with them
- participate in decisions to seek psychotherapy
- express a sense of control and mastery over the present situation and its outcome.

Interventions

1. Assess for physical symptoms of vicarious traumatization, such as headaches, fatigue, palpitations, nausea, and abdominal distress.

2. Identify any psychological and behavioral responses, such as emotional lability, crying, mood swings, and feelings of inadequacy or incompleteness.

3. Determine the degree of disorganization in thinking and coping.

Rationales

1. These symptoms must be identified and differentiated from symptoms of other problems so that appropriate treatment can be initiated.

2. Emotional responses to vicarious traumatization can vary; however, they must be acknowledged and managed in an adaptive manner to prevent ineffective coping behaviors.

3. The degree of disorganization determines the necessary level of intervention.

NURSING DIAGNOSIS

Powerlessness related to inadequate problem-solving and coping skills and overwhelming anxiety

Nursing priority

Help the health care professional to regain a sense of control over feelings and behaviors.

Patient outcome criteria

As treatment progresses, the health care professional should be able to:
• use individual clinical supervision to manage countertransference issues and to obtain support
• participate in group clinical supervision with peers
• identify feelings and effective methods to cope with them
• participate in decisions to seek psychotherapy
• express a sense of control and mastery over the present situation and its outcome.

Interventions

1. Determine the health care professional's previous coping abilities and level of mastery.

2. Explore cultural or religious beliefs that support helpless behavior.

3. Collaborate with the health care professional to establish an effective plan of care that includes realistic and achievable goals.

4. Help the health care professional identify feelings of powerlessness and the factors that contribute to such feelings.

5. Instruct the health care professional about strategies to combat stress and escalating anxiety. Provide opportunities for practice and feedback.

Rationales

1. Reminding the health care professional of previous success enhances self-confidence, acknowledges options, and promotes self-control.

2. Exploring these beliefs lets the health care professional acknowledge their ability to instill shame and guilt.

3. Active involvement in treatment can enhance the health care professional's sense of control and mastery over a stressful situation.

4. Awareness of these feelings and their causes can promote positive coping.

5. Strategies for managing stress and anxiety, such as using deep-breathing exercises, suspending thought, using refocusing techniques, and seeking counsel from a trusted colleague or friend, provide alternative coping skills and increase the ability to manage feelings.

6. Encourage the health care professional to participate in individual and group clinical supervision.

6. Individual clinical supervision provides the health care professional an ongoing opportunity to deal with secondary trauma within a safe relationship. Group clinical supervision allows the health care professional to learn and share with peers who have also experienced secondary trauma and its consequences.

Nursing diagnosis

Sleep pattern disturbance related to recurrent nightmares or dreams of personal death and fear of their recurrence

Nursing priority

Promote sleep by reducing the incidence of intrusive thoughts and dreams.

Patient outcome criteria

As treatment progresses, the health care professional should be able to:
• identify and use safe, effective measures to promote sleep.

Interventions

1. Determine the health care professional's normal and current sleep patterns. Ask the client to describe any changes.

2. Assess usual sleep routines.

3. Instruct the health care professional in effective sleep hygiene measures.

4. Help the health care professional arrange a restful sleep environment that is neither too warm nor too bright. Suggest using a night-light or having a light switch next to the bed.

5. Suggest that the health care professional develop an individualized relaxation program or refer the client to an appropriate program. Encourage practice of the techniques learned.

Rationales

1. Subjective and objective information provides baseline assessment of the sleep disturbance and focuses interventions.

2. Sedatives can interfere with the ability to fall asleep and disrupt normal sleep cycles, reducing refreshment from sleep.

3. Changing behaviors to promote sleep can help decrease anxiety about sleeplessness. Effective sleep hygiene measures may include retiring and rising at the same times, avoiding naps and time spent awake in bed (such as reading in bed), eliminating caffeine and alcohol intake before bedtime and, if unable to fall asleep in 15 minutes, performing a quiet activity outside the bedroom.

4. A comfortable environment promotes sleep. A readily available source of light helps promote orientation should the client awaken suddenly from a nightmare.

5. Relation techniques, such as self-hypnosis, visualization and imagery, or progressive muscle relaxation, can produce mental and physical relaxation, thus promoting sleep and providing a means of control over nightmares.

Selected references

Diagnostic and Statistical Manual of Mental Disorders, 4th ed. Washington, D.C.: American Psychiatric Association, 1994.

Dyregrov, A. "The Process of Psychological Debriefings," *Journal of Traumatic Stress Studies* 10(4):589-605, 1997.

Hatlendorf, J., and Tollerud, T. "Domestic Violence: Counseling Strategies that Minimize the Impact of Secondary Victimization," *Perspectives in Psychiatric Care* 33:14, 1997.

Nader, K. *Trauma and Dreams.* Cambridge, Mass.: Harvard University Press, 1996.

Saakvitne, K.W., and Pearlman, L.A. *Transforming the Pain: A Workbook on Vicarious Traumatization.* New York: W.W. Norton & Co., 1996.

Stahlmiller, C.M. *Rescuers of Cypress: Learning from Disaster.* Vol. 2 of International Healthcare Ethics Series. New York: Peter Lang, 1996.

Ursano, B.C., et al., eds. *Individual and Community Responses to Trauma and Disaster: The Structure of Human Chaos.* Cambridge: Cambridge University Press, 1996.

Part 14

Assessment tools

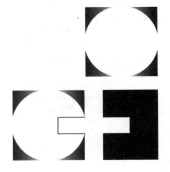

Assessment of extrapyramidal effects

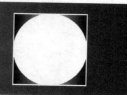

Regular evaluation for extrapyramidal effects is extremely important to the care of a client receiving psychotropic medications. However, maintaining consistency in assessment from one health care professional to another can be difficult. An assessment tool can reduce variation between examiners as well as reduce the influence of subjective observation. Two such tools are presented here: the Simpson Neurologic Rating Scale (SNRS) and the Abnormal Involuntary Movement Scale (AIMS).

The SNRS examines 10 distinct areas of neuromuscular function, assessing the degree of rigidity, resistance, tremor, salivation, and general restlessness. The AIMS helps identify movements that result from specific psychotropic medications; it examines facial and oral movements, extremity movements, trunk movements, and global judgments. The AIMS can be especially helpful in assessing a client's response to medication given to reduce extrapyramidal effects.

Simpson Neurologic Rating Scale (SNRS)

Conduct the examination in a room where the subject can walk a sufficient distance to get into a natural rhythm (at least 15 paces).

Examine each side of the body; if one side shows more pronounced pathology than the other, record more severe pathology.

Cogwheel rigidity may be palpated when the examination is carried out for items 3, 4, 5, and 6. It is not rated separately and is merely another way to detect rigidity. Cogwheel rigidity requires a minimum score of 2.

1. Gait: The subject is examined walking into the examining room—gait, swing of the arms, and general posture form the basis for an overall score for this item.
1 = Normal
2 = Mild diminution in swing while the subject is walking
3 = Obvious diminution in swing suggesting shoulder rigidity
4 = Stiff gait with little or no armswing noticeable
5 = Rigid gait with arms slightly pronated or stooped, shuffling gait with propulsion and repropulsion
9 = Not ratable

2. Arm dropping: The subject and the examiner both raise their arms to shoulder height and let them fall to their sides. In a normal subject, a stout slap is heard as the arms hit the sides. In the subject with extreme Parkinson's syndrome, the arms fall very slowly.
1 = Normal, free fall with loud slap and rebound
2 = Fall slowed slightly with less audible contact and little rebound
3 = Fall slowed, no rebound
4 = Marked slowing, no slap at all
5 = Arms fall as though against resistance or as though through glue
9 = Not ratable

3. Shoulder shaking: The subject's arms are bent at a right angle at the elbow and are taken one at a time by the examiner, who grasps one hand and also clasps the other around the subject's elbow. The subject's upper arm is pushed to and fro and the humerus is externally rotated. The degree of resistance from normal to extreme rigidity is scored as detailed. The procedure is repeated with one hand palpating the shoulder cuff while rotation takes place.
1 = Normal
2 = Slight stiffness and resistance
3 = Moderate stiffness and resistance
4 = Marked rigidity with difficulty in passive movement
5 = Extreme stiffness and rigidity with almost a frozen joint
9 = Not ratable

4. Elbow rigidity: The elbow joints are bent separately at right angles and passively extended and flexed, with the subject's biceps observed and simultaneously palpated. The resistance to this procedure is rated.
1 = Normal
2 = Slight stiffness and resistance
3 = Moderate stiffness and resistance
4 = Marked rigidity with difficulty in passive movement
5 = Extreme stiffness and rigidity with almost a frozen joint
9 = Not ratable

5. Wrist rigidity: The wrist is held in one hand and the fingers held by the examiner's other hand, with the wrist moved to extension, flexion, and ulnar and radial deviation; or the extended wrist is allowed to fall under its own weight; or the arm can be grasped above the wrist and shaken to and fro. A score of 1 would be a hand that extends easily, falls loosely, or flaps easily upward and downward.
1 = Normal
2 = Slight stiffness and resistance
3 = Moderate stiffness and resistance
4 = Marked rigidity with difficulty in passive movement
5 = Extreme stiffness and rigidity with almost a frozen wrist
9 = Not ratable

6. Head rotation: The subject sits or stands and is told that the examiner is going to move the subject's head from side to side, that it will not hurt, and to relax. (Questions about pain in the cervical area or difficulty in moving the head should be obtained to avoid causing any pain.) Clasp the subject's head between the two hands with the fingers on the back of the neck. Gently rotate the head in a circular motion three times and evaluate the muscular resistance to this movement.
1 = Loose, no resistance
2 = Slight resistance to movement although the time to rotate may be normal
3 = Resistance is apparent and the time of rotation is shortened
4 = Resistance is obvious and rotation is slowed
5 = Head appears stiff and rotation is difficult to carry out
9 = Not ratable

7. Glabellar tap: Subject is told to open eyes wide and not to blink. The glabellar region is tapped at a steady, rapid speed. Note the number of times the subject blinks in succession. Take care to stand behind the subject so that the movement of the tapping finger is not observable. A full blink need not be observed; there may be contraction of the infraorbital muscle producing a twitch each time a stimulus is delivered. Vary the speed of tapping to ensure that muscle contraction is related to the tap.
1 = 0 to 5 blinks
2 = 6 to 10 blinks
3 = 11 to 15 blinks
4 = 16 to 20 blinks
5 = 21 or more blinks
9 = Not ratable

8. Tremor: Subject is observed walking into examination room and then is reexamined for this item with arms extended at right angles to the body and the fingers spread out as far as possible.
1 = Normal
2 = Mild finger tremor, obvious to sight and touch
3 = Tremor of hand or arm occurring spasmodically
4 = Persistent tremor of one or more limbs
5 = Whole body tremor
9 = Not ratable

9. Salivation: The subject is observed while talking and then asked to open the mouth and elevate the tongue.
1 = Normal
2 = Excess salivation so that pooling takes place if mouth is open and tongue raised
3 = Excess salivation is present and might occasionally result in difficulty in speaking
4 = Speaking with difficulty because of excess salivation
5 = Frank drooling
9 = Not ratable

10. Akathisia: The subject is observed for restlessness. If restlessness is noted, ask, "Do you feel restless or jittery inside? Is it difficult to sit still?" A response is not necessary for scoring, but the subject's report can help make the assessment.
1 = No restlessness reported or observed
2 = Mild restlessness observed, such as occasional jiggling of the foot when the subject is seated
3 = Moderate restlessness observed; for example, jiggles foot, crosses and uncrosses legs, or twists a body part on several occasions
4 = Restlessness is observed frequently; for example, the foot or legs move most of the time
5 = Restlessness persistently observed; for example, subject cannot sit still, may get up and walk
9 = Not ratable

Assement tools

Abnormal Involuntary Movement Scale (AIMS)

Instructions: Complete examination procedure.
Movement Ratings: Rate highest severity observed. Rate movements that occur upon activation 1 point less than those observed spontaneously.
0 = None
1 = Minimal, may be extreme normal
2 = Mild
3 = Moderate
4 = Severe

Examination procedure

Either before or after completing the examination procedure, observe the client unobtrusively at rest such as in the waiting room. The chair used in this examination should be a hard, firm one without arms.

1. Ask the client to remove shoes and socks.
2. Ask the client to remove any gum or candy from the mouth.
3. Ask about the current condition of the client's teeth. Ask if the client wears dentures and if the teeth or dentures currently bother the client.
4. Ask whether the client notices any movements in the mouth, face, hands, or feet. If yes, ask for a description and to what extent they currently bother the client or interfere with activities.

5. Have the client sit in the chair with hands on knees, legs slightly apart, and feet flat on the floor. Look at the entire body for movements while in this position.
6. Ask the client to sit with hands hanging unsupported between the legs or, if the client is wearing a dress, hanging over the knees. Observe the hands and other body areas.
7. Ask the client to open the mouth. Observe the tongue at rest within the mouth. Do this twice.
8. Ask the client to protrude the tongue. Observe abnormalities of tongue movement.
9. Ask the client to tap the thumb with each finger as rapidly as possible for 10 to 15 seconds, first with the right hand, then with left hand. Observe facial and leg movements.
10. Flex and extend the client's left and right arms, one at a time. Note any rigidity.
11. Ask the client to stand up. Observe in profile. Observe all body areas again, including the hips.
12. Ask the client to extend both arms outstretched in front with palms down. Observe the trunk, legs, and mouth.
13. Have the client walk a few paces, turn, and walk back to the chair. Observe the hands and gait. Do this twice.

	(Circle One)
Facial and oral movements	
1. Muscles of facial expression (such as movements of forehead, eyebrows, periorbital area, and cheeks; include frowning, blinking, smiling, and grimacing)	0 1 2 3 4
2. Lips and perioral area (such as puckering, pouting, and smacking)	0 1 2 3 4
3. Jaw (such as biting, clenching, chewing, mouth opening, and lateral movement)	0 1 2 3 4
4. Tongue (rate only increase in movement both in and out of mouth, *not* inability to sustain movement)	0 1 2 3 4
Extremity movements	
5. Upper: arms, wrists, hand, fingers (include choreic movements, such as rapid, objectively purposeless, irregular, or spontaneous; and athetoid movements, such as slow, irregular, complex, or serpentine)	0 1 2 3 4
6. Lower: legs, knees, ankles, toes (such as lateral knee movement, foot tapping, heel dropping, foot squirming, or inversion and eversion of foot)	0 1 2 3 4
Trunk movements	
7. Neck, shoulders, and hips (such as rocking, twisting, squirming, or pelvic gyrations)	0 1 2 3 4
Global judgments	
8. Severity of abnormal movements	0 None, normal
	1 Minimal
	2 Mild
	3 Moderate
	4 Severe

9. Incapacitation resulting from abnormal movements

0 None, normal
1 Minimal
2 Mild
3 Moderate
4 Severe

10. Client's awareness of abnormal movements (rate only client's report)

0 No awareness
1 Aware, no distress
2 Aware, mild distress
3 Aware, moderate distress
4 Aware, severe distress

Dental status

11. Current problems with teeth or dentures

1 No
2 Yes

12. Does the client usually wear dentures?

1 No
2 Yes

Barry Psychosocial Assessment Interview

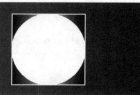

This comprehensive assessment tool uses Gordon's functional health patterns to facilitate the data-gathering process and to promote the identification of corresponding nursing diagnoses.

The assessment categories include the following patterns:
- Health perception–health management
- Nutritional-metabolic
- Elimination
- Activity-exercise
- Sleep-rest
- Cognitive-perceptual
- Self-perception–self-concept
- Role-relationship
- Sexuality-reproductive
- Coping–stress tolerance
- Value-belief

These categories help the nurse focus on specific aspects of the assessment and identify problem areas. Problem areas are then clarified through a focused assessment.

Assess all boxed questions subjectively, rather than asking the client directly. Bold italic statements advise the nurse how to proceed.

Name _____ Age _____ Date of admission _____

Marital status S _____ M _____ W _____ D _____ How long? _____

Occupation _____ Years of education completed _____

Date of assessment _____ Admitting diagnosis _____

Health perception–health management

What was the original problem that caused you to come to the hospital? _____

On what date did you first become ill? _____

What caused this illness? _____

How do you feel about being in a hospital? _____

How can the physicians and nurses help you most? _____

How will this illness affect you when you are out of the hospital? _____

Do you think it will cause any changes in your life? _____

How will it affect your family? _____

Potential for noncompliance? Yes ____ No ____ Possible ____

Related to:

____ Anxiety
____ Negative side effects of treatment

____ Unsatisfactory relationship with caregiving environment or caregivers
____ Other

Explain:

Potential for injury? Yes ____ No ____ Possible ____

Explain:

Nutritional-metabolic

How does your current appetite compare with your normal appetite?

Same _____ Increased _____ Decreased _____

How long has it been different? _____

Has your weight fluctuated by more than 5 lb in the last several weeks?_____

Yes _____ No _____ How many pounds? _____

What is your normal fluid intake per day? ml* _____ Your current intake? ml _____

*Nurse can substitute estimate of milliliters for client's reported fluid intake.

Aspects of client's illness or condition that could contribute to organic mental disorder? No _____ Yes_____

Delirium type _____ Dementia type_____

Possible cause:
_____ Metabolic
_____ Electrolytes
_____ Other metabolic or endocrine condition
_____ Arterial disease
_____ Mechanical disease

_____ Electrical disorder
_____ Infectious disease
_____ Neoplastic disease
_____ Nutritional disease
_____ Degenerative (chronic) brain disease
_____ Drug toxicity

Elimination

What is your current pattern of bowel movements?

Constipated _____ Diarrhea _____ Incontinent _____

How does this compare to normal? _____

Same _____ Different _____

Explain:

What is your current pattern of urination? _____

How does this compare to normal?

Same _____ Different _____

Explain:

Possibility that emotional distress may be contributing to any change?

High _____ Moderate _____ Low _____

Activity-exercise

What is your normal energy level?

High _____ Moderate _____ Low _____

Has it changed in the past 6 months? Yes _____ No _____

To what do you attribute the cause? _____

How would you describe your normal activity level? _____

High _____ Moderate _____ Low _____

How may it change following this hospitalization? _____

What types of activities do you normally pursue outside the home? _____

What recreational activities do you enjoy? _____

Do you anticipate your ability to manage your home will be changed following your hospitalization? _____

Explain:

Current self-care deficits?

Feeding _____ Bathing _____ Dressing _____ Toileting _____

Anticipated deficits following hospitalization? _____

Current impairment in mobility? _____

Anticipated immobility following hospitalization? _____

Alterations in the following?

Airway clearance   How? _____

Breathing patterns How? _____

Cardiac output   How? _____

Respiratory function How? _____

Potential for altered tissue perfusion as manifested by altered cognitive-perceptual patterns? _____

Sleep-rest

Normal sleeping pattern

How many hours do you normally sleep per night?   From what hour to what hour? _____ to _____

Changes in normal sleeping pattern

Do you have difficulty falling asleep? _____

Do you awaken in the middle of night? _____

Do you awaken early in the morning? _____

Are you sleeping more or fewer hours than normal? _____ How many? _____

Cognitive-perceptual

Are you feeling pain now? _____ How severe? _____ How often? _____ What relieves the pain? _____

What information does this client need to know to manage this illness or health state? _____

Ability to comprehend this information?

Good _____ Moderate _____ Poor _____

If poor, explain:

Mental status examination

Level of awareness and orientation _____

Appearance and behavior _____

Speech and communication _____

Affect (mood) _____

Thinking process _____

Related to: Inability to evaluate reality _____ Aging _____ Other _____

Explain:

If there is a distortion of the thought process, a focused assessment is indicated.

Perception _____

Abstract thinking _____

Social judgment _____

Memory _____

Impairment in short-term memory _____ Long-term memory _____

Is there evidence of unilateral neglect? Yes _____ No _____ Does not apply _____

Self-perception

Does the client describe feelings of anxiety or uneasiness? _____

Is he able to identify a cause? Yes_____ No_____

Cause? _____

If the client feels anxious but cannot identify a cause, assess for the major coping risks of physical illness below.

Assessment tools

Is there anything you are frightened of during this hospitalization or illness?

Yes _____ No _____ What is it? _____

How will this illness affect your future plans? _____

Normally, do you believe that you control what happens to you (internal locus of control) or do you believe that other people or events control what happens to you (external locus of control)?

Internal locus of control _____ External locus of control _____

Will this illness affect the way you feel about yourself? _____

How? _____ About your body _____

Psychosocial risks of illness

What are the major issues of this illness for this client? _____

For this family? _____

Use the following space to record client and family comments illustrating how they are coping with these issues.

Trust   Client _____

                Family _____

Self-esteem   Client _____

                Family _____

Body image   Client _____

                Family _____

Control   Client _____

                Family _____

Loss   Client _____

                Family _____

Guilt   Client _____

Intimacy   Family _____

Could one or more of these issues be contributing to feelings of anxiety, hopelessness, powerlessness, or disturbance in self-concept?

Yes _____ No _____ Possible _____

If so, explain which ones and proceed with a focused assessment.

Role-relationship

What is your occupation? _____

How many years have you been in this occupation?_____

Do you anticipate that this illness will have an effect on your ability to work? Yes _____No _____How _____

With whom do you live?_____ Are they supportive? _____

Who are the most important people in your life? _____

Do you ever feel socially isolated? Yes _____ No _____

Explain:

> Is there any indication in this history of social isolation or impaired social interaction? Yes _____ No _____
>
> Explain:
>
> Ability to communicate
>
> Within normal limits _____ Impaired _____
>
> Describe:

Family history

Who are the members of your immediate family? What are their ages and how are they related to you? Please include deceased members and when they died.

Name of family member _____ Relationship to you _____ Age _____ Date of death _____

_____   _____   _____   _____

_____   _____   _____   _____

_____   _____   _____   _____

_____   _____   _____   _____

What is your position in relation to your brothers and sisters? For example, are you the second oldest, the youngest?_____

How often do you see your immediate family members? _____

What goes on in your family when something bad happens?_____

What do most of the members do? _____

Have any of your relationships within your immediate and extended family changed recently?_____

Which ones? _____

How have they changed?_____

Is there any change in the way you parent your children? Yes _____ No_____

If so, to what do you attribute the cause?

_____ New baby

_____ Death of other family member

_____ Illness in other family member

_____ Change in residence (describe reason for change)

_____ Other (describe)

What is your normal role within your family?_____

What role do the significant other people in your family play?_____

Potential for disruption of these roles by this illness? High _____ Moderate _____ Low _____

Explain:

While the client is describing the family, is there any indication of uncontrolled anger or rage? Yes _____ No _____

Related to a specific issue or person?_____

Explain:

Open (trusting) or closed (untrusting) communication style in family? (Can be initially determined by statements and

emotional expression of client.) _____

Developmental stage of family

_____ Early married

_____ Married with no children

_____ Active childbearing

_____ Preschool or school age children

_____ Adolescent children and children leaving home

_____ Middle-aged children no longer at home

_____ Elderly, well-functioning

_____ Elderly, infirm

Is there any other aspect of your family or the way your family normally operates that you think should be added here? What is it?

If any item discussed in this section appears to be a current stressor for this client or family, it can be assessed using a focused approach with the other items under coping-stress tolerance pattern.

Interpersonal style

_____ Dependent

_____ Controlled

_____ Dramatizing

_____ Suspicious

_____ Self-sacrificing

_____ Superior

_____ Uninvolved

_____ Mixed (usually two styles predominate)

_____ No predominant personality style

Write a brief sentence explaining your choice. _____

Response to you as the interviewer: Guarded? _____ Open? _____

Is the client able to maintain good eye contact? _____

Sexuality-reproductive

Have you experienced any recent change in your sexual functioning? Yes _____ No _____

How? _____ For how long? _____

Do you associate your change in sexual functioning with some event in your life? _____

Do you think this illness could change your normal pattern of sexual functioning? _____

How? _____

Is this change in sexuality patterns related to:

____ Ineffective coping

____ Change or loss of body part

____ Prenatal or postpartum changes

____ Changes in neurovegetative functioning related to depression

Explain:

Use focus assessment if necessary.

Assessment tools

Coping–stress tolerance

Level of stress during year before admission

How long have you been out of work with this illness? _____

Have you experienced any recent change in your job? _____

Have you been under any unusual job stress during the past year? _____

What was the cause?

_____ Retirement   _____ Same job, but new boss or working relationship

_____ Fired   _____ Promotion or demotion

Other. Explain:

Do you expect the stress will be present when you return to work? _____

The preceding questions should be adapted for students to a school situation.

Have there been changes in your family during the last 2 years?

Which family members are involved? Include dates.

Death _____

Was this someone you were close to? _____

Divorce _____

Child leaving home _____

Cause? _____

Other _____

Has there been any other unusual stress during the last year that is still affecting you?

Describe:

Any unusual stress in your family?

Describe:

Normal coping ability

When you go through a very difficult time, how do you handle it?

_____ Talk it out with someone	_____ Become depressed
_____ Drink	_____ Get angry and yell
_____ Ignore it	_____ Get angry and clam up
_____ Become anxious	_____ Get angry and hit or throw something
_____ Withdraw from others	_____ Other (explain)

How often do you experience feelings of depression? _____

In the past, what is the longest period of time this feeling has lasted? _____

Have you felt depressed during the past few weeks? Yes _____ No _____

To what do you attribute the cause? _____

If rape trauma is the cause of this admission, do not explore the psychological reaction with the client until reading the report of the rape crisis counselor, who should have met with the client within 1 hour of arrival at the emergency department. Either follow the recommendations on the report for ongoing assessment or proceed with gentle questioning about current feelings.

What is the most serious trauma you have experienced? _____

What was the most difficult time you have experienced in your life? _____

How long did it take you to get over it? _____

What did you do to cope with it? _____

Potential for self-harm

This part of the assessment should be included if moderate to severe depression is present.

Have you ever thought of committing suicide? Yes _____ No _____

If yes, continue on.

What would you do to end your life? No plan _____ Plan _____

Describe:

What would prevent you from committing suicide? _____

Substances that may be used as stress relievers

Smoking history

Do you smoke? _____ How long have you been smoking? _____ How many packs per day? _____

Alcohol use history

Do you drink? _____ How often? _____ How much? _____

Is there a history of alcoholism in your family? _____ Who?_____

Drug use

What prescribed medications are you currently using?

Name of medications _____

Dose or schedule _____ Prescribing physician _____

Are you currently using any other drugs? Yes _____ No _____

What are they? _____

How long have you been using them? _____

What is the usual amount? _____ How often _____

Have you ever been treated for substance abuse? _____

Value-belief

What is your religious affiliation? _____

Do you consider yourself active or inactive in practicing your religion? Active _____ Inactive _____

Is your religious leader a supportive person? Yes _____ No _____

Explain:

What does this illness mean to you? _____

Are you experiencing spiritual distress? Yes _____ No _____

Explain:

What would you consider to be the primary cause of this spiritual distress (actual, possible, or potential)?

_____ Inability to practice spiritual rituals   _____ Crisis of illness, suffering, or death

_____ Conflict between religious, spiritual, or cultural beliefs   _____ Other (explain)
and prescribed health regimen

Do you expect there will be any disparity in your caregivers' approach that could present a problem to you?_____

Any problems in the areas of:

_____ Spiritual rituals   _____ Communication

_____ Cause of illness   _____ Problem solving

_____ Perception of illness and sick role   _____ Nutrition

_____ Health maintenance   _____ Family response

Explain:

How has this illness affected your relationship with God or the supreme being of your religion?

Explain:

The 11 functional health patterns were named by Marjorie Gordon in *Nursing Diagnosis: Process and Application,* New York: McGraw-Hill Book Co., 1987.

Adapted with permission from Barry, P.D. *Psychosocial Nursing: Assessment and Intervention,* 3rd ed. Philadelphia: Lippincott-Raven Pubs. 1996.

Modified Overt Aggression Scale

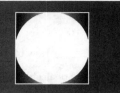

The Modified Overt Aggression Scale (MOAS) is a psychometric tool for determining the severity of aggression. The MOAS can be used to describe the nature and prevalence of aggression in an inpatient psychiatric population. The MOAS assesses four categories of aggression: verbal aggression, aggression against property, autoaggression, and physical aggression.

Scoring is based on a 5-point rating system that represents increasing levels of severity. Each section has a weighted score that reflects the overall severity of aggression (the higher the score, the more severe the aggression). The total score is determined by multiplying the four individual scales by their specific weights and then adding the four weighted scores.

Client's name _____ Sex _____ Date _____

Rater _____ Unit _____ Shift _____ Hospital No. _____

Period of observation _____

Directions: For each category of aggressive behavior, check the highest applicable rating point to describe the most serious act of aggression committed by the client during the specified observation period.

Verbal aggression
Verbal hostility, such as statements or invectives that seek to inflict psychological harm on another through devaluation or degradation, and threats of physical attack.
0 = No verbal aggression
1 = Shouts angrily, curses mildly, or makes personal insults
2 = Curses viciously, is severely insulting, has temper outbursts
3 = Impulsively threatens violence toward others or self
4 = Threatens violence toward others or self repeatedly or deliberately (such as to gain money or sex)

Autoaggression
Physical injury toward oneself, such as self-mutilation or suicide attempt.
0 = No autoaggression
1 = Picks or scratches skin, pulls out hair, hits self (without injury)
2 = Bangs head, hits fists into walls, throws self on floor
3 = Inflicts minor cuts, bruises, burns, or welts on self
4 = Inflicts major injury on self or makes a suicide attempt

Aggression against property
Wanton and reckless destruction of unit paraphernalia or others' possessions.
0 = No aggression against property
1 = Slams door angrily, rips clothing, urinates on floor
2 = Throws objects down, kicks furniture, defaces walls
3 = Breaks objects, smashes windows
4 = Sets fires, throws objects dangerously

Physical aggression
Violent action intended to inflict pain, bodily harm, or death upon another.
0 = No physical aggression
1 = Makes menacing gestures, swings at people, grabs at clothing
2 = Strikes, kicks, pushes, scratches, pulls hair of others (without injury)
3 = Attacks others, causing mild injury (such as bruises, sprains, or welts)
4 = Attacks others, causing serious injury (such as fracture, loss of teeth, deep cuts, or loss of consciousness)

Rating summary

Scale	Scaled score		Weighted score
Verbal aggression	_____	× 1 =	_____
Aggression against property	_____	× 2 =	_____
Autoaggression	_____	× 3 =	_____
Physical aggression	_____	× 4 =	_____
			_____ Total weighted score

Adapted with permission from Kay, S.R., et al. "Profiles of Aggression among Psychiatric Patients," *Journal of Nervous and Mental Disease* 176(9):539-46, 1988.

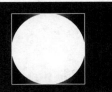

Overt Agitation Severity Scale

Intensity score	Behavior	Not present	Rarely	Some of the time	Most of the time	Always present	Severity score
A.	**Vocalizations and oral/facial movements**						
1 ×	Whimpering, whining, moaning, grunting, crying	0	1	2	3	4	=____
2 ×	Smacking or licking of lips, chewing, clenching jaw, licking, grimacing, spitting	0	1	2	3	4	=____
3 ×	Rocking, twisting, banging of head	0	1	2	3	4	=____
4 ×	Vocal perseverating, screaming, cursing, threatening, wailing	0	1	2	3	4	=____
B.	**Upper torso and upper extremity movements**						
1 ×	Tapping fingers, fidgeting, wringing of hands, swinging or flailing arms	0	1	2	3	4	=____
2 ×	Task perseverating (e.g., opening and closing drawers, folding and unfolding clothes, picking at objects, clothes, or self)	0	1	2	3	4	=____
3 ×	Rocking (back and forth), bobbing (up and down), twisting or writhing of torso; rubbing self or masturbating	0	1	2	3	4	=____
4 ×	Slapping, swatting, hitting at objects or others	0	1	2	3	4	=____
C.	**Lower extremity movements**						
1 ×	Tapping or clenching toes; tapping heel; extending, flexing, or twisting foot	0	1	2	3	4	=____
2 ×	Shaking legs, tapping knees and/or thighs, thrusting pelvis	0	1	2	3	4	=____
3 ×	Pacing, wandering	0	1	2	3	4	=____
4 ×	Thrashing legs, kicking at objects or others	0	1	2	3	4	=____

Total OASS =____
Subtract baseline OASS =____
Revised OASS =____

Instructions for completing form

Step one: For each behavior, circle the corresponding frequency.
Step two: For every behavior <u>exhibited</u>, multiply the intensity score by the frequency and record as the Severity Score.
Step three: For the Overt Agitation Severity Score (OASS), total all severity scores and record as Total OASS.
Step four: Does this patient have a neuromuscular disorder (i.e., Parkinson's disease, tardive dyskinesia) affecting Total OASS?
☐ Yes   ☐ No
If yes, please establish baseline OASS in nonagitated state and subtract from above Total OASS for Revised OASS.

Comments:
Name of patient: _____

Sex of patient: Male (1) Female (2)

Diagnosis: _____

Age: _____ Race: _____

Name of rater: _____

Time of observation: from ____ am/pm to ____ am/pm

Date: __ __ __ __ __ __
　　　M　M　D　D　Y　Y

Case ID: _____

Adapted with permission from Yudofsky, S.C. The American Psychiatric Press Textbook of Psychopharmacology. Washington, D.C. American Psychiatric Press, 1994.

Suicide risk assessment

The following assessment tool was developed by the Los Angeles Suicide Prevention Center to help identify clients at risk for suicide. Scores are given in each of several categories, then totaled and averaged based on the number of categories rated. An average score of 1 or 2 indicates that the client is at low risk for suicide; a score of 3 to 6, at medium risk; and a score of 7, 8, or 9, at high risk.

Name _____ Age _____ Sex _____ Date _____

Rater _____ Evaluation _____

	Low	Medium	High
	1 2	3 4 5 6	7 8 9

Suicide potential

Age and sex _____   Resources _____   Total _____

Symptoms _____   Prior suicidal behavior _____

Stress _____   Medical status _____   Number of categories related _____

Acute versus chronic _____   Communication aspects _____

Suicidal plan _____   Reaction of significant other _____   Average _____

Rating for category

Age and sex (1-9) _____
Male
Age 50 plus (7-9) _____
Ages 35-49 (4-6) _____
Ages 15-34 (1-3) _____
Female
Age 50 plus (5-7) _____
Ages 35-49 (3-5) _____
Ages 15-34 (1-3) _____

Symptoms (1-9) _____
Severe depression: sleep disorder, anorexia, weight loss, withdrawal, despondent, loss of interest, apathy (7-9) _____
Feelings of hopelessness, helplessness, exhaustion (7-9) _____
Delusions, hallucination, loss of contact, disorientation (6-8) _____
Compulsive gambler (6-8) _____
Disorganization, confusion, chaos (5-7) _____
Alcoholism, drug addiction, homosexuality (4-7) _____
Agitation, tension, anxiety (4-6) _____
Guilt, shame, embarrassment (4-6) _____
Feelings of rage, anger, hostility, revenge (4-6) _____
Poor impulse control, poor judgment (4-6) _____
Frustrated dependency (4-6) _____
Other (describe):

Rating for category

Stress (1-9) _____
Loss of loved person by death, divorce, separation (5-9) _____
Loss of job, money, prestige, status (4-8) _____
Sickness, serious illness, surgery, accident, loss of limb (3-7) _____
Threat of prosecution, criminal involvement, exposure (4-6) _____
Changes in life, environment, setting (4-6) _____
Success, promotion, increased responsibilities (2-5) _____
No significant stress (1-3) _____
Other (describe):

Acute versus chronic (1-9) _____
Sharp, noticeable, and sudden onset of specific symptoms (1-9) _____
Recurrent outbreak of similar symptoms (4-9) _____
Recent increase in long-standing traits (4-7) _____
No specific recent change (1-4) _____
Other (describe):

Suicidal plan (1-9)
Lethality of proposed method: gun, jump, hanging, drowning, knife, poison, pills, aspirin (1-9) _____
Availability of means in proposed method (1-9) _____

	Rating for category		Rating for category

Suicidal plan (1-9)   *(continued)*
Specific detail and clarity in organization of plan (1-9)   _____
Specificity in time planned (1-9)   _____
Bizarre plans (4-6)   _____
Rating of previous suicide attempts(s) (1-9)   _____
No plans (1-3)   _____
Other (describe):

Resources (1-9)   _____
No sources of support (family, friends, agencies, employment) (7-9)   _____
Family and friends available, unwilling to help (4-7)   _____
Financial problem (4-7)   _____
Available professional help, agency, or therapist (2-4)   _____
Family or friends willing to help (1-3)   _____
Stable life history (1-3)   _____
Physician or clergy available (1-3)   _____
Employed (1-3)   _____
Finances no problem (1-3)   _____
Other (describe):

Prior suicidal behavior (1-7)   _____
One or more prior attempts of high lethality (6-7)   _____
One or more prior attempts of low lethality (4-5)   _____
History of repeated threats and depression (3-5)   _____
No prior suicidal or depressed history (1-3)   _____
Other (describe):

Medical status (1-7)   _____
Chronic debilitating illness (5-7)   _____
Pattern of failure in previous therapy (4-6)   _____
Many repeated unsuccessful experiences with doctors (4-6)   _____
Psychosomatic illness (such as asthma, ulcer) (2-4)   _____
Chronic minor illness complaints, hypochondria (1-3)   _____
No medical problems (1-2)   _____
Other (describe):

Communication aspects (1-7)   _____
Communication broken with rejection of efforts to reestablish by both client and others (5-7)   _____
Communications have internalized goal (such as to cause guilt in others or to force behavior) (2-4)   _____

Communications directed toward world and people in general (3-5)   _____
Communications directed toward one or more specific persons (1-3)   _____
Other (describe):

Reaction of significant other (1-7)   _____
Defensive, paranoid, rejected, punishing attitude (5-7)   _____
Denial of own or client's need for help (5-7)   _____
No feelings of concern about the client; does not understand the client (4-6)   _____
Indecisiveness, feelings of helplessness (3-5)   _____
Alternation between feelings of anger and rejection and feelings of responsibility and desire to help (2-4)   _____
Sympathy and concern plus admission of need for help (1-3)   _____
Other (describe):

Adapted with permission from Los Angeles Suicide Prevention Center. *Assessment of Suicidal Potentiality.* Los Angeles: The Center, 1980.

Assessment tools

Alcohol withdrawal assessment

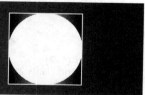

Clinical Institute Withdrawal Assessment — Alcohol (revised) [CIWA-Ar Scale]

Temperature _____ Pulse _____ Blood alcohol level (BAL) _____

Blood Pressure _____ Respirations _____

Nausea and vomiting
0 None
1 Mild nausea with no vomiting
4 Intermittent
7 Nausea, dry heaves, vomiting

Tremor (arms extended, fingers spread)
0 No tremor
1 Not visible—an be felt fingertip to fingertip
4 Moderate with arms extended
7 Severe even with arms not extended

Sweating (observation)
0 No sweat visible
1 Barely perceptible, palms sweats
4 Beads of sweat visible
7 Drenching sweats

Tactile disturbances
0 None
1 Very mild itching, pins and needles or numbness
2 Mild itching or pins and needles, burning or numbness
3 Moderate itching, pins and needles, burning or numbness
4 Moderately severe hallucinations
5 Severe hallucinations
6 Extremely severe hallucinations
7 Continuous hallucinations

Visual disturbances (ask)
Does the light appear to be too bright? Is its color different? Does it hurt your eyes? Are you seeing anything that is disturbing to you. Are you seeing things you know are not there?
0 Not present
1 Very mild sensitivity
2 Mild sensitivity
3 Moderate sensitivity
4 Moderately severe hallucinations (intermittently fused)
5 Severe hallucinations
6 Extremely severe hallucinations
7 Continuous hallucinations

Auditory disturbances (ask)
Are you more aware of sounds around you? Are they harsh? Do they frighten you? Are you hearing anything that is disturbing to you? Are you hearing things you know are not there?
0 Not present
1 Very mild harshness or ability to frighten
2 Mild harshness or ability to frighten
3 Moderate harshness or ability to frighten
4 Moderately severe hallucinations (occasionally fused)
5 Severe hallucinations
6 Extremely severe hallucinations
7 Continuous hallucinations

Orientation and clouding of sensorium (ask)
What day is this? What is this place?
0 Oriented and can do serial additions
1 Cannot do serial additions or is uncertain about dates
2 Disoriented for date by no more that 2 calendar days
3 Disoriented for date by more than 2 calendar days
4 Disoriented for place or person
Reorient to time, place, and person if necessary

Anxiety (observation; ask)
Do you feel nervous?
0 No anxiety, at ease
1 Mildly anxious
4 Moderately anxious or guarded (anxiety inferred)
7 Equivalent to panic states as seen in severe delirium, acute schizophrenic reactions

Agitation (observation)
0 Normal activity
1 Somewhat more than normal activity
4 Moderately fidgety and restless
7 Pacing, or thrashing about constantly

Headache, fullness in head (ask)
Does your head feel different? Does it feel like a band around your head? (Do not rate for dizziness or light-headedness. Otherwise, rate severity.)
0 Not present
1 Very mild
2 Mild
3 Moderate
4 Moderately severe
5 Severe
6 Very severe
7 Extremely severe

Total score _____
Maximum possible score: 67

SCORING:
0 to<8 No evidence of active withdrawal symptoms. Continue to monitor with regular vital signs.
8 to <15 Stage 1: Early stage of withdrawal: monitor with increased frequency. Begin medication.
15 to <20 Stage 2: Moderate signs of withdrawal. Monitor with CIWA-Ar hourly and medicate until score is <8 for 3 hours.
20 State 3: Severe withdrawal. At risk for developing delirium tremens or seizures. Increase monitoring and medications every 30 minutes until CIWA-Ar score is <8 for 2 hours.

NAME_____

DATE _____

Last drink - Date _____ Time _____ Day # _____

CIWA-Ar assessment tool adapted with permission from Sullivan, J.T., et al. "Assessment of Alcohol Withdrawal: The Revised Clinical Institute Withdrawal Assessment for Alcohol Scale (CIWA-Ar)," *British Journal of Addiction* 84:1353-57, 1989.

Scoring and monitoring recommendations adapted with permission from Krupnick, S.W., et al. "Alcohol Withdrawal Syndrome: An Evidence-Based Clinical Assessment and Intervention Practice Protocol," Springfield, Mass.: Baystate Healthcare System, 1998.

Assessment of opiate withdrawal symptoms

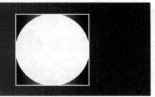

Assessment of opiate withdrawal syndrome symptoms is important in the care of the individual who is experiencing opiate withdrawal. Assessment tools that use objective and subjective measures to quantify the symptoms can provide guidance in the treatment of acute withdrawal. The Subjective Opiate Withdrawal Scale (SOWS) and the Objective Opiate Withdrawal Scale (OOWS) represent two tools that can be used together to provide the clinician with quantified assessment of the client's withdrawal.

Subjective Opiate Withdrawal Scale (SOWS)

Instructions: Answer the following statements as accurately as you can. Circle the answer that best fits the way you feel now.

1 = Not at all
2 = A little
3 = Moderately
4 = Quite a bit
5 = Extremely

1. I feel anxious.	1 2 3 4 5	9. I have cold flashes.	1 2 3 4 5
2. I feel like yawning.	1 2 3 4 5	10. My bones and muscles ache.	1 2 3 4 5
3. I am perspiring.	1 2 3 4 5	11. I feel restless.	1 2 3 4 5
4. My eyes are tearing.	1 2 3 4 5	12. I feel nauseous.	1 2 3 4 5
5. My nose is running.	1 2 3 4 5	13. I feel like vomiting	1 2 3 4 5
6. I have gooseflesh.	1 2 3 4 5	14. My muscles twitch.	1 2 3 4 5
7. I am shaking.	1 2 3 4 5	15. I have cramps in my stomach.	1 2 3 4 5
8. I have hot flashes.	1 2 3 4 5	16. I feel like shooting up now.	1 2 3 4 5

Total SOWS score: _____

Objective Opiate Withdrawal Scale (OOWS)

Instructions: Rate the patient on the basis of what you observe during a timed 10-minute period.

Item score Points
1 point for each item if:

1. Yawning **present** _____
2. Rhinorrhea **3 or more** _____
3. Piloerection (observe client's arm or chest) **present** ____
4. Perspiration **present** _____
5. Lacrimation **present** _____
6. Mydriasis **present** _____
7. Tremors **present**_____
8. Hot and cold flashes (shivering or huddling **present** __for warmth)
9. Restlessness (frequent shifts of position) **present**_____
10. Vomiting **present**_____

11. Muscle twitches **present**_____
12. Abdominal cramps (holding stomach) **present** _____
13. Anxiety (observable manifestations: **present** _____
finger tapping, fidgeting, agitation)

Total OOWS score: _____
(Sum of items 1-13)

SOWS and OOWS adapted with permission from Rounsaville, B. *Diagnostic Source Book on Drug Abuse Research and Treatment*. NIH Publication No. 93-3508. Rockville, Md.: National Institutes of Health, 1993.

Benzodiazepine withdrawal assessment

Clinical Institute Withdrawal Assessment — Benzodiazepine (CIWA-B)

For each of the following items, circle the number that best describes the severity of each sign or symptom.

1. Observe behavior for restlessness and agitation.
   - 0 None, normal activity
   - 1
   - 2 Restless
   - 3
   - 4 Paces back and forth, unable to sit still

2. Ask patient to extend arms with fingers apart; observe for tremor.
   - 0 No tremor
   - 1 Not visible; can be felt in fingers
   - 2 Visible but mild
   - 3 Moderate with arms extended
   - 4 Severe, with arms not extended

3. Observe for sweating; feel palms.
   - 0 No sweating visible
   - 1 Rare perceptible sweating; palms moist
   - 2 Palms and forehead moist; reports armpit sweating
   - 3 Beads of sweat on forehead
   - 4 Severe drenching sweats

For each of the following items, please circle the number which best describes how you feel.

	Scale		**Scale**
4. Do you feel irritable?	0 1 2 3 4 5	14. Do you feel upset?	0 1 2 3 4 5 (not at all) (very much so)
5. Do you feel fatigued?	0 1 2 3 4 5	15. How restful was your sleep last night?	0 1 2 3 4 5 (very restful) (not at all)
6. Do you feel tense?	0 1 2 3 4 5		
7. Do you have difficulty concentrating?	0 1 2 3 4 5 (no difficulty) (unable to concentrate)	16. Do you feel weak?	0 1 2 3 4 5 (not at all) (very much so)
8. Do you have any loss of appetite?	0 1 2 3 4 5 (no loss) (no appetite)	17. Do you think you had enough sleep last night?	0 1 2 3 4 5 (yes, very much so) (not at all)
9. Have you any numbness or burning sensation on your face hands or feet?	0 1 2 3 4 5 (no numbness) (intense burning or numbness)	18. Do you have any visual disturbances? (light sensitivity or blurred vision)	0 1 2 3 4 5 (not at all) (very sensitive, blurred vision)
10. Do you feel your heart racing? (palpitations)	0 1 2 3 4 5 (no disturbance) (constant racing)	19. Are you fearful?	0 1 2 3 4 5 (not at all) (very much so)
11. Does your head feel full or achy?	0 1 2 3 4 5 (not at all) (severe headache)	20. Have you been worrying about possible misfortunes lately?	0 1 2 3 4 5 (not at all) (very much so)
12. Do you feel muscle aches or stiffness?	0 1 2 3 4 5 (not at all) (severe stiffness or pain)	21. How many hours of sleep do you think you had last night?	0 1 2 3 4 5
13. Do you feel anxious, nervous or jittery?	0 1 2 3 4 5 (not at all) (very much so)	22. How many minutes do you think it took you to fall asleep last night?	0 1 2 3 4 5

Total score: _____
Sum of items 1-22 and add together:

Adapted with permission from Busto, U.E., et al. "A Clinical Scale to Assess Benzodiazepine Withdrawal," *Journal of Clinical Psychopharmacology* 9(4):412-16, 1989.

Culturally specific care in psychiatric nursing

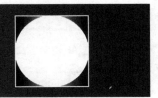

Cultural and ethnic assessment

Culture is the totality of learned, socially transmitted beliefs, values, and behaviors that are derived from members' interpersonal transactions. All cultural groups have established sets of values, beliefs, and patterns of behavior. Conceptions of what it means to be mentally ill are vastly different from one group to another, and these notions may clash with those of the psychiatric–mental health professional. In some cultures, people view mental illness as a condition that requires either punishment or exclusion from the group; however, other cultures are more tolerant of mental illness and believe that family and community members are crucial to their care, treatment, and recovery.

For treatment to be effective, caregivers need to understand and try to change the client's, and even the community's, attitudes, beliefs, and values. For these things to occur, the client's cultural and social background must be thoughtfully incorporated into the collaborative plan of care. It is important to conduct at least a brief cultural assessment of the client as he enters your treatment, no matter what the type of facility. Although this requires some additional effort, it will save time and effort later on by helping to avoid misunderstandings that may lead to failed interventions. Some cultural assessment questions include the following:
• What is the client's ethnic background and does the client identify with that ethnic group?
• What specific attitudes, beliefs, and values regarding health, illness, and health care will influence or impact on this health care situation (for example, praying, coining, bedside chanting rituals, specific dietary customs)?
• How does the client define the family within his cultural and ethnic background? Who in the family serves as the spokesperson or decision maker? Who must be included in all health care decisions?
• How does the client explain the illness? Is it due to "bad nerves," "possession by spirits," "somatic complaints," or possibly "inexplicable misfortune" or "God's decision?"
• What language(s) does the client speak and which (if more than one) is the client most comfortable speaking and hearing?
• Are there any cultural taboos (prohibitions) that we need to know about to make this hospitalization less stressful or uncomfortable?

• Explore cultural factors related to the client's social environment and support network: social stressors; accessibility and availability of social support network; current functional capacity level; any type of disability present, and how that disability is perceived within his culture; the role of religion within his culture and for him; stressors in the client's social environment; and family, residence, and community.

Culture-bound syndrome and ethnic pharmacology

In psychiatric–mental health nursing, a few critical issues are being raised and researched, including the need to maintain diagnostic objectivity in cross-cultural health care situations and identifying and understanding culture-bound syndromes. We must bear in mind that illness and disease occur within cultural and social structures. The types of mental illness seen within a given culture reflect the way that individuals within that culture express anxiety, depression, fear, and grief. Specific syndromes that appear to express certain cultural ideologies and that are not shared across cultures are termed *culture-bound syndromes*. (See *Overview of culture-bound syndrome*, pages 300 and 301.)

A newly emerging specialty, ethnic pharmacology, investigates the variant responses to pharmaceuticals manifested by clients of different ethnic groups. This field is important for psychiatric nurses because the medications they are using may be effective for some clients but detrimental, and even life-threatening, for others due to their differing genetic heritage. Two examples will illuminate this point: Hispanics tend to experience adverse effects of tricyclic antidepressants at about one-half the dosage that would cause the same problem in eastern Europeans. (Most drug trials are conducted on European-American men). Clients of Ashkenazic Jewish descent who take the neuroleptic agent clozapine (Clozaril) for schizophrenia are much more likely to experience agranulocytosis (20%) as an adverse effect than clients from among the general population (1%).

(*Text continues on page 302.*)

Overview of culture-bound syndromes

Culture-bound syndromes are described below. These are syndromes that express certain cultural ideologies that are not shared across all cultures.

Disorder	Region or ethnic group	Presentation
Amok	Laos, Malaysia, Philippines, Papua New Guinea, Polynesia, Puerto Rico, Navajo	• Brooding followed by outbursts of violent, aggressive, or homicidal behavior directed at people and objects • Accompanied by persecutory ideas, automation, amnesia, and exhaustion
Ataque de nervios	Caribbean, Latin American, Latin Mediterranean	• Uncontrollable shouting, attacks of crying, trembling, heat in chest rising into head, verbal or physical aggression • Sometimes dissociative experiences, seizure-like or fainting episodes, and suicidal gestures
Bilis and Colera (referred to as muina)	Latino	• Anger or rage as underlying emotion • Acute nervous tension, headache, trembling, screaming, stomach disturbances • Loss of consciousness (in severe cases) • Chronic fatigue (from acute episode)
Bouefée delirante	Haiti, West Africa	• Sudden outburst of agitated or aggressive behavior, marked confusion, and psychomotor excitement, possibly accompanied by visual or auditory hallucinations or paranoia • Can resemble an episode of brief psychotic disorder
Dhat	India, Sri Lanka, China	• Severe anxiety and hypochondriacal concerns associated with the discharge of semen, whitish discoloration of the urine, feelings of weakness and exhaustion
Falling out or black-out	Caribbean, Southern United States	• Sudden collapse, with or without warning • Inability to see, despite eyes being open • Ability to hear and understand what is occurring, but person feels powerless to move
Ghost or ghost sickness	Native American tribes	• Preoccupation with death and the deceased • Bad dreams, weakness, fear, anxiety, hallucinations, feelings of danger, loss of consciousness, confusion, loss of appetite, dizziness, fainting, and a sense of suffocation
Hwa-byung (anger syndrome)	Korea	• Suppression of anger • Insomnia, fatigue, panic, fear of impending death, dysphoric affect, indigestion, anorexia, dyspnea, palpitations, generalized aches and pains, feeling of epigastric mass
Koro: skukyong and suoyang, jinjinia bemar, rok-joo	Malaysia, South Asia, East Asia, China, Assam, Thailand	• Episode of sudden and intense anxiety that one's penis (males) or vulva or nipples (females) will recede into the body and cause death
Latah	Indonesia, Japan, Malaysia, Philippines, Siberia, Thailand	• Hypersensitivity to sudden fright, with echopraxia, echolalia, command obedience, and dissociative or trancelike behavior
Locura	Latinos (American), Latin America	• Severe form of chronic psychosis • Incoherence, agitation, auditory or visual hallucinations, inability to follow rules of social interaction, agitation, possible violence
Mal de ojo (Evil eye)	Mediterranean cultures	• Infants and children at risk • Fitful sleep, crying without apparent cause, diarrhea, vomiting, fever
Nervios	Latinos (American), Latin America	• Emotional distress, somatic disturbances, inability to function • Headaches, irritability, sleep disturbances, nervousness, easy tearfulness, inability to concentrate, trembling, tingling sensations • Awakened in a terrified state, unable to move, with a sensation of weight on chest

Overview of culture-bound syndromes *(continued)*

Disorder	Region or ethnic group	Presentation
Pibloktoq	Inuit (Arctic and Subarctic)	• Dissociative episode accompanied by extreme excitement followed by convulsive seizures and coma • Tendency during attack to tear off clothes, break furniture, shout obscenities, eat feces, flee from protective environment
Qi-gong psychotic reaction	China	• Acute, time-limited episode characterized by dissociative, paranoid, or other psychotic or nonpsychotic symptoms that can occur after participating in the Chinese health-enhancing practice of qi-gong
Rootwork	Southern United States, African American, European American, Caribbean Cultures, Latino cultures (puesto or brujeria)	• Generalized anxiety, GI complaints (nausea, vomiting, diarrhea), weakness, fear of being poisoned or of being killed (voodoo death) • Belief that spells or hexes can be put on another person
Sangue dormido (sleeping blood)	Portuguese Cape Verde Islanders	• Pain, numbness, tremor, paralysis, convulsions, stroke, blindness, heart attack, infection, miscarriage • GI problems, sexual dysfunction, irritability, and disturbances of autonomic nervous system
Shejing shuairuo (Neurasthenia)	China	• Diagnosis is included in the *Chinese Classification of Mental Disorders,* 2nd ed. (CCMD-2) • Physical and mental fatigue, dizziness, headaches, pain, concentration difficulties, sleep disturbances, and memory loss
Shen-k'vei	Taiwan, China	• Symptoms attributed to excessive semen loss from frequent intercourse, masturbation, nocturnal emission, or passing white turbid urine. Excessive semen loss is feared because it represents loss of one's vital essence and can be a threat to life. • Dizziness, headache, fatigability, general weakness, insomnia, frequent dreams, sexual dysfunction
Shin-byung	Korean	• Anxiety, somatic complaints including weakness, dizziness, fear, anorexia, insomnia, GI problems, with associated dissociation, and possession by ancestral spirits
Spell	African Americans, European Americans (in Southern United States)	• Trance state in which individuals communicate with deceased relatives or with spirits
Susto (fright or soul loss)	Latino (American), Mexico, Central America, South America	• Illness attributed to a frightening event that causes the soul to leave the body, resulting in unhappiness and sickness. It is believed that in extreme cases *susto* may result in death. • Symptoms include appetite disturbances, inadequate or excessive sleep, dreams, sadness, feelings of low self-worth or dirtiness.
Taijin kyofusho	Japan	• Intense fear that one or more body parts or body functions displease, embarrass, or offend other people related to appearance, odor, facial expressions, or movements • Distinctive phobia resembling social phobia in *DSM-IV* and included in the Japanese Diagnostic System for Mental Disorders
Windigo psychosis	Native Americans	• Severe depression in which the fears of cannibalism color the depressive delusions
Zar	Egypt, Ethiopia, Iran, Middle Eastern countries, North Africa, Somalia, Sudan	• Dissociative episodes that may include shouting, laughing, hitting the head against a wall, singing, and weeping • Apathy, withdrawal, refusal to eat or participate in activities of daily living

Assessment tools

SELECTED REFERENCES

Axelson, J., and McGrath, P. *Counseling and Development of a Multicultural Society.* Belmont, Calif.: Wadsworth Publishing Co., 1998.

Cultural Competence Standards in Managed Mental Health Care for Four Underserved/Underrepresented Racial/Ethnic Groups. Bethesda, Md.: Center for Mental Health Services, 1997.

McGoldrick, M., et al. *Ethnicity and Family Therapy,* 2nd ed. New York: Guilford Press, 1996.

Mezzich, J.E., et al. *Culture and Psychiatric Diagnosis: A DSM-IV Perspective.* Washington, D.C.: American Psychiatric Association, 1996.

Ruiz, P. "Issues in the Psychiatric Care of Hispanics," *Psychiatric Services* 48:539, 1997.

Sharts-Hopko, N. "Health and Illness Concepts for Cultural Competence with Japanese Clients," *Journal of Cultural Diversity* 3(3):74-9, 1996.

Appendices
and index

Appendix A: *DSM IV* classification: Multiaxial system

Axis I Clinical disorders
Other conditions that may be a focus of clinical attention
Axis II Personality disorders
Mental retardation
Axis III General medical conditions
Axis IV Psychosocial and environmental problems
Axis V Global assessment of functioning

NOS = Not otherwise specified

Disorders usually first diagnosed in infancy, childhood, or adolescence

Mental retardation
Note: These are coded on Axis II.
317   Mild mental retardation
318.0   Moderate mental retardation
318.1   Severe mental retardation
318.2   Profound mental retardation
319   Mental retardation, severity unspecified

Learning disorders
315.00   Reading disorder
315.1   Mathematics disorder
315.2   Disorder of written expression
315.9   Learning disorder NOS

Motor skills disorder
315.4   Developmental coordination disorder

Communication disorders
315.31   Expressive language disorder
315.31   Mixed receptive-expressive language disorder
315.39   Phonological disorder
307.0   Stuttering
307.9   Communication disorder NOS

Pervasive developmental disorders
299.00   Autistic disorder
299.80   Rett's disorder
299.10   Childhood disintegrative disorder
299.80   Asperger's disorder
299.80   Pervasive developmental disorder NOS

Attention-deficit and disruptive behavior disorders
314.xx   Attention-deficit/hyperactivity disorder
314.01   Combined type
314.00   Predominantly inattentive type
314.01   Predominantly hyperactive-impulsive type
314.9   Attention-deficit/hyperactivity disorder NOS
312.8   Conduct disorder
Specify type: Childhood-onset or adolescent-onset

313.81   Oppositional defiant disorder
312.9   Disruptive behavior disorder NOS

Feeding and eating disorders of infancy or early childhood
307.52   Pica
307.53   Rumination disorder
307.59   Feeding disorder of infancy or early childhood

Tic disorders
307.23   Tourette's disorder
307.22   Chronic motor or vocal tic disorder
307.21   Transient tic disorder
       Specify if: Single episode or recurrent
307.20   Tic disorder NOS

Elimination disorders
___.__   Encopresis
787.6   With constipation and overflow incontinence
307.7   Without constipation and overflow incontinence
307.6   Enuresis (not due to a general medical condition)
       Specify type: Nocturnal only, diurnal only, or nocturnal and diurnal

Other disorders of infancy, childhood, or adolescence
309.21   Separation anxiety disorder
       Specify if: Early onset
313.23   Selective mutism
313.89   Reactive attachment disorder of infancy or early childhood
       Specify if: Inhibited type or disinhibited type
307.3   Stereotypic movement disorder
       Specify if: With self-injurious behavior
313.9   Disorder of infancy, childhood, or adolescence NOS

Delirium, dementia, and amnestic and other cognitive disorders

Delirium
293.0   Delirium due to (*indicate the general medical condition*)
___.__   Substance intoxication delirium (*refer to Substance-related disorders for substance-specific codes*)
___.__   Substance withdrawal delirium (*refer to Substance-related disorders for substance-specific codes*)
___.__   Delirium due to multiple etiologies (*code each of the specific etiologies*)
780.09   Delirium NOS

Dementia

290.xx   Dementia of the Alzheimer's type, with early onset (*also code 331.0 Alzheimer's disease on Axis III*)
290.10   Uncomplicated
290.11   With delirium
290.12   With delusions
290.13   With depressed mood
          Specify if: With behavioral disturbance
290.xx   Dementia of the Alzheimer's type, with late onset (*also code 331.0 Alzheimer's disease on Axis III*)
290.0   Uncomplicated
290.3   With delirium
290.20   With delusions
290.21   With depressed mood
          Specify if: With behavioral disturbance
290.xx   Vascular dementia
290.40   Uncomplicated
290.41   With delirium
290.42   With delusions
290.43   With depressed mood
          Specify if: With behavioral disturbance
294.9   Dementia due to HIV disease (*also code 043.1 HIV infection affecting central nervous system on Axis III*)
294.1   Dementia due to head trauma (*also code 854.00 head injury on Axis III*)
294.1   Dementia due to Parkinson's disease (*also code 332.0 Parkinson's disease on Axis III*)
294.1   Dementia due to Huntington's disease (*also code 333.4 Huntington's disease on Axis III*)
290.10   Dementia due to Pick's disease (*also code 331.1 Pick's disease on Axis III*)
290.10   Dementia due to Creutzfeldt-Jakob disease (*also code 046.1 Creutzfeldt-Jakob disease on Axis III*)
294.1   Dementia due to (*indicate the general medical condition not listed above and code general medical condition on Axis III*)
____.__   Substance-induced persisting dementia (*refer to Substance-related disorders for substance-specific codes*)
____.__   Dementia due to multiple etiologies (*code each of the specific etiologies*)
294.8   Dementia NOS

Amnestic disorders

294.0   Amnestic disorder due to (*indicate the general medical condition*)
          Specify if: Transient or chronic
____.__   Substance induced persisting amnestic disorder (*refer to Substance-related disorders for substance-specific codes*)
294.8   Amnestic disorder NOS

Other cognitive disorders

294.9   Cognitive disorder NOS

Mental disorders due to a general medical condition not elsewhere classified

239.89   Catatonic disorder due to (*indicate the general medical condition*)
310.1   Personality change due to (*indicate the general medical condition*)
          Specify type: Labile, disinhibited, aggressive, apathetic, paranoid, other, combined, unspecified
293.9   Mental disorder NOS due to (*indicate the general medical condition*)

Substance-related disorders

[a]*The following specifiers may be applied to substance dependence:* With physiological dependence or without physiological dependence; early full remission, early partial remission, sustained full remission,or sustained partial remission; and on agonist therapy or in a controlled environment.

The following specifiers may be applied to substance-induced disorders as noted: [I]With onset during intoxication or [W]with onset during withdrawal.

Alcohol-related disorders

Alcohol use disorders
303.90   Alcohol dependence[a]
305.00   Alcohol abuse

Alcohol-induced disorders
303.00   Alcohol intoxication
291.8   Alcohol withdrawal
          Specify if: With perceptual disturbances
291.0   Alcohol intoxication delirium
291.0   Alcohol withdrawal delirium
291.2   Alcohol-induced persisting dementia
291.1   Alcohol-induced persisting amnestic disorder
291.x   Alcohol-induced psychotic disorder
291.5   With delusions[I,W]
291.3   With hallucinations[I,W]
291.8   Alcohol-induced mood disorder[I,W]
291.8   Alcohol-induced anxiety disorder[I,W]
291.8   Alcohol-induced sexual dysfunction I
291.8   Alcohol-induced sleep disorder[I,W]
291.9   Alcohol-related disorder NOS

Amphetamine (or amphetamine-like) related disorders

Amphetamine use disorders
304.40   Amphetamine dependence[a]
305.70   Amphetamine abuse

Amphetamine-induced disorders
292.89   Amphetamine intoxication
          Specify if: With perceptual disturbances
292.0   Amphetamine withdrawal
292.81   Amphetamine intoxication delirium

292.xx   Amphetamine-induced psychotic disorder
292.11   With delusions[I]
292.12   With hallucinations[I]
292.84   Amphetamine-induced mood disorder[I,W]
292.89   Amphetamine-induced anxiety disorder[I]
292.89   Amphetamine-induced sexual dysfunction[I]
292.89   Amphetamine-induced sleep disorder[I,W]
292.9   Amphetamine-related disorder NOS

Caffeine-related disorders

Caffeine-induced disorders
305.90   Caffeine intoxication
292.89   Caffeine-induced anxiety disorder[I]
292.89   Caffeine-induced sleep disorder[I]
292.9   Caffeine-related disorder NOS

Cannabis-related disorders

Cannabis use disorders
304.30   Cannabis dependence[a]
305.20   Cannabis abuse

Cannabis-induced disorders
292.89   Cannabis intoxication
         Specify if: With perceptual disturbances
292.81   Cannabis intoxication delirium
292.xx   Cannabis-induced psychotic disorder
292.11   With delusions[I]
292.12   With hallucinations[I]
292.89   Cannabis-induced anxiety disorder[I]
292.9   Cannabis-related disorder NOS

Cocaine-related disorders

Cocaine use disorders
304.20   Cocaine dependence[a]
305.60   Cocaine abuse

Cocaine-induced disorders
292.89   Cocaine intoxication
         Specify if: With perceptual disturbances
292.0   Cocaine withdrawal
292.81   Cocaine intoxication delirium
292.xx   Cocaine-induced psychotic disorder
292.11   With delusions[I]
292.12   With hallucinations[I]
292.84   Cocaine-induced mood disorder[I,W]
292.89   Cocaine-induced anxiety disorder[I,W]
292.89   Cocaine-induced sexual dysfunction I
292.89   Cocaine-induced sleep disorder[I,W]
292.9   Cocaine-related disorder NOS

Hallucinogen-related disorders

Hallucinogen use disorders
304.50   Hallucinogen dependence[a]
305.30   Hallucinogen abuse

Hallucinogen-induced disorders
292.89   Hallucinogen intoxication
292.89   Hallucinogen persisting perception
         disorder (flashbacks)
292.81   Hallucinogen intoxication delirium
292.xx   Hallucinogen-induced psychotic disorder
292.11   With delusions[I]

292.12   With hallucinations[I]
292.84   Hallucinogen-induced mood disorder[I]
292.89   Hallucinogen-induced anxiety disorder[I]
292.9   Hallucinogen-related disorder NOS

Inhalant-related disorders

Inhalant use disorders
304.60   Inhalant dependence[a]
305.90   Inhalant abuse

Inhalant-induced disorders
292.89   Inhalant intoxication
292.81   Inhalant intoxication delirium
292.82   Inhalant-induced persisting dementia
292.xx   Inhalant-induced psychotic disorder
292.11   With delusions[I]
292.12   With hallucinations[I]
292.84   Inhalant-induced mood disorder[I]
292.89   Inhalant-induced anxiety disorder[I]
292.9   Inhalant-related disorder NOS

Nicotine-related disorders

Nicotine use disorder
305.10   Nicotine dependence[a]

Nicotine-induced disorder
292.0   Nicotine withdrawal
292.9   Nicotine-related disorder NOS

Opioid-related disorders

Opioid use disorders
304.00   Opioid dependence[a]
305.50   Opioid abuse

Opioid-induced disorders
292.89   Opioid intoxication
         Specify if: With perceptual disturbances
292.0   Opioid withdrawal
292.81   Opioid intoxication delirium
292.xx   Opioid-induced psychotic disorder
292.11   With delusions[I]
292.12   With hallucinations[I]
292.84   Opioid-induced mood disorder[I]
292.89   Opioid-induced sexual dysfunction[I]
292.89   Opioid-induced sleep disorder[I,W]
292.9   Opioid-related disorder NOS

Phencyclidine (or phencyclidine-like) related disorders

Phencyclidine use disorders
304.90   Phencyclidine dependence[a]
305.90   Phencyclidine abuse

Phencyclidine-induced disorders
292.89   Phencyclidine intoxication
         Specify if: With perceptual disturbances
292.81   Phencyclidine intoxication delirium
292.xx   Phencyclidine-induced psychotic disorder
292.11   With delusions[I]
292.12   With hallucinations[I]
292.84   Phencyclidine-induced mood disorder[I]
292.89   Phencyclidine-induced anxiety disorder[I]
292.9   Phencyclidine-related disorder NOS

Sedative-, hypnotic-, or anxiolytic-related disorders

Sedative, hypnotic, or anxiolytic use disorders
304.10　Sedative, hypnotic, or anxiolytic dependence[a]
305.40　Sedative, hypnotic, or anxiolytic abuse

Sedative-, hypnotic-, or anxiolytic-induced disorders
292.89　Sedative, hypnotic, or anxiolytic intoxication
292.0　　Sedative, hypnotic, or anxiolytic withdrawal
　　　　Specify if: With perceptual disturbances
292.81　Sedative, hypnotic, or anxiolytic intoxication delirium
292.81　Sedative, hypnotic, or anxiolytic withdrawal delirium
292.82　Sedative-, hypnotic-, or anxiolytic-induced persisting dementia
292.83　Sedative-, hypnotic-, or anxiolytic-induced persisting amnestic disorder
292.xx　Sedative-, hypnotic-, or anxiolytic-induced psychotic disorder
292.11　　With delusions [1,W]
292.12　　With hallucinations[1,W]
292.84　Sedative-, hypnotic-, or anxiolytic-induced mood disorder[1,W]
292.89　Sedative-, hypnotic-, or anxiolytic-induced anxiety disorder[W]
292.89　Sedative-, hypnotic-, or anxiolytic-induced sexual dysfunction[1]
292.89　Sedative-, hypnotic-, or anxiolytic-induced sleep disorder[1,W]
292.9　　Sedative-, hypnotic-, or anxiolytic-related disorder NOS

Polysubstance-related disorder
304.80　Polysubstance dependence[a]

Other (or unknown) substance-related disorders

Other (or unknown) substance use disorders
304.90　Other (or unknown) substance dependence[a]
305.90　Other (or unknown) substance abuse

Other (or unknown) substance-induced disorders
292.89　Other (or unknown) substance intoxication
　　　　Specify if: With perceptual disturbances
292.0　　Other (or unknown) substance withdrawal
　　　　Specify if: With perceptual disturbances
292.81　Other (or unknown) substance-induced delirum
292.82　Other (or unknown) substance-induced persisting dementia
292.83　Other (or unknown) substance-induced persisting amnestic disorder
292.xx　Other (or unknown) substance-induced psychotic disorder
292.11　　With delusions[1,W]
292.12　　With hallucinations[1,W]
292.84　Other (or unknown) substance-induced mood disorder[1,W]
292.89　Other (or unknown) substance-induced anxiety disorder[1,W]

292.89　Other (or unknown) substance-induced sexual dysfunction[1]
292.89　Other (or unknown) substance-induced sleep disorder[1,W]
292.9　　Other (or unknown) substance-related disorder NOS

Schizophrenia and other psychotic disorders
295.xx　Schizophrenia
The following Classification of Longitudinal Course applies to all subtypes of schizophrenia: Episodic with interepisode residual symptoms (*specify if:* With prominent negative symptoms) or episodic with no interepisode residual symptoms (*specify if:* With prominent negative symptoms); single episode in partial remission (*specify if:* With prominent negative symptoms) or single episode in full remission; and other or unspecified pattern.
295.30　　Paranoid type
295.10　　Disorganized type
295.20　　Catatonic type
295.90　　Undifferentiated type
295.60　　Residual type
295.40　Schizophreniform disorder
　　　　Specify if: Without good prognostic features or with good prognostic features
295.70　Schizoaffective disorder
　　　　Specify if: Bipolar type or depressive type
297.1　　Delusional disorder
　　　　Specify type: erotomanic, grandiose, jealous, persecutory, somatic, mixed, or unspecified
298.8　　Brief psychotic disorder
　　　　Specify if: With marked stressor(s), without marked stressor(s), or with postpartum onset
297.3　　Shared psychotic disorder
293.xx　Psychotic disorder due to (*indicate the general medical condition*)
293.81　　With delusions
293.82　　With hallucinations
——.——　Substance-induced psychotic disorder (*refer to Substance-related disorders for substance-specific codes*)
　　　　Specify if: With onset during intoxication or with onset during withdrawal
298.9　　Psychotic disorder NOS

Mood disorders
Code current state of major depressive disorder or bipolar I disorder in fifth digit:
　　　　1 = Mild
　　　　2 = Moderate
　　　　3 = Severe without psychotic features
　　　　4 = Severe with psychotic features
　　　　　Specify: Mood-congruent psychotic features or mood-incongruent psychotic features
The following specifiers apply (for current or most recent episode) to mood disorders as noted: [a]Severity, psychotic,

Appendices

or remission specifiers; [b]chronic; [c]with catatonic features; [d]with melancholic features; [e]with atypical features; [f]with postpartum onset.

The following specifiers apply to mood disorders as noted: [g]with or without full interepisode recovery, [h]with seasonal pattern, or [i]with rapid cycling.

Depressive disorders
296.xx   Major depressive episode
296.2x   Single episode[a,b,c,d,e,f]
296.3x   Recurrent[a,b,c,d,e,f,g,h]
300.4   Dysthymic disorder
         Specify if: Early or late onset
         Specify: With atypical features
311   Depressive disorder NOS

Bipolar disorders
296.xx   Bipolar I disorder
296.0x   Single manic episode[a,c,f]
         Specify if: Mixed
296.40   Most recent episode hypomanic[g,h,i]
296.4x   Most recent episode manic[a,c,f,g,h,i]
296.6x   Most recent episode mixed[a,c,f,g,h,i]
296.5x   Most recent episode depressed[a,b,c,d,e,f,g,h,i]
296.7   Most recent episode unspecified[g,h,i]
296.89   Bipolar II disorder[a,b,c,d,e,f,g,h,i]
         Specify (current or most recent episode):
         Hypomanic or depressed
301.13   Cyclothymic disorder
296.80   Bipolar disorder NOS
293.83   Mood disorder due to (*indicate the general medical condition*)
         Specify if: With depressive features, with major depressive-like episode, with manic features, or with mixed features
___.___ Substance-induced mood disorder (*refer to Substance-related disorders for substance-specific codes*)
         Specify type: With depressive features, with manic features, or with mixed features.
         Specify if: With onset during intoxication or with onset during withdrawal
296.90   Mood disorder NOS

Anxiety disorders
300.01   Panic disorder without agoraphobia
300.21   Panic disorder with agoraphobia
300.22   Agoraphobia without history of panic disorder
300.29   Specific phobia
         Specify type: Animal, natural environment, blood-injection-injury, situational, or other
300.23   Social phobia
         Specify if: Generalized
300.3   Obsessive compulsive disorder
         Specify if: With poor insight
309.81   Posttraumatic stress disorder
         Specify if: Acute or chronic and with delayed onset
308.3   Acute stress disorder
300.02   Generalized anxiety disorder

293.89   Anxiety disorder due to (*indicate the general medical condition*)
         Specify if: With generalized anxiety, with panic attacks, or with obsessive-compulsive symptoms
___.___ Substance-induced anxiety disorder (*refer to Substance-related disorders for substance-specific codes*)
         Specify if: With generalized anxiety, with panic attacks, with obsessive-compulsive symptoms, or with phobic symptoms and with onset during intoxication or with onset during withdrawal
300.00   Anxiety disorder NOS

Somatoform disorders
300.81   Somatization disorder
300.81   Undifferentiated somatoform disorder
300.11   Conversion disorder
         Specify type: With motor symptom or deficit, with sensory symptom or deficit, with seizures or convulsions, or with mixed presentation
307.xx   Pain disorder
307.80   Associated with psychological factors
307.89   Associated with both psychological factors and a general medical condition
         Specify if: Acute or chronic
300.7   Hypochondriasis
         Specify if: With poor insight
300.7   Body dysmorphic disorder
300.81   Somatoform disorder NOS

Factitious disorders
300.xx   Factitious disorder
300.16   With predominantly psychological signs and symptoms
300.19   With predominantly physical signs and symptoms
300.19   With combined psychological and physical signs and symptoms
300.19   Factitious disorder NOS

Dissociative disorders
300.12   Dissociative amnesia
300.13   Dissociative fugue
300.14   Dissociative identity disorder
300.6   Depersonalization disorder
300.15   Dissociative disorder NOS

Sexual and gender identity disorders
Sexual dysfunctions
The following specifiers apply to all primary sexual dysfunctions: Lifelong type, acquired type, generalized type, situational type, due to psychological factors, or due to combined factors.

Sexual desire disorders
302.71   Hypoactive sexual desire disorder
302.79   Sexual aversion disorder

Sexual arousal disorders
302.72　Female sexual arousal disorder
302.72　Male erectile disorder

Orgasmic disorders
302.73　Female orgasmic disorder
302.74　Male orgasmic disorder
302.75　Premature ejaculation

Sexual pain disorders
302.76　Dyspareunia (not due to a general medical condition)
306.51　Vaginismus (not due to a general medical condition)

Sexual dysfunction due to a general medical condition
625.8　Female hypoactive sexual desire disorder due to (_indicate the general medical condition_)
608.89　Male hypoactive sexual desire disorder due to (_indicate the general medical condition_)
607.84　Male erectile disorder due to (_indicate the general medical condition_)
625.0　Female dyspareunia due to (_indicate the general medical condition_)
608.89　Male dyspareunia due to (_indicate the general medical condition_)
625.8　Other female sexual dysfunction due to (_indicate the general medical condition_)
608.89　Other male sexual dysfunction due to (_indicate the general medical condition_)
___.__　Substance-induced sexual dysfunction (_refer to Substance-related disorders for substance-specific codes_)
　　　Specify if: With impaired desire, with impaired arousal, with impaired orgasm, or with sexual pain and with onset during intoxication
302.70　Sexual dysfunction NOS

Paraphilias
302.4　Exhibitionism
302.81　Fetishism
302.89　Frotteurism
302.2　Pedophilia
　　　Specify if: Sexually attracted to males, sexually attracted to females, or sexually attracted to both; limited to incest; and exclusive type or nonexclusive type
302.83　Sexual masochism
302.84　Sexual sadism
302.3　Transvestic fetishism
　　　Specify if: With gender dysphoria
302.82　Voyeurism
302.9　Paraphilia NOS

Gender identity disorders
302.xx　Gender identity disorder
302.6　In children
302.85　In adolescents or adults
　　　Specify if: Sexually attracted to males, sexually attracted to females, sexually attracted to both, or sexually attracted to neither

302.6　Gender identity disorder NOS
302.9　Sexual disorder NOS

Eating disorders
307.1　Anorexia nervosa
　　　Specify type: Restricting or binge-eating and purging
307.51　Bulimia nervosa
　　　Specify type: Purging or nonpurging
307.50　Eating disorder NOS

Sleep disorders

Primary sleep disorders

Dyssomnias
307.42　Primary insomnia
307.44　Primary hypersomnia
　　　Specify if: Recurrent
347　Narcolepsy
780.59　Breathing related sleep disorder
307.45　Circadian rhythm sleep disorder
　　　Specify type: Delayed sleep phase, jet lag, shift work, or unspecified
307.47　Dyssomnia NOS

Parasomnias
307.47　Nightmare disorder
307.46　Sleep terror disorder
307.46　Sleepwalking disorder
307.47　Parasomnia NOS

Sleep disorders related to another mental disorder
307.42　Insomnia related to (_indicate the Axis I or Axis II disorder_)
307.44　Hypersomnia related to (_indicate the Axis I or Axis II disorder_)

Other sleep disorders
780.xx　Sleep disorders due to (_indicate the general medical condition_)
780.52　Insomnia type
780.54　Hypersomnia type
780.59　Parasomnia type
780.5　Mixed type
___.__　Substance-induced sleep disorder (_refer to Substance-related disorders for substance-specific codes_)
　　　Specify type: Insomnia, hyersomnia, parasomnia, or mixed
　　　Specify if: With onset during intoxication or with onset during withdrawal

Impulse-control disorders not elsewhere classified
312.34　Intermittent explosive disorder
312.32　Kleptomania
312.33　Pyromania
312.31　Pathological gambling
312.39　Trichotillomania
312.30　Impulse-control disorder NOS

Adjustment disorders
309.xx Adjustment disorder
309.0 With depressed mood
309.24 With anxiety
309.28 With mixed anxiety and depressed mood
309.3 With disturbance of conduct
309.4 With mixed disturbance of emotions and conduct
309.9 Unspecified
  Specify if: Acute or chronic

Personality disorders
Note: These are coded on Axis II.
301.0 Paranoid personality disorder
301.20 Schizoid personality disorder
301.22 Schizotypal personality disorder
301.7 Antisocial personality disorder
301.83 Borderline personality disorder
301.50 Histrionic personality disorder
301.81 Narcissistic personality disorder
301.82 Avoidant personality disorder
301.6 Dependent personality disorder
301.4 Obsessive-compulsive personality disorder
301.9 Personality disorder NOS

Other conditions that may be a focus of clinical attention

Psychological factors affecting medical condition
316 *(Specify psychological factor)* affecting *(indicate the general medical condition)*
  Choose name based on nature of factors:
  Mental disorder affecting medical condition
  Psychological symptoms affecting medical condition
  Personality traits or coping style affecting medical condition
  Maladaptive health behaviors affecting medical condition
  Stress-related physiological response affecting medical condition
  Other or unspecified psychological factors affecting medical condition

Medication-induced movement disorders
332.1 Neuroleptic-induced parkinsonism
333.92 Neuroleptic malignant syndrome
333.7 Neuroleptic-induced acute dystonia
333.99 Neuroleptic-induced acute akathisia
333.82 Neuroleptic-induced tardive dyskinesia
333.1 Medication-induced postural tremor
333.90 Medication-induced movement disorder NOS

Other medication-induced disorder
995.2 Adverse effects of medication NOS

Relational problems
V61.9 Relational problem related to a mental disorder or a general medical condition
V61.20 Parent-child relational problem
V61.1 Partner relational problem
V61.8 Sibling relational problem
V62.81 Relational problem NOS

Problems related to abuse or neglect
V61.21 Physical abuse of child *(code 995.5 if focus of attention is on victim)*
V61.21 Sexual abuse of child *(code 995.5 if focus of attention is on victim)*
V61.21 Neglect of child *(code 995.5 if focus of attention is on victim)*
V61.1 Physical abuse of adult *(code 995.81 if focus of attention is on victim)*
V61.1 Sexual abuse of adult *(code 995.81 if focus of attention is on victim)*

Additional conditions that may be a focus of clinical attention
V15.81 Noncompliance with treatment
V65.2 Malingering
V71.01 Adult antisocial behavior
V71.02 Child or adolescent antisocial behavior
V62.89 Borderline intellectual functioning
  Note: This is coded on Axis II.
780.9 Age-related cognitive decline
V62.82 Bereavement
V62.3 Academic problem
V62.2 Occupational problem
313.82 Identity problem
V62.89 Religious or spiritual problem
V62.4 Acculturation problem
V62.89 Phase of life problem

Additional codes
300.9 Unspecified mental disorder (nonpsychotic)
V71.09 No diagnosis or condition on Axis I
799.9 Diagnosis or condition deferred on Axis I
V71.09 No diagnosis or condition on Axis II
799.9 Diagnosis deferred on Axis II

Adapted with permission from *Diagnostic and Statistical Manual of Mental Disorders,* 4th ed. Washington, D.C.: American Psychiatric Association, 1994.

Below is a list of the North American Nursing Diagnosis Association's (NANDA) approved diagnostic categories arranged according to Gordon's functional health patterns.

Health perception–Health management pattern
- Altered health maintenance (specify)
- Altered protection (specify)
- Delayed surgical recovery
- Effective management of therapeutic regimen: Individual
- Energy field disturbance
- Health-seeking behaviors (specify)
- Ineffective management of therapeutic regimen (Individuals)
- Ineffective management of therapeutic regimen: Community
- Ineffective management of therapeutic regimen: Family
- Latex allergy
- Noncompliance (specify)
- Risk for infection
- Risk for injury
- Risk for latex allergy
- Risk for perioperative positioning injury
- Risk for poisoning
- Risk for suffocation
- Risk for trauma

Nutritional-metabolic pattern
- Adult failure to thrive
- Altered dentition
- Altered oral mucous membrane (specify alteration)
- Altered nutrition: More than body requirements (exogenous obesity)
- Altered nutrition: Risk for more than body requirements (risk for obesity)
- Altered nutrition: Less than body requirements (nutritional deficit-specify type)
- Effective breast-feeding
- Feeding self-care deficit
- Fluid volume deficit
- Fluid volume excess
- Hyperthermia
- Hypothermia
- Impaired skin integrity
- Impaired swallowing (uncompensated)
- Impaired tissue integrity
- Ineffective breast-feeding
- Interrupted breast-feeding
- Ineffective infant feeding pattern
- Ineffective thermoregulation
- Nausea
- Risk for altered body temperature
- Risk for aspiration
- Risk for fluid volume deficit
- Risk for fluid volume imbalance
- Risk for impaired skin integrity (or risk for skin breakdown)

Elimination pattern
- Altered urinary elimination
- Bowel incontinence
- Colonic constipation
- Constipation
- Diarrhea
- Functional urinary incontinence
- Perceived constipation
- Reflex urinary incontinence
- Risk for constipation
- Risk of urinary urge incontinence
- Stress incontinence
- Urge incontinence
- Toileting self-care deficit
- Total incontinence
- Urinary retention

Activity-exercise pattern
- Activity intolerance (specify level)
- Altered growth and development
- Altered tissue perfusion (specify)
- Bathing or hygiene self-care deficit (specify level)
- Decreased cardiac output
- Disorganized infant behavior
- Diversional activity deficit
- Dressing or grooming self-care deficit (specify level)
- Dysfunctional ventilatory weaning response (DVWR)
- Dysreflexia
- Fatigue
- Impaired bed mobility
- Impaired gas exchange
- Impaired home maintenance management (mild, moderate, severe, potential, chronic)
- Impaired physical mobility (specify level)
- Impaired walking
- Impaired wheelchair mobility
- Impaired wheelchair transfer ability
- Inability to sustain spontaneous ventilation
- Ineffective airway clearance
- Ineffective breathing pattern
- Potential for enhanced organized infant behavior
- Risk for activity intolerance
- Risk for autonomic dysreflexia
- Risk for disorganized infant behavior
- Risk for disuse syndrome
- Risk for peripheral neurovascular dysfunction

Sleep-rest pattern
- Sleep deprivation
- Sleep pattern disturbance

Cognitive-perceptual pattern
- Acute confusion
- Altered thought processes
- Chronic confusion
- Chronic pain (specify type and location)
- Decisional conflict (specify)
- Decreased adaptive capacity: Intracranial
- Impaired environmental interpretation syndrome
- Impaired memory
- Knowledge deficit (specify area)
- Pain
- Sensory-perceptual alteration (specify)
- Unilateral neglect

Self-perception–self-concept pattern
- Anxiety
- Body-image disturbance
- Chronic low self-esteem
- Fear (specify focus)
- Hopelessness
- Personal identity disturbance
- Powerlessness
- Risk for loneliness
- Risk for self-mutilation
- Self-esteem disturbance
- Situational low self-esteem

Role-relationship pattern
- Altered family processes
- Altered family processes: Alcoholism
- Altered growth and development (specify)
- Altered parenting (specify alteration)
- Altered role performance (specify)
- Anticipatory grieving
- Caregiver role strain
- Dysfunctional grieving
- Impaired social interaction
- Impaired verbal communication
- Parental role conflict
- Relocation stress syndrome
- Risk for altered development
- Risk for altered growth
- Risk for altered parent-infant-child attachment
- Risk for altered parenting
- Risk for caregiver role strain
- Risk for violence: Self-directed or directed at others
- Social isolation

Sexual-reproductive pattern
- Altered sexuality patterns
- Rape-trauma syndrome
- Rape-trauma syndrome: Compound reaction
- Rape-trauma syndrome: Silent reaction
- Sexual dysfunction

Coping–stress tolerance pattern
- Chronic sorrow
- Death anxiety
- Defensive coping
- Family coping: Potential for growth
- Impaired adjustment
- Ineffective community coping
- Ineffective denial
- Ineffective family coping: Compromised
- Ineffective family coping: Disabling
- Ineffective individual coping
- Post-trauma syndrome
- Potential for enhanced community coping
- Rape-trauma syndrome
- Risk for post-trauma syndrome

Value-belief pattern
- Potential for enhanced spiritual well-being
- Spiritual distress (distress of human spirit)
- Risk for spiritual distress

Adapted with permission from Gordon, M. *Manual of Nursing Diagnosis: 1997-1998.* St. Louis: Mosby–Year Book., Inc., 1997.

Appendix C: Commonly prescribed medications associated with sexual adverse effects and dysfunction

Drug	Reported sexual adverse effect
acetazolamide (Diamox)	loss of libido, ↓ potency
Alcohol (ethanol)	impotence
alprazolam (Xanax)	inhibited orgasmic function, delayed or no ejaculation, ↓ libido
amiloride (Midamor)	↓ libido, impotence
aminocaproic acid (Amicar)	dry ejaculation
amiodarone (Cardarone)	↓ libido
amitriptyline (Elavil, Endep)	loss of libido, impotence, no ejaculation
amoxapine (Asendin)	loss of libido, impotence, ejaculatory problems
Amphetamines	chronic use in males: impotence, delayed or no ejaculation chronic use in females: anorgasmic
amyl nitrite (Amyl nitrate)	↓ libido, impotence
atenolol (Tenormin)	impotence
atropine (Isopto Atropine)	impotence
baclofen (Lioresal)	impotence, no ejaculation
Barbiturates	↓ libido, impotence
benztropine (Cogentin)	impotence
bromocriptine (Parlodel)	painful clitoral tumescence, impotence
bupropion (Wellbutrin)	↓ libido, impotence, priapism
buspirone (BuSpar)	priapism
Cannabis (THC, marijuana)	↑ libido
captopril (Capoten)	ejaculatory problems, impotence
carbamazepine (Tegretol)	impotence
carbidopa-levodopa	↑ libido, priapism
chlordiazepoxide (Librium)	↓ libido
chlorothiazide (Diuril)	impotence, ejaculatory and libidinal problems
chlorpromazine (Thorazine)	↓ libido, impotence, no ejaculation, priapism
cimetidine (Tagamet)	↓ libido, impotence
clomipramine (Anafranil)	↓ libido, impotence, retarded, painful or no ejaculation or no orgasm, orgasm precipitated by yawning
clonidine (Catapres)	↓ libido, impotence, delayed or retrograde ejaculation
clozapine (Clozaril)	priapism
Cocaine	priapism
cyclophosphamide (Cytoxan)	impotence
danazol (Danocrine)	↓ libido or ↑ libido
desipramine (Norpramin, Pertofrane)	↓ libido, impotence, painful orgasm
diazepam (Valium)	↓ libido, delayed ejaculation, erectile problems, retarded or no orgasm (in females)
digitalis glycoside (Digoxin)	↓ libido, impotence
diphenhydramine (Benadryl)	impotence
disopyramide (Norpace)	impotence
disulfiram (Antabuse)	impotence
doxepin (Sinequan)	↓ libido, ejaculatory problems
Estrogen products	↓ libido or ↑ libido
ethosuximide (Zarontin)	↑ libido

Drug	Reported sexual adverse effect
ethoxyzolamide	↓ libido
famotidine (Pepcid)	impotence
Fat emulsion products	priapism
fluoxetine (Prozac)	anorgasmia, delayed or spontaneous orgasm, ejaculatory problems, penile anesthesia, ↓ libido
fluphenazine (Prolixin,Permitil)	↓ libido, erectile problems, inhibited ejaculation, priapism
fluvoxamine (Luvox)	delayed ejaculation, inhibited orgasm, ↑ libido
guanethidine (Ismelin)	↓ libido, impotence, delayed, retrograde or no ejaculation
guanfacine (Tenex)	impotence
haloperidol (Haldol)	impotence, painful ejaculation
Heroin	↓ libido or ↑ libido, ejaculatory problems
hydralazine (Ser-Ap-Es)	impotence, priapism
hydrochlorothiazide (Esidrix)	impotence, ejaculatory and libidinal problems
hydroxyzine (Vistaril)	impotence
imipramine (Adapin, Tofranil)	↓ libido, impotence, painful, delayed ejaculation, delayed orgasm (females)
indapamide (Lozol)	↓ libido, impotence
indomethacin (Indocin)	impotence, ↓ libido
interferon- α (Roferon-A)	↓ libido, impotence
isocarboxazid (Marplan)**	impotence, delayed ejaculation, no orgasm (females)
ketoconazole (Nizoral)	impotence, ↓ libido
labetalol (Normadyne)	priapism, impotence, delayed or no ejaculation, ↓ libido
levodopa (Larodopa)	↑ libido
lithium (Eskalith, Lithane, Lithobid)	↓ libido, impotence
lorazepam (Ativan)	loss of libido
Lysergic acid (LSD)	↓ libido or ↑ libido, ejaculatory and erectile problems
maprotiline (Ludiomil)	↓ libido, impotence
mazindol (Sanorex)	impotence, spontaneous ejaculation, painful testes
mesoridazine (Serentil)	no ejaculation, impotence, priapism
methadone (Dolophine)	↓ libido, impotence, on orgasm, retarded ejaculation
methotrexate (Rheumatrex)	impotence, erectile problems
methyldopa (Aldomet)	↓ libido, impotence, delayed or no ejaculation, delayed or no orgasm (females)
metoclopramide (Reglan)	↓ libido, impotence
metoprolol (Toprol Xl)	impotence
metyrosine (Demser)	impotence, no ejaculation
mexiletine (Mexitil)	↓ libido, impotence
midazolam (Versed)	sexual fantasies (females)
molindone (Moban)	priapism
morphine (Duramorph)	↓ libido, impotence
nadolol ((Corgard)	↓ libido, impotence, ejaculatory problems
naltrexone (Trexan)	delayed ejaculation, ↓ potency
naproxen (Naprosyn)	impotence, no ejaculation
nifedipine (Adalat)	priapism
nortriptyline (Pamelor, Aventyl)	impotence, ↓ libido
omeprazole (Prilosec)	painful nocturnal erections
papaverine (Cerebid)	priapism
pargyline (Eutonyl)	no ejaculation, impotence
paroxetine (Paxil)	delayed ejaculation, inhibited orgasm

Drug	Reported sexual adverse effect
pergolide (Permax)	hypersexuality, priapism, spontaneous ejaculation
perphenazine (Trilafon)	↓ or no ejaculation
phencyclidine (PCP)	↓ libido or ↑ libido, erectile and ejaculatory problems
phenelzine (Nardil)	impotence, retarded or no ejaculation, delayed or no orgasm, priapism
phentolamine (Regitine)	impotence
phenytoin (Dilantin)	↓ libido, impotence, priapism
pimozide (Orap)	↓ libido, impotence, no ejaculation
pindolol (Visken)	impotence
prazosin (Minipress)	impotence, priapism
procarbazine (Matulane)	↓ libido, impotence, dyspareunia
Progestins	impotence
propofol (Diprivan)	sexual disinhibition
propranolol (Inderal)	loss of libido, impotence
protriptyline (Vivactil)	loss of libido, impotence, painful ejaculation
risperidone (Risperidal)	erectile dysfunction, delayed ejaculation, abnormal orgasm
scopolamine (Transderm Scop)	impotence
selegeline (Eldepryl)	transient anorgasmia, ↓ penile sensation
sertindole (Serlect)	abnormal or dry ejaculation
sertraline (Zoloft)	delayed ejaculation, inhibited orgasm
spironolactone (Aldactone)	↓ libido, impotence
Steroids	↓ libido or ↑ libido
tamoxifen (Nolvadex)	priapism
terazosin (Hytrin)	impotence
testosterone	priapism
Thiazide diuretics	impotence
thioridazine (Mellaril)	impotence, priapism, delayed, decreased, painful, retrograde or no ejaculation, anorgasmia
thiothixene (Navane)	spontaneous ejaculation, impotence, priapism
timolol (Timoptic)	↓ libido, impotence
tranylcypromine (Parnate)	impotence, painful or retarded ejaculation
trazodone (Desyrel)	priapism, clitoral priapism, ↑ libido, retrograde or no ejaculation, anorgasmia
trifluoperazine (Stelazine)	painful or spontaneous ejaculation
trimpramine (Surmontil)	↓ libido, impotence, anorgasmia
venlafaxine (Effexor)	↓ libido, impotence, abnormal ejaculation, delayed orgasm
verapamil (Calan, Isoptin, Verelan)	impotence
vinblastine (Velban)	↓ libido, impotence, dyspareunia

Appendices

** No longer available in United States

Appendix D: Managing adverse effects of psychotropic medications

The chart below presents nursing interventions aimed at managing adverse effects of antipsychotics (APS), tricyclic antidepressants (TCA), monoamine oxidase inhibitors (MAOI), anticholinergics (ACH), lithium (LITH), selective serotonin reuptake inhibitors (SSRI), selective serotonin-norepinephrine reuptake inhibitors (SSNRI), and benzodiazepines (BENZ). For adverse effects preceded by an asterisk, collaborate with the doctor or nurse practitioner to consider use of 1% solution of pilocarpine (cholinergic agonist) as a mouthwash three times a day or bethanechol (cholinergic agonist) 10 to 30 mg once or twice a day.

System	Adverse effects	Class of drug	Nursing interventions
Cardiovascular	Orthostatic hypotension	•APS •TCA •MAOI •ACH	•Instruct the client to rise slowly from a lying position to a sitting or standing position. •Keep side rails up for hospitalized clients. •Suggest that the client call for assistance when getting up until he has learned to manage the problem. •Suggest elastic or support stockings. •Instruct the client to avoid hot showers or baths, because they may cause vasodilation and aggravate the problem. •Monitor client's blood pressure when drug therapy is started and during periods of dosage adjustment.
	Tachycardia	•TCA •ACH •LITH	•Monitor client's pulse two to four times daily until stable. •Withhold the dose if the resting pulse before a dose is 110 or greater (follow institutional policy regarding this). •Teach the client and family to record the pulse regularly at home. •Instruct the client to avoid excessive caffeine intake.
Endocrine and metabolic	Weight gain	•APS •TCA •MAOI	•Weigh the client weekly; instruct the client to monitor and record weight at home on a weekly basis. •Provide dietary instruction about nutritious but low-calorie meal planning. •Help in the development of a regular exercise program.
	Hyperglycemia and hypoglycemia	•TCA •APS	•Monitor blood sugar carefully and frequently in diabetic clients. Consult the doctor or nurse practitioner about modifications in prescribed diet, insulin dose, or dose of oral hypoglycemic agent, as necessary.
	Increased or decreased libido, changes in ability to ejaculate or maintain erection	•APS •TCA •LITH •SSRI •SSNRI	•Conduct sexual history. •Provide emotional support to client and spouse as appropriate. •Alter the drug dose or switch medications. •Collaborate with the doctor or nurse practitioner to consider treatment with yohimbine (Yocon), an α_2-adrenergic antagonist, or neostigmine (Prostigmin) 7.5 to 15 mg 30 minutes before sexual intercourse.
	Menstrual irregularities	•APS	•Refer women for gynecologic examination, if appropriate.
	Amenorrhea, galactorrhea, false pregnancy	•TCA	•Advise the use of birth control measures to avoid unplanned pregnancy.
Gastrointestinal	Gastric irritation	•TCA •LITH	•Alter the prescribed times for taking doses to coincide with meals. •Decrease the size of the dose and administer more frequently. •Change the medication form (for example, switch to liquid from tablets).
	Anorexia	•SSRI •SSNRI	•Instruct the client to keep a daily food journal.
	Nausea and vomiting	•SSRI •SSNRI •TCA	•Administer the medication with meals. •Decrease the dose. •Collaborate with the doctor in considering cisapride 5 mg twice a day for nausea from an SSRI.
Hematologic	Leukopenia, thrombocytopenia, agranulocytosis	•TCA •TCA •APS	•Continue to monitor closely. •Discontinue the drug immediately. •Manage medically. •Educate the client about reverse isolation. •Try a medication from a different chemical structural group.

System	Adverse effects	Class of drug	Nursing interventions
Hepatic	Jaundice: increased temperature, malaise, abnormal liver function tests, abdominal pain	•APS •TCA	•Discontinue the medication. •Switch to another chemical structural group. •Monitor liver function tests. •Instruct the client about a high-protein, high-carbohydrate diet.
Neurologic	Drowsiness and sedation	•APS •TCA •MAOI •ACH •BENZ •SSRI	•Caution the client to avoid driving or other dangerous activities requiring mental alertness until the degree of drowsiness can be evaluated. (With some medications or with some clients, drowsiness may be a desirable effect.) •Increase the nighttime dose or give the entire day's dosage at bedtime if daytime drowsiness persists. (Persistent drowsiness may indicate the need to change the medication or dose; this requires careful clinical judgment. Drowsiness may lessen with time. Encourage the client to continue the medication for several weeks at least.)
	* Anticholinergic dry mouth	•APS •TCA •MAOI •ACH •SSRI	•Encourage the client to take frequent sips of water or other beverages; because weight gain is often a problem, low-calorie beverages are preferred. •Suggest that the client suck on hard candy or mints or chew gum; low-calorie or sugarless forms are preferred. •Frequent toothbrushing or rinsing the mouth with a pleasant mouthwash or other solution may help eliminate a bad taste in the mouth. •Commercially prepared saliva substitutes are available; consult a pharmacist.
	* Constipation	•APS •TCA •MAOI •ACH	•Monitor and record the frequency of bowel movements. •Encourage the client to increase the dietary intake of bran, fresh fruits, or prunes. Collaborate with a nutritionist. •Have the client increase fluid intake to 2,500 to 3,000 ml per day if not contraindicated by other medical conditions. •Encourage the client to increase level of activity (walking or engaging in other forms of exercise) within any functional limits. •Consult with the doctor or nurse practitioner about prescribing stool softeners or bulk-forming agents.
	* Blurred vision	•APS •TCA •MAOI •ACH •BENZ	•Caution the client to avoid driving or operating hazardous equipment until the blurring clears. •If blurred vision persists, notify the doctor or nurse practitioner, because it may indicate a need to change drugs or reduce dosages. •Encourage the client to see an ophthalmologist.
	* Urine retention	•APS •TCA	•Although this adverse effect is possible at any age, it is more prevalent in elderly and immobilized clients and in men with enlarged prostate glands. •Monitor intake and output. Assess the client for difficulty voiding and subjective complaints of incomplete bladder emptying. Notify the doctor or nurse practitioner if retention is suspected; catheterization may be necessary. •Suggest that the client void before taking ordered doses of the medication. •Teach the client to notify the health care provider if retention is suspected.
	Anticholinergic diaphoresis	•TCA •SSRI	•Maintain adequate fluid intake (usually 2,500 to 3,000 ml per day), depending on cardiopulmonary function. •Assess for electrolyte imbalance and monitor serum electrolytes. •Encourage good hygiene. •Suggest cotton clothing.
	Seizures	•APS •TCA	•Decrease the dose. •Change to a high-potency antipsychotic.
	Insomnia	•SSRI •SSNRI	•Administer the medication early in the day. •Lower the dose. •Instruct the client in sleep hygiene measures. •Decrease or delete caffeine.

Adapted with permission from S. Lego, *Psychiatric Nursing: A Comprehensive Reference*, 2nd ed. Philadelphia: Lippincott-Raven Pubs., 1996.

Appendices

Appendix E: Resources for clients and families

Addictive illnesses

Dual Diagnosis Web Site
http://www.erols.com/ksciacca

Web of Addictions
http://www.well.com/user/woa/

Aging

American Association of Retired Persons
601 E St., NW
Washington, DC 20049
1-202-434-2277

American Society on Aging
833 Market St.
Rm 516
San Francisco, CA 94103-1824
1-415-974-9600

Children of Aging Parents
1609 Woodbourne Rd.
Suite 302 A
Levittown, PA 19057
1-800-227-7294

Gerontological Society of America
1275 K St., NW
Suite 350
Washington, DC 20005
1-202-842-1275

National Association of Area Agencies on Aging
1112 16th St., NW
Suite 100
Washington, DC 20036
1-202-296-8130

National Council on the Aging, Inc.
409 3rd St., NW
Suite 200
Washington, DC 20024
1-202-479-1200

National Institute on Aging
Public Information Office
Federal Bldg. Rm 5C27
Bldg. 31
9000 Rockville Pkwy.
Bethesda, MD 20892
1-301-496-4000

Social Security Administration
6325 Security Blvd.
Baltimore, MD 21207
Medicare Hotline 1-800-2345-SSA

AIDS and HIV

AIDS Project Los Angeles, Inc.
7362 Santa Monica Blvd.
West Hollywood, CA 90046
1-213-876-8951

AIDS-Related Information (NIH)
gopher://odie.niaid.nih.gov/11/aids

AIDS Virtual Library
http://www.actwin.com/aids/vl.html

Growth House, Inc. (AIDS and HIV links)
http://www.growthhouse.org/hivlinks.html

MedWeb: AIDS and HIV
http://www.gen.emory.edu/medweb/medweb.aids.html

New York State AIDS Information
AIDS Drug Assistance Program
1-800-542-2437
General Information:
1-800-541-AIDS

Positives Anonymous
World Services Office
25 Saint Marks Place
New York, NY 10003
1-212-732-6879

The World Wide Web Virtual Library: AIDS
http://planetq.com/aidvl/index/html

Yahoo Index: AIDS/HIV
http://www.yahoo.com/Health/Diseases-and-Conditions/AIDS-HIV/

Alcoholism

African American Services Institute on Black Chemical Abuse
2616 Nicollet Ave. S.
Minneapolis, MN 55408
1-612-871-7878

Al-Anon Family Group Headquarters
P.O. Box 862
Midtown Station
New York, NY 10018-0862
1-212-254-7230
Fax: 1-212-869-3757

Alcoholics Anonymous
465 Park Ave.
New York, NY 10016
1-212-686-1100

California Hispanic Commission on Alcohol and Drug Abuse
2101 Capital Ave.
Sacramento, CA 95816
1-916-443-5473

Catholic Alcoholics—
Calix Society
7601 Wayzata Blvd.
2nd Floor
Minneapolis, MN 55426
1-612-546-0544

Children of Alcoholics Foundation
Phoenix House
33 W. 60th St.
New York, NY 10023
1-212-757-2100
1-800-359-2623

Lesbian, Gay, Bisexual and Transgender Specialty Center
Lesbian, Gay Community Services
208 W. 13th St.
New York, NY 10011
1-212-620-7310

National Association for Children of Alcoholics
1426 Rockville Pike
Suite 100
Rockville, MD 20852
1-301-468-0985
Fax: 1-301-468-0987

National Association of Lesbian and Gay Alcoholism Professionals
1147 South Alvarado St.
Los Angeles, CA 90006
1-213-381-8524
Fax: 1-213-381-8525

National Association of Native American Children of Alcoholics
1402 3rd Ave.
Suite 1110
Seattle, WA 98101
1-206-467-7686
Fax: 1-206-467-7689

Substance and Alcohol Intervention Services for the Deaf
Rochester Institute of Technology
115 Lomb Memorial Dr.
Rochester, NY 14623-5608
1-716-475-4978 (voice and TTY)
1-716-475-4979 (TTY)

Women for Sobriety, Inc.
P.O. Box 618
Quakertown, PA 18951
1-215-536-8026

Alzheimer's disease
Alzheimer's Association Home Page
http://www.alz.org/

Alzheimer's Disease and Related Disorders Association
70 E. Lake St.
Chicago, IL 60601
1-312-853-3060
1-800-272-3900

Alzheimer's Disease International
12 S. Michigan Ave.
Chicago, IL 60603
1-312-335-5777

Alzheimer's Foundation
877 South Harvard
M/C-114
Tulsa, OK 74137
1-918-631-3665

Alzheimer's Web
http://werple.mira.net.au/-dhs/ad.html

BGRECC Alzheimer Website
(Bedford Geriatric Research Education Clinical Center, Bedford, MA)
http://med-www.bu.edu/Alzheimer/home.html

Family Caregiver Alliance
http://www.caregiver.org

Amyotropic lateral sclerosis
The ALS Association
21021 Ventura Blvd., #321
Woodland Hills, CA 91364
1-818-340-7500

Anger management
http://www.kumu.com/"grhoades

Anxiety and obsessive-compulsive disorders
Anxiety Disorders Association of America
6000 Executive Blvd.
Suite 200
Rockville, MD 20852
1-301-231-9350

Emotions Anonymous International Offices
2233 University Ave. W.
Saint Paul, MN 55114
1-612-647-9712

National Anxiety Foundation
3135 Custer Dr.
Lexington, KY 40517
1-606-272-7166

NPAD News: National Panic/Anxiety Disorder News
http://www.npadnews.com

Obsessive-Compulsive Disorder Foundation
P.O. Box 70
Milford, CT 06460-0070
1-800-639-7462
1-203-878-5669

Attention deficit hyperactivity disorder
Attention Deficit Disorder WWW Archive
http://homepage.seas.upenn.edu/-mengwong/add/

C.H.A.D.D. (Children and Adults with Attention Deficit Disorders)
http://www.chadd.org/

Birth defects
March of Dimes Foundations
1275 Mamaroneck Ave.
White Plains, NY 10605
1-914-428-7100

Brain tumors
Association for Brain Tumor Research
2720 River Rd.
Suite 146
Des Plaines, IL 60018
1-708-827-9910

Cancer
American Cancer Society
1-800-227-2345 (ACS-2345)

Cancer Care, Inc.
New York City Central Office
1180 Ave. of the Americas
New York, NY 10035
1-212-221-3300

Children and adolescents
American Professional Society on the Abuse of Children
407 S. Dearborn
Suite 1300
Chicago, IL 60605
1-312-554-0166

Children's and Youth Emotions Anonymous
P.O. Box 4245
St. Paul, MN 55104
1-612-647-9712

Child Welfare League of America
440 First St., NE
Suite 310
Washington, DC 20001-2085
1-202-638-2952

Clearinghouse on Child Abuse and Neglect Information
Box 1182
Washington, DC 20013
1-703-385-7565

National Resource Center on Child Sexual Abuse
107 Lincoln St.
Huntsville, AL 34801
1-205-534-6868

Crisis, bereavement, and loss
Crisis Brings Grief
http://www.dgsys.com/-tgolden/1grief/html

Crisis, Grief and Healing
http://www.webhealing.com

Physical Loss, Chronic Illness and Bereavement: A Guide to Internet Resources
gopher://una.hh.lib.umich.edu/00/inetdirstacks/emotsupport%3ajunpow

Cultural care and cultural diversity
Association of Multiethnic Americans
1060 Tennessee St.
San Francisco, CA 94107

Blacks Educating Blacks About Sexual Health Issues
1319 Locust St.
Philadelphia, PA 19107
1-215-546-4140

Coalition of Hispanic Health and Human Service Organizations
1030 15th St., NW
Washington, DC 20005
1-202-371-2100

Culturgram (Information
about different cultures)
Brigham Young University
David Kennedy Center for
International Studies
Publication Series
280 HRCB
Provo, UT 84602
1-801-387-6528

Holt International
Children's Services
P.O. Box 2880
Eugene, OR 98402
1-541-687-2202

Multicultural Prevention
Resource Center
1540 Market St.
Suite 320
San Francisco, CA 94102
1-415-861-2142

Multiethnic Unity Effort
c/o Cheryl Paxson
P.O. Box 522
Waukegan, IL 60079
1-708-367-1782

National Alliance of the
Mentally Ill
Minority Group
Community Resources
200 N. Gleeb Rd.
Suite 1015
Arlington, VA 22203-3754
1-703-524-7600

National Coalition to End
Racism in American Child
Care System, Inc.
(Support for transcultural
adoption)
22075 Koths
Taylor, MI 48180
1-313-295-0257

Office of Minority Health
Resource Center
P.O. Box 37337
Washington, DC 20013-
7337
1-213-385-1474

Outreach to African-
American and Hispanic
Families
Thresholds National
Research and Training
Center
2001 N. Clybrain Ave.
Suite 302
Chicago, IL 60614
1-312-348-5522

Down syndrome
Down's Syndrome
Congress
1605 Chantilly Dr.
Suite 250
Atlanta, GA 30324
1-800-232-6372

Drug abuse
American Lung
Association
National Headquarters
1740 Broadway
New York, NY
10019-4374
1-212-315-8700

Cocaine Anonymous
World Service Office, Inc.
3740 Overland Ave.
Suite G
Culver City, CA 90034
1-310-559-5833
1-800-347-8998 (24-hour
referral line)
Fax: 1-310-559-2554

Narcotics Anonymous
World Service Office, Inc
P.O. Box 9999
Van Nuys, CA 91409
1-818-780-3951
Fax: 1-818-785-0923

Office on Smoking and
Health
1600 Clifton Rd., NE
Mail Stop K-50
Atlanta, GA 30333
1-404-488-5705
1-404-488-5708
Fax: 1-404-332-2552

Smokers Anonymous
World Services
P.O. Box 591777
San Francisco, CA 94123
1-415-750-0328

Eating disorders
American Anorexia and
Bulimia Association, Inc.
165 West 46th St.
Suite 1108
New York, NY 10036
1-212-575-6200

Anorexia Nervosa and
Bulimia Association
http://qlink.queensu.ca/
"4map/anabhome.htm

National Association of
Anorexia Nervosa and
Associated Disorders
P.O. Box 7
Highland Park, IL 60035
1-847-831-3438

National Eating Disorders
Organization
6655 S. Yale Ave.
Tulsa, OK 74136
1-918-481-4044

Overeaters Anonymous
World Services Office
6075 Zenith Ct., NE
Rio Rancho, NM 87124-
6424
1-505-891-2664

Epilepsy
Epilepsy Foundation of
America
451 Garden City Dr.
Landover, MD 20785
1-301-459-3700

**Family and interperson-
al violence**
Abuse Survivor's Resource
http://www.tezczt.com/
"tinal/psych.html

AYUDA Clinical Legal
Latina
1736 Columbia Rd., NW
Washington, DC 20009
1-202-387-0424

Center to Prevent
Handgun Violence
1225 Eye St., NW
Suite 1100
Washington, DC. 20005
1-202-289-7319

Family Violence
Prevention Fund
383 Rhode Island St.
San Francisco, CA 94103-
5133
1-415-252-8900

National Coalition Against
Domestic Violence
P.O. Box 34103
Washington, DC
20043-4103
1-303-839-1852

National Coalition on
Television Violence
P.O. Box 2157
Champaign, IL 61825
1-810-439-3177

National Organization for
Victims Assistance
1757 Park Rd., NW
Washington, DC 20010
1-800-TRY-NOVA

Safety Net: Domestic
Violence Information and
Resources
http://www.cybergrr.com/
dv.html

Trauma Foundation
Bldg. One
Room 306
San Francisco General
Hospital
San Francisco, CA 94110
1-415-821-8209
Fax: 1-415-282-2363

Victim Assistance
Network
Mt. Vernon Center
8119 Holland Rd.
Alexandria, VA 22306

Family support groups
Alliance for the Mentally
Ill/Friend and Advocates
of Mentally Ill
http://www.schizophrenia.
com/ami/

Codependents
Anonymous
P.O. Box 33577
Phoenix, AZ 85067-3577
1-602-277-7991

Codependents of Sex
Addicts
Twin Cities COSA
P.O. Box 14537
Minneapolis, MN 55414
1-612-537-6904

Families Anonymous, Inc.
14553 Delano St.
Van Nuys, CA 91411
1-818-989-7841

Federation of Families for
Children's Mental Health
1021 Prince St.
Alexandria, VA 22314-
2971
1-703-684-7710

Help! A Consumers Guide
to Mental Health
Information
http://www.io.org/-mad-
magic/help/help.
html#about

National Alliance for the
Mentally Ill
2101 Wilson Blvd.
Suite 302
Arlington, VA 22203-3754
1-703-524-7600
http://www.nami.org

Parents Anonymous
5 Foothill Blvd.
Suite 220
Claremont, CA 91711

Parents Without Partners,
Inc.
8807 Colesville Rd.
Silver Spring, MD 20910
1-301-588-9354

Step Family Foundation,
Inc.
333 West End Ave.
New York, NY 10023
1-212-877-3244

Tough Love
P.O. Box 1069
Doylestown, PA 18901
1-215-348-7090 or
1-800-333-1069

General information
HANDITEL: Mental
Health
http://www.santel.lu/
HANDITEL/wwwlinks/
mental.html

Healthy People 2000:
Mental Health and Mental
Disorders Resource List
http://nhic-nt.health.org/
nmp/hr2kpage/6mental2.
htm

Medical and Mental
Health Resources
http://www.realtime.net/
-mmjw/

Mental Health Info Link
http://www.onlinepsych.
com/treat/mh.htm

Mental Health Net
http://www.cmhc.com/

National Empowerment
Center
20 Ballard Rd.
Lawrence, MA 01843
1-800-POWER-2-U

National Health
Information Center Web
Server
U.S. Department of Health
and Human Services
http://nhic-nt.health.org

National Self-Help
Clearinghouse
Graduate School
University Center
City University of New
York
33 W. 42nd St.
New York, NY 10036

National Stigma
Clearinghouse
275 Seventh Ave.
16th Floor
New York, NY 10001

The KEY: National Mental
Health Consumer's Self
Help Clearinghouse
(newsletter)
Community Support
Programs
Center for Mental Health
Services
SAMSHA
311 Juniper St., Suite
1000
Philadelphia, PA 19107
1-800-553-4539

Headache and migraine
National Migraine
Foundation
5252 Northwestern Ave.
Chicago, IL, 60625

**Head injury (Brain
injury)**
The National Head Injury
Foundation
333 Turnpike Rd.
Southboro, MA 01772
1-617-485-4183

**Hereditary (genetic) dis-
eases**
Hereditary Disease
Foundation
1427 7th St.
Suite 2
Santa Monica, CA 90401
1-213-458-4183

Hotlines
Alateen
(Children/Teenagers of
Alcoholics)
1-800-344-2666

Covenant House Nineline
1-800-999-9999

National Child Abuse
Hotline
1-800-422-4453

National Runaway Hotline
1-800-231-6946

National Sexually
Transmitted Diseases
Hotline
1-800-227-8922

National Youth Crisis
Hotline
1-800-HIT-HOME

National Youth Suicide
Hotline
1-800-621-4000

Pregnancy Hotline
1-800-238-4269

Rainbows (Children griev-
ing loss, death, divorce)
1-708-310-1880

Students Against Drunk
Drivers
1-508-481-3568

Huntington's disease
Huntington's Disease
Society of America
140 West 22nd St.
6th Floor
New York, NY 10011-
2420
1-212-242-1968

Huntington's Disease
Society of Canada
Box 333
Cambridge, Ontario
CANADA NiR 5T8

Hypertension
American Heart
Association
1-800-242-8721 (AHA-
USA1)

Mental retardation
Learning Disabilities of
America
4156 Library Rd.
Pittsburgh, PA 15234
1-412-341-1515

Mood disorders
Beyond Stigma: ECT and
Depression
http://www.frii.com/
"hageseth/

Depression After Delivery
P.O. Box 1282
Morrisville, PA 19067
1-215-295-3994

Depression Sucks!
http://www.duke.edu/
~ntd/depression.html

Internet Depression
Resources List
http://www.execpc.com/
~corbeau/

Mood Disorders
http://avocado.pc.helsinki.
fi/~janne/mood/mood.html

National Depressive and
Manic-Depressive
Association
730 North Franklin
Suite 501
Chicago, IL 60610
1-312-642-0049

National Foundation for
Depressive Illness, Manic
and Depressive Support
Group, Inc.
P.O. Box 2257
New York, NY 10116
1-212-370-7190

Pendulum's Bipolar
Disorder/Manic-
Depression Page
http://www.pendulum.org

**Multiple personality and
dissociative disorder**
Multiple Personality
Disorder and Dissociative
Disorder
http://members.tripod.
com/-fsvival/index.htm

Multiple sclerosis
National Multiple
Sclerosis Society
205 E. 42nd St.
New York, NY 10017-
5706
1-212-986-3240

Muscular dystrophy
Muscular Dystrophy
Association
810 Seventh Ave.
New York, NY 10019
1-212-586-0808

Myasthenia gravis
The Myasthenia Gravis
Foundation
52 W. Jackson Blvd.
Suite 909
Chicago, IL 60604
1-312-427-6252

Pain
Chronic Pain Outreach
Association, Inc.
822 Wycliff Court
Manassas, VA 22110
1-703-368-7357

National Chronic Pain
Outreach Association, Inc.
4922 Hampden Ln.
Bethesda, MD 20814
1-301-652-4948

**Panic and phobic disor-
ders**
Freedom From Fear
Network
308 Seaview Ave.
Staten Island, NY 10305
1-718-351-1717

Phobia and Stress
Treatment Group
1460 Old Mill Rd.
Upper Marlboro, MD
1-301-952-0128 or 9680

Parkinson's disease
American Parkinson's
Disease Association
116 John St.
Suite 417
New York, NY 10038
1-212-685-2741

National Parkinson
Foundation
1501 NW Ninth Ave.
Miami, FL 33136
1-945-938-2137

Parkinson's Disease
Foundation
Wm. Black Medical Bldg.
710 W. 168th St.
New York, NY 10032
1-212-923-4700

Parkinson's Educational
Program
1800 Park Newport,
302
Newport Beach, CA
92660
1-714-640-0218

United Parkinson
Foundation
360 W. Superior St.
Chicago, IL 60610
1-312-664-2344

**Personality and dissocia-
tive disorders**
BPD Central: Borderline
Personality Disorder
http://members.aol.com/
BPDcentral/index.html

BPD Page
http://www.cmhc.com/
disorders/sx10t.htm

International Society for
the Study of Multiple
Personality and
Dissociation
5700 Old Orchard Rd.
1st Floor
Skokie, IL 60077-1024

Psychopharmacology
Psychopharmacology and
Drug References on the
Mental Health Net
http://www.cmhcsys.com/
guide/pro22.htm#A

Psychopharmacology TIPS
http://uhs.bsd.uchicago.
edu/-bhsiung/tips/

**Schizophrenia and
severe-persistent mental
illness**
International Association
of Psychosocial
Rehabilitation Services
10025 Governor Warfield
Pkwy.
Colombia, MD 21044
1-410-730-7190

NARSAD: National
Alliance for Research on
Schizophrenia and
Depression
http://www.mhsource.
com/narsad.html

National Alliance for the
Mentally Ill
200 N. Gleeb Rd.
Suite 1015
Arlington, VA 22203-3754
1-703-524-7600

National Association of
Psychiatric Survivors
P.O. Box 618
Sioux Falls, SD 57101-
0618
1-605-334-4067

National Crisis Prevention
Institute
3315-K N. 124th St.
Brookfield, WI 53005
1-800-558-8976
1-414-783-5787

National Mental Health
Association
1021 Prince St.
Alexandria, VA
22314-2971
1-703-684-7722

Recovery, Inc.: The
Association of Nervous
and Former Mental
Patients
116 S. Michigan Ave.
Chicago, IL 60603
1-312-337-5661

Schizophrenia
Anonymous
1209 California Rd.
Eastchester, NY 10709
1-914-337-2252

Schizophrenia Home Page
http://www.schizophrenia.
com

**Sexual disorders, sexual
abuse, and violence**
Impotents Anonymous
119 S. Ruth St.
Maryville, TN 37801
1-615-983-6064

Incest Survivors
Anonymous
P.O. Box 5613
Long Beach, CA
90805-0613
1-213-428-5599

Parents United (incest)
P.O. Box 952
San Jose, CA 95108
1-408-280-5055

Resolve, Inc. (problems of
infertility)
1310 Broadway
Somerville, MA 02144
1-617-623-0744

Sex and Love Addicts
Anonymous
Augustine Fellowship
P.O. Box 119
Newtown Branch
Boston, MA 02258
1-617-332-1845

Sex Information and
Education Council of the
United States
New York University
130 W. 42nd St.
Suite 2500
New York, NY 10036
1-212-819-9770

Sexual Dysfunction
Program
University of Minnesota
School of Medicine
2630 University Ave., S.E.
Minneapolis, MN 55414
1-612-627-4360

Survivors of Incest
Anonymous
World Service Office
P.O. Box 21817
Baltimore, MD
21222-6817
1-301-282-3400

Sexuality
Healthy Sexuality
http://www.uiuc.edu/
departments/mck...health-
info/sexual/intro/intro.htm

Homosexuality: Questions
and Statements Answered
http://www.geocites.com/
WestHollywood/1348/

Sleep
American Narcolepsy
Association
P.O. Box 1187
San Carlos, CA 94070
1-415-591-7979

Sleep Disorders Yahoo!
http://www.yahoo.com/
Health/Diseases-and-
Conditions/Sleep-
Disorders/

The Sleep Well
http://www-leland.
stanford.edu/-dement/

Spinal cord injuries
American Paralysis
Association
500 Morris Ave.
Springfield, NJ 07081
1-800-225-0292

National Spinal Cord
Injury Association
2 Rehabilitation Way
Woburn, MA 01801
1-781-933-8666

Spinal Cord Society
Wendell Rd.
Fergus Falls, MN 56537
1-218-739-5252

Stalking
Stalking Victims Sanctuary
http://www.ccon.com/
stalkvictim/

Survivors of Stalking, Inc.
http://www.soshelp.org/

**Stroke (cerebrovascular
injury)**
American Heart
Association
7320 Greenville Ave.
Dallas, TX 75231
1-214-750-5300

National Information for
Neurology Disorders
Building 31, Room 8A-16
Bethesda, MD 20205
1-301-496-5751

National Stroke
Association
300 E. Hampden Ave.
Suite 240
Englewood, CO 80110-
2622
1-303-762-9922

**Suicide and suicidal
behavior**
American Association of
Suicidology
2459 S. Ash
Denver, CO 80222
1-303-692-0985
http://www.cyberpsych.
org/aas.htm

Suicide Awareness/Voices
of Education
http://www.save.org

Suicide Prevention Center,
Inc.
184 Salem Ave.
Dayton, OH 45406
1-513-297-4777

Tardive dystonia
Tardive Dyskinesia/Tardive
Dystonia National
Association
4244 University Way, NE
P.O. Box 45732
Seattle, WA 98145-0732
1-206-522-3166

Tremor
International Tremor
Foundation
360 W. Superior St.
Chicago, IL 60610
1-312-664-2344

Appendices

Index